Tumours of the Mediastinum

Current Histopathology

Consultant Editor
Professor G. Austin Gresham, TD, ScD, MD, FRCPath.
Professor of Morbid Anatomy and Histology, University of Cambridge

Volume Nineteen

TUMOURS OF THE MEDIASTINUM

BY

J. M. VERLEY, MD
Chief, Department of Surgical Pathology,
Chargée de Recherche at the National Institute of Medical Research (INSERM),
Surgical Centre Marie Lannelongue,
Le Plessis Robinson, Paris, France

and

K. H. HOLLMANN, MD
Professor of Oncology,
Directeur de Recherche at the National Centre for Scientific Research (CNRS),
Surgical Centre Marie Lannelongue,
Le Plessis Robinson, Paris, France

KLUWER ACADEMIC PUBLISHERS
DORDRECHT / BOSTON / LONDON

Distributors

for the United States and Canada: Kluwer Academic Publishers, PO Box 358, Accord Station, Hingham, MA 02018-0358, USA
for all other countries: Kluwer Academic Publishers Group, Distribution Center, PO Box 322, 3300 AH Dordrecht, The Netherlands

Published in the United Kingdom by Kluwer Academic Publishers, PO Box 55, Lancaster, UK.

Kluwer Academic Publishers BV incorporates the publishing programmes of D. Reidel, Martinus Nijhoff, Dr W. Junk and MTP Press.

Typeset and originated by Speedlith Photo Litho Ltd., Stretford, Manchester M32 0JT
Printed and bound in Great Britain by Redwood Press Ltd., Melksham, Wilts.

British Library Cataloguing in Publication Data

A catalogue record for this book is available from the British Library.

ISBN 0-7923-8986-7

Library of Congress Cataloging-in-Publication Data

Verley, J.M.
Tumours of the mediastinum / by J.M. Verley and K.H. Hollman.
p. cm. — (Current histopathology; v. 19)
Includes bibliographical references and index.
ISBN 0-7923-8986-7 (casebound)
1. Mediastinum—Tumours—Histopathology.
I. Hollman, K.H. II. Title. III. Series.
[DNLM: 1. Mediastinal Neoplasms—pathology.
W1 CU88JBA v. 19 / WF 900 V521t]
RC280.M35V47 1992
616.99'22707—dc20
DNLM/DLC
for Library of Congress 91-35327
CIP

Contents

Current Histopathology Series

Already published in this series:

Volume 1 Atlas of Lymph Node Pathology
Volume 2 Atlas of Renal Pathology
Volume 3 Atlas of Pulmonary Pathology
Volume 4 Atlas of Liver Pathology
Volume 5 Atlas of Gynaecological Pathology
Volume 6 Atlas of Gastrointestinal Pathology
Volume 7 Atlas of Breast Pathology
Volume 8 Atlas of Oral Pathology
Volume 9 Atlas of Skeletal Muscle Pathology
Volume 10 Atlas of Male Reproductive Pathology
Volume 11 Atlas of Skin Pathology
Volume 12 Atlas of Cardiovascular Pathology
Volume 13 Atlas of Experimental Toxicological Pathology
Volume 14 Atlas of Serous Fluid Cytopathology
Volume 15 Atlas of Bone Marrow Pathology
Volume 16 Atlas of Ear, Nose and Throat Pathology
Volume 17 Atlas of Fungal Pathology
Volume 18 Atlas of Synovial Fluid Cytopathology

Other volumes currently scheduled in this series include the following titles

Atlas of AIDS Pathology

Atlas of Bone Tumours

Atlas of Non-Tumour Bone Pathology

Atlas of Neuropathology

Atlas of Endocrine Pathology

Atlas of Ocular Pathology

Atlas of Paediatric Tumours

Atlas of Parasitic Pathology

Atlas of Renal Transplantation Pathology

Atlas of Soft Tissue Pathology

Consultant Editor's Note

At the present time books on morbid anatomy and histopathology can be divided into two broad groups: extensive textbooks often written primarily for students and monographs on research topics.

This takes no account of the fact that the vast majority of pathologists are involved in an essentially practical field of general diagnostic pathology providing an important service to their clinical colleagues. Many of these pathologists are expected to cover a broad range of disciplines and even those who remain solely within the field of histopathology usually have single and sole responsibility within the hospital for all this work. They may often have no chance for direct discussion on problem cases with colleagues in the same department. In the field of histopathology, no less than in other medical fields, they have been extensive and recent advances, not only in new histochemical techniques but also in the type of specimen provided by new surgical procedures.

There is great need for the provision of appropriate information for this group. This need has been defined in the following terms:

1. It should be aimed at the general clinical pathologist or histopathologist with existing practical training but should also have value for the trainee pathologist.
2. It should concentrate on the practical aspects of histopathology taking account of the new techniques which should be within the compass of the worker in a unit with reasonable facilities.
3. New types of material, e.g. those derived from endoscopic biopsy, should be covered fully.
4. There should be an adequate number of illustrations on each subject to demonstrate the variation in appearance that is encountered.
5. Colour illustrations should be used wherever they aid recognition.

The present concept stemmed from this definition but it was immediately realised that these aims could only be achieved within the compass of a series, of which this volume is one. Since histopathology is, by its very nature, systemized, the individual volumes deal with one system or where this appears more appropriate with a single organ.

New methods of radiological and other diagnostic procedures have led to the finding of conditions sometimes unsuspected. 50% of mediastinal tumours are diagnosed by various forms of scanning and they are often sampled by needle biopsy. This volume fulfils a need arising from modern diagnostic procedures. It is a comprehensive account of abnormal masses that occur in the mediastinum describing macroscopic and microscopic appearances and the clinical and therapeutic problems associated with them. There is also an extensive bibliography. It will be a useful bench manual for the diagnostic histopathologist.

G. A. Gresham

Preface

In the past decade tremendous progress has been made in the diagnosis and treatment of tumours of the mediastinum.

For diagnostic purposes the advent of immunohistochemistry and molecular biology has significantly improved our knowledge of lymphomas, and they have become important aids in the identification of all other tumour types. The generalized use of the electron microscope in surgical pathology is another step forward. A better knowledge of tumour markers and their systematic study in any mediastinal tumour has drastically modified the diagnostic approach of germ-cell tumours, in numerous cases superseding surgical biopsy for their recognition. Advances in investigative radiology, such as computerized tomographic (CT) scan and magnetic resonance imaging (MRI), have facilitated better identification of the lesions, and the extensive use of mediastinoscopy has achieved a positive histological diagnosis in numerous cases.

Thus, the classification of the tumours of the mediastinum has become more clear and accurate, and the old confusions due to multiplication of proposed definitions and terminologies have disappeared.

These diagnostic advances explain the difficulties encountered in comparing the older with the new statistical data, and allow appreciation of the frequency of the different types of mediastinal tumours. In reports prior to the 1980s thymomas seem to be the most frequent of all primary tumours of the mediastinum, whereas lymphomas, mostly non-Hodgkin's lymphomas, today seem as frequent, or even predominant. This is due not to an increase of non-Hodgkin's lymphomas but to better recognition of these tumours.

At the same time modern therapy – including megavoltage radiotherapy and combination chemotherapy, and better strategies sometimes alternating surgery, radiotherapy and chemotherapy – has given remarkable results with improved survival, particularly in malignant germ-cell tumours, in certain neurogenic tumours, and in lymphomas. The identification of patients at risk will, in the future, lead to more aggressive strategies and to a more thoroughly combined therapy.

ACKNOWLEDGEMENTS

The authors wish to thank the staff of the Surgical Centre Marie Lannelongue for providing surgical material and clinical information about their patients, and Mrs C. Rochepeau, A. Perrin and S. Planté, and Mr D. Petraz, for their technical assistance. The authors are also very grateful to Dr E. Dulmet for her personal support. Gilla von Titanero provided her indefatigable encouragement and love.

Introduction 1

Tumours of the mediastinum are common thoracic lesions but are relatively infrequent in the general population. These include all mediastinal swellings except:

1. those of inflammatory and parasitic origin;
2. tumours of the trachea, oesophagus, heart, and great vessels.

The mediastinum is the part of the thoracic cavity which is bounded by the pleural cavities. It extends antero-posteriorly from the sternum to the spine and in the apico-caudal direction from the thoracic inlet to the diaphragm. The mediastinal space is divided into either three or four compartments, according to the authors. In this book the mediastinum is treated as divided into four compartments: superior, anterior, middle and posterior. The anterior and posterior compartments are sometimes subdivided into a superior and an inferior part (Fig. 1.1).

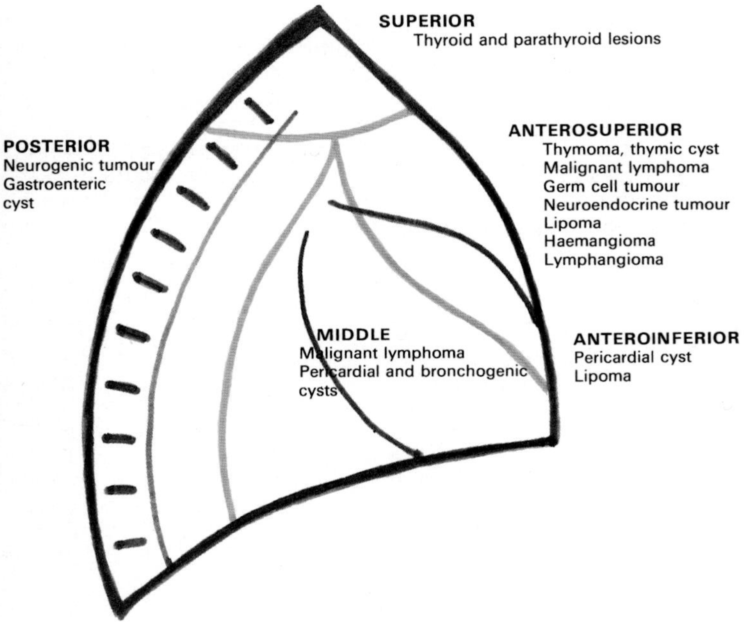

Figure 1.1 Predominant location of mediastinal tumours and cysts

The anterior compartment is anteriorly bounded by the body of the sternum, posteriorly by the heart, by the superior mediastinal space superiorly, and by the diaphragm below. It contains the thymus gland, the adipose and mesenchymal tissues, lymphatics, and the thyroid and parathyroid glands on occasion.

The posterior compartment is bounded posteriorly by the ribs and anteriorly by the line drawn along the anterior borders of the bodies of the vertebrae. It contains the oesophagus, the descending aorta, and the sympathetic and peripheral nerves.

The middle mediastinum is the remaining area between the anterior and posterior compartments, which contains the trachea and the main bronchi, with their lymph nodes.

The superior mediastinum is the narrow upper portion of the mediastinum limited by the thoracic inlet superiorly, the upper manubrium sterni anteriorly and the fourth thoracic vertebra posteriorly. It contains the upper portion of the trachea, the superior vena cava, and occasionally the thyroid, parathyroid and thymus glands.

CLASSIFICATION OF MEDIASTINAL TUMOURS

The thymus is the most common site of origin of mediastinal neoplasms. The classification of thymic tumours has long been debated, but it is now well established that thymomas and thymic carcinomas originate from the epithelial component of the thymus. Tumours of the thymus composed of elements other than thymic epithelium are delineated as distinct entities. These include malignant lymphomas, germ-cell tumours, neuroendocrine tumours, and others. Thus, the most generally accepted classification of mediastinal tumours and cysts is the following:

1. epithelial tumours of the thymus, including thymoma and thymic carcinoma;
2. malignant lymphomas (Hodgkin's disease and non-Hodgkin's lymphoma);
3. germ-cell tumours;
4. neurogenic and neuroendocrine tumours;
5. endocrine tumours (thyroid and parathyroid tumours);
6. tumour-like conditions of the mediastinum:
   thymic hyperplasia, thymolipoma and thymic cysts,
   Castleman's disease,
   cysts (other than thymic);
7. mesenchymal tumours, metastases and miscellaneous.

SITE AND FREQUENCY

Studies surveying large numbers of cases give a good indication of the relative incidence and distribution of mediastinal tumours. Table 1.1 shows the distribution in two large collective series (Morrison, 1958; Davis *et al.*, 1987), compared with our own series (1980 to 1989) (unpublished data).

Most of the tumours of the mediastinum have a predilection for one mediastinal compartment over the others, and the predominant location is of great diagnostic help

Table 1.1 Primary tumours of the mediastinum

Tumour	*Morrison (1958)**		*Davis* et al. *(1987)**		*Our series (1980–89)*	
Thymic[1]	114	(11%)	458	(19%)	200	(26%)
Lymphoma[2]	106	(10%)	301	(13%)	196	(26%)
Neurogenic[3]	305	(29%)	496	(21%)	119	(16%)
Germ-cell tumour	171	(16%)	239	(10%)	44	(6%)
Endocrine[4]	72	(7%)	154	(6%)	77	(10%)
Mesenchymal	84	(8%)	143	(6%)	26	(4%)
Carcinoma			111	(5%)	8	(1%)
Cysts	203	(19%)	439	(18%)	81	(11%)
Other			58	(2%)		
Total	1055		2399		751	

* Collective review. There is an overlapping between the two collective reviews that both include the work of Sabiston and Scott (1952) dealing with 101 cases
[1] Thymoma, thymic cyst and hyperplasia; [2] Hodgkin's and non-Hodgkin's lymphomas; [3] including neuroendocrine tumours; [4] thyroid and parathyroid tumours

(Fig. 1.1). The anterosuperior mediastinal compartment is the most commonly involved site (54%), followed by the posterior mediastinum (26%) and the middle mediastinum (20%). Nevertheless, the tumours as they grow, particularly the malignant ones, encroach on more than one compartment and may invade the whole mediastinum. Thus, their origin becomes difficult to establish with certainty. This is the case of malignant lymphomas (Hodgkin's or non-Hodgkin's lymphomas) and malignant neuroendocrine carcinomas, the origin of which from the thymus gland or from the middle mediastinal lymph nodes may become impossible to assess. The proportion of malignancy among all tumours and tumour-like lesions, including cysts, is about 25% and the percentage among only the neoplasms about 40%. Anterosuperior masses are more likely to be malignant (59%) than lesions in the middle mediastinum (29%) or the posterior mediastinum (16%, Davis *et al.*, 1987). There is no distinctive sex pattern in the overall distribution of mediastinal tumours, except for specific types of malignant germ-cell tumours known to occur virtually only in males (Morrison, 1958; Luosto *et al.*, 1978).

In the anterior mediastinal compartment the relative incidence of tumours differs in children as opposed to adults (Mullen and Richardson, 1986). Thymic lesions and lymphomas are the most frequent in adults. Endocrine and germ-cell tumours are roughly equal in occurrence, although their incidence is differently appreciated in various series (Table 1.2). In infants, lymphomas largely predominate. Germ-cell neoplasms are the second most prevalent tumours, followed by thymic lesions and mesenchymal tumours. Thymic lesions consist primarily of hyperplasia and cysts, and thymomas are very infrequent. Endocrine tumours are almost non-existent in children (Table 1.3). Whereas Davis *et al.* (1987) state that children have the highest percentage of benign neoplasms if the whole mediastinum is considered, Mullen and Richardson (1986) consider that children are more likely to have a malignancy than are adults.

Table 1.2 Primary anterior mediastinal tumours in adults

Tumour	*Morrison (1958)**		*Mullen and Richardson (1986)**		*Davis* et al. *(1987)*		*Our series (1980–89)*	
Thymic	114	(25%)	327	(46%)	67	(36%)	200	(39%)
Lymphoma	106	(23%)	160	(23%)	62	(34%)	196	(38%)
Germ-cell	171	(37%)	103	(15%)	42	(23%)	44	(8%)
Endocrine	72	(15%)	112	(16%)	12	(7%)	77	(15%)
Total	463		702		183		517	

* Collective review

Table 1.3 Primary anterior mediastinal tumours in children

Tumour	*Mullen and Richardson (1986) (collective review)*	
Thymic lesions*	30	(17%)
Lymphoma	80	(45%)
Germ-cell	43	(24%)
Mesenchymal	26	(14%)

* Including thymic cysts, thymic hyperplasia and thymoma

In the posterior mediastinum, neurogenic tumours predominate in both adults and children.

GENERAL FEATURES OF MEDIASTINAL NEOPLASMS

The mediastinal tumours are often asymptomatic and about 50% of the tumours are detected at routine chest X-ray, the proportion of incidental findings varying in different series from 35% to 61%. When present, the symptoms that appear to be particularly common are chest pain, dyspnoea, cough, and, in highly invasive tumours, superior vena caval obstruction. The presence of symptoms in a patient with a mediastinal tumour clearly has prognostic importance because malignant lesions are more often symptomatic than benign ones, but presence of symptoms does not imply that the patient has a malignant tumour, since 60–70% of the malignant tumours, and 30–40% of the benign ones are symptomatic. According to Davis *et al.* (1987) there is an increasing number of asymptomatic patients with malignant lesions in the past 20 years, and benign neoplasms are detected when substantially smaller. This is due to the increased use of chest roentgenograms in clinical practice and screening, and increased imaging sensitivity. Myasthenia gravis is also a presenting symptom that has increased the number of thymomas discovered during systematic thymectomy.

Chest roentgenography remains the primary initial diagnostic examination giving information concerning anatomical location, size of the neoplasm, presence of calcification and whether cystic or solid. Newer techniques such as radioisotopic scanning, CT scans and MRI greatly enhance the accuracy of the radiographic preoperative diagnosis. Iodine scintigraphy is of interest when an intrathoracic goitre is suspected. The use of fine-needle aspiration with CT guidance increases the accuracy of preoperative histological diagnoses. Finally, in the rare cases of human choriogonadotrophic hormone (HCG) or alphafetoprotein (AFP) secreting malignant germ-cell tumour, hormonal measurements by radioimmunoassay or by scintigraphy after injection of isotope-labelled specific antibodies to the patients may allow a definite diagnosis of the tumour. Nevertheless, a final diagnosis can usually be made only by surgery. Mediastinoscopy is particularly helpful in unilateral or bilateral hilar lesions and in obviously large unresectable anterior or superior mediastinal tumours (Best *et al.*, 1987); otherwise thoracotomy is advocated.

References

Best, L.-A., Munichor, M., Ben-Shakhar, M., Lemer, J., Lichtig, C. and Peleg, H. (1987). The contribution of anterior mediastinotomy in the diagnosis and evaluation of diseases of the mediastinum and lung. *Ann. Thorac. Surg.*, **43**, 78–81

Davis, R. D., Oldham, H. N. and Sabiston, D. C. (1987). Primary cysts and neoplasms of the mediastinum: recent changes in clinical presentation, methods of diagnosis, management, and results. *Ann. Thorac. Surg.*, **44**, 229–237

Luosto, R., Koikkalainen, K., Jyrälä, A. and Franssila, K. (1978). Mediastinal tumours. A follow-up study of 208 patients. *Scand. J. Thorac. Cardiovasc. Surg.*, **12**, 253–259

Morrison, I. M. (1958). Tumours and cysts of the mediastinum. *Thorax*, **13**, 294–307

Mullen, B. and Richardson, J. D. (1986). Primary anterior mediastinal tumors in children and adults. *Ann. Thorac. Surg.*, **42**, 338–345

Sabiston, D. C. and Scott, H. W. (1952). Primary neoplasms and cysts of the mediastinum. *Ann. Surg.*, **136**, 777–797

Tumours and tumour-like conditions of the thymus

2

THE THYMUS GLAND

The thymus is an epithelial organ that develops from the third pair of endodermal pouches and ectodermal clefts. The two epithelial buds proliferate, migrate towards the anterior mediastinum, lose their cervical connection by the eighth week and finally join, but do not completely fuse. By the end of the second month the epithelial thymic anlage is colonized by lymphoblasts which will acquire their functional maturity from precursor to effector T cells. The intrathymic differentiation of T progenitors involves three steps: (a) irreversible commitment towards the T cell lineage and T cell differentiation, (b) selection of the T cell repertoire towards self major histocompatibility complex antigens, and (c) diversification into functional subsets (Stutman, 1978, 1985; Sprent *et al.*, 1988). Thymic epithelial cells play a fundamental role in this process of differentiation and maturation of T cells. This includes direct cell-to-cell contact between thymocytes and thymic epithelial cells, and local production of thymic hormones. Most studies indicate morphological, phenotypic and functional heterogeneity within the thymic epithelial cell population distinguishing between epithelial cells of the subcapsular, cortical, and medullary areas.

The adult thymus is composed of lobules bordered and separated from each other by a basement membrane which penetrates into the parenchyma around the vessels. Each vessel is thus surrounded by two basement membranes, vascular and epithelial, separated by a perivascular space.

The thymic lobules are divided into cortical and medullary areas. The cortex consists of a network of large epithelial cells with stellate outlines, and long, prominent cellular processes, encircling lymphocytes. The epithelial cells have round to oval nuclei, with finely dispersed chromatin and prominent central nucleoli. Their cytoplasms are ill-defined. The cortex is rich in lymphocytes, accounting for its dark-staining appearance. In the subcapsular region the lymphocytes are large blast cells, often in mitosis. Deeper in the cortex the lymphocytes are smaller with a round nucleus, condensed chromatin and a thin rim of cytoplasm (Janossy *et al.*, 1989).

The medulla is formed of closely associated epithelial cells containing few thymocytes. The epithelial cells are small to medium-sized, often spindle-shaped cells, with scant eosinophilic cytoplasm, and thin cellular processes. The nuclei are oval to fusiform, with coarser chromatin structure and inconspicuous nucleoli. Lymphocytes are of the mature thymocyte type. A characteristic feature of the medulla is the presence of Hassall's corpuscles. The corpuscles are composed of concentrically arranged mature and keratinizing epithelial cells, which are continuous with the epithelium of the medulla. Occasionally Hassall's corpuscles are cystic.

In addition to epithelial and lymphoid cells the thymus contains histiocytes, rare plasma cells and eosinophils. Interdigitating cells are present mainly in the medulla. Myoid cells are observed in proximity to Hassall's corpuscles in infants, but disappear in adults. The presence of neuroendocrine cells in human thymus is not well established. Cysts of microscopic size lined by mucin-secreting and ciliated epithelium are common.

Thymic epithelial cells contain a wide range of keratin subunits from low to high molecular mass. The use of a panel of monoclonal anti-keratin antibodies identified three distinct patterns of keratin subunit expression (Čolić *et al.*, 1988). Cytokeratin of large molecular mass (53–68 kD) is present in almost all epithelium including Hassall's corpuscles. Anti-cytokeratin of molecular mass 45 kD strongly labels most of the cortical epithelium, excluding subcapsular, subtrabecular epithelial cell layer and cortical perivascular epithelium. It also stains a subpopulation of medullary epithelium. Anti-cytokeratin of molecular mass either 40 or 54 kD binds to the subcapsular/subtrabecular epithelial cell layer, cortical perivascular epithelial cells and a subpopulation of medullary thymic epithelial cells, but no Hassall's corpuscles. Such complexity could be related to the specific embryonic origin of the thymus, and it has been suggested that subcapsular and medullary epithelium could be of ectodermal origin, whereas the internal cortex could derive from the endodermal portion of the thymus anlage.

References

Čolić, M., Matanović, D., Hegediš, L. and Dujić, A. (1988). Heterogeneity of rat thymic epithelium defined by monoclonal anti-keratin antibodies. *Thymus*, **12**, 123–130

Janossy, G., Campana, D. and Akbar, A. (1989). Kinetics of T lymphocyte development. *Curr. Top. Pathol.*, **79**, 59–99

Sprent, J., Lo, D., Gao, E.-R. and Ron, Y. (1988). T cell selection in the thymus. *Immunol. Rev.*, **101**, 173–190

Stutman, O. (1978). Intrathymic and extrathymic T cell maturation. *Immunol. Rev.*, **42**, 138–184

Stutman, O. (1985). Ontogeny of T cells. *Clin. Immunol. Allergy*, **5**, 191–234

THYMOMA AND THYMIC CARCINOMA

Thymoma and thymic carcinoma are tumours originating from the epithelial component of the thymus, accompanied by a variable number of non-neoplastic lymphocytes (Rosai and Levine, 1976). They are characterized by a remarkable morphological heterogeneity and variable clinical behaviour. Despite an impressive number of studies, considerable confusion and controversy persists in their classification and the relationship between histological characteristics and the clinical course of the neoplasm.

Classification

The most widely used classification is that proposed by Levine and Rosai (1978; Table 2.1). This classification takes into account the histological aspect of the tumour and the biological behaviour determined by the degree of invasiveness at surgery. Although the separation into histological subtypes is rather subjective, it is useful in differential diagnosis.

The use of the term thymoma is restricted to thymic epithelial tumours with minimal or no cytological atypia. Well-encapsulated non-invasive tumours are postulated to be benign. Tumours locally invasive or associated with lymphatic or haematogenous spread are classified as malignant thymoma. All the tumours are composed of thymic epithelial cells with a variable admixture of lymphocytes. According to the size and shape of epithelial cells and the ratio of lymphocytes to epithelial cells, thymomas are further subdivided as predominantly lym-

Table 2.1 Classification of thymoma and thymic carcinoma

I. Benign thymoma
  - No or minimal cytological atypia
  - Encapsulated, not invasive
    - Epithelial (polygonal or spindle)
    - Lymphocytic
    - Mixed epithelial and lymphocytic

II. Malignant thymoma
  - No or minimal cytological atypia
  - (a) Locally invasive (usual form)
  - (b) With lymphatic or haematogenous spread (rare)
    - Epithelial (mostly polygonal)
    - Lymphocytic (rare)
    - Mixed epithelial and lymphocytic

III. Thymic carcinoma
  - Cytologically malignant
  - Usually invasive, or with lymphatic or haematogenous spread
    - Squamous-cell carcinoma
    - Lymphoepithelioma-like carcinoma
    - Clear-cell carcinoma
    - Sarcomatoid carcinoma
    - Undifferentiated carcinoma
    - Mucoepidermoid carcinoma

Modified from Levine and Rosai, 1978

phocytic, predominantly epithelial, or mixed. Predominantly epithelial tumours with prominent fusiform cells, or spindle-cell thymomas, are considered as a special entity.

Tumours displaying obvious histological malignancy are more appropriately termed thymic carcinoma. Although cytological abnormalities of the neoplastic epithelial cells alone are not considered as predictive of malignancy, thymic carcinoma is more likely to be invasive and to metastasize.

A more descriptive classification, based only on histological criteria, was proposed by us (Verley and Hollmann, 1985) distinguishing four histological types of increasing malignancy:

Type 1: Spindle- and oval-cell thymoma, simulating the epithelium of resting thymus, irrespective of the number of lymphocytes.
Type 2: Lymphocyte-rich thymoma, with few small, round or star-like epithelial cells, resembling those of the normal thymus.
Type 3: Differentiated epithelial thymoma, with well-differentiated cellular and architectural patterns. This corresponds to the epithelial, and to the mixed lympho-epithelial type of Rosai and Levine, predominantly composed of large, round or polygonal epithelial cells.
Type 4: Undifferentiated epithelial thymoma, corresponding to thymic carcinoma.

This histological typing largely correlates with invasiveness, but histology appears as a distinct parameter with separate prognostic significance. Thus, spindle-cell thymomas and lymphocyte-rich thymomas are essentially benign in nature, whereas differentiated epithelial thymomas are potentially aggressive, and undifferentiated epithelial thymomas are truly malignant. As a consequence this typing is useful for the pathologist in establishing a prognosis (Table 2.2).

The classification proposed by Marino and Müller-Hermelink (1985) is an interesting approach, based on both morphology and immunohistochemistry, and relating thymomas to the different subsets of normal thymic epithelial cells and their functional activity.

In the normal thymus the thymic epithelial cells regulate the proliferation and differentiation of the immature precursors of the T-cell lineage into mature peripheral T lymphocytes. In most thymomas the proliferation and maturation of T cells is maintained, at least partially, by neoplastic cells which in addition give rise to certain structural features resembling the normal tissue, e.g. lobular growth pattern, occurrence of perivascular spaces or differentiation into Hassall's corpuscles. According to the prevalent epithelial cell type and the pattern of lymphoid infiltration, the authors describe three subtypes of thymoma.

Cortical thymomas are related to the outer thymic cortex. They consist of large epithelial cells with stellate outlines, and long prominent cellular processes. Lymphocytes are usually abundant, often with a blastic appearance.
Medullary thymomas derive from medullary epithelial cells. They are composed of small to medium-sized, often spindle-shaped, epithelial cells. Lymphocytes, generally present in small numbers, are of the mature thymocyte type.
Mixed thymomas are also described and characterized by the proliferation of both cortical and medullary epithelial cells, intermingled with a variable number of lymphocytes. They are further divided into three subgroups: the mixed common type, mixed with cortical predominance, and mixed with medullary predominance.

The three subtypes correlate well with surgical stage of the tumours, biological behaviour and long-term prognosis. The medullary type and the mixed type are mostly benign in nature. The cortical type and the predominant cortical type are often invasive and of poorer prognosis. They are frequently associated with myasthenia gravis. Pure epithelial tumours correspond either to a high degree of monophasic benign epithelial differentiation in medullary spindle-cell thymoma, or to the loss of normal functional differentiation in thymic carcinoma.

In morphometric studies Nomori *et al.* (1988, 1989) confirm that the epithelial cell nuclei of cortical thymomas are larger than those of medullary thymomas, and that cortical thymomas are more frequently invasive and associated with myasthenia gravis, and have a higher malignant grade than the medullary and mixed types.

Table 2.2 Relationship between clinical stages and histological types in 200 patients with thymoma

		Histological type					
Clinical stage	*No. of patients*	*1*	*2*	*Total benign*	*3*	*4*	*Total malignant*
Non-invasive	133	54	52	106 (80%)	26	1	27 (20%)
Invasive	67	6	7	13 (19.5%)	41	13	54 (80.5%)

Type 1: Spindle-cell thymoma; type 2: lymphocyte-rich thymoma; type 3: differentiated epithelial thymoma; type 4: undifferentiated epithelial thymoma or thymic carcinoma. From Verley and Hollmann, 1985

Evaluation of the degree of maturation of thymoma lymphocytes by flow cytometry and monoclonal antibodies was investigated by Ito *et al.* (1988). From the viewpoint of lymphocyte subsets, thymomas can be divided into three types: thymus lymphocyte type (immature thymocyte; $CD1^+ > 50\% > CD3^+$), peripheral lymphocyte type (mature thymocyte predominantly of $CD3^+$ phenotype; $CD1^+ < 10\% < CD3^+$), and intermediate type ($10\% > CD1^+ < 30\%$).

There is a close relationship between histological features of thymoma and results of lymphocyte subset analysis. All polygonal large-cell thymomas are infiltrated by immature $CD1^+$ thymocytes, whereas spindle-cell thymomas contain various types of lymphocyte subsets. In the immature $CD1^+$ thymus lymphocyte type, lymphocytes are numerous and intermingled with the epithelial tumour cells. In the mature predominantly $CD3^+$ peripheral lymphocyte type, lymphocytes are scarce and aggregate along the margins of the tumour cell foci. In most cases there is a predominance of $CD1^+$ cells, suggesting that most of the thymoma cells have properties resembling those of thymic cortical epithelial cells.

From these studies a new approach in the classification of thymomas emerges, taking into account the histogenesis, morphology and immunohistochemistry of the neoplastic epithelial component, and the degree of maturation of the non-neoplastic lymphocytes related to functional activity of the epithelial cells. Unfortunately, the different classifications do not always correlate (Table 2.3). Some need sophisticated immunohistochemical or morphometric techniques. The distinction between the different subtypes described by Marino and Müller-Hermelink appears subtle and somewhat arbitrary, and the main drawback of their classification is the difficulty for surgical pathologists to use it with confidence. The classification of Levine and Rosai is also deceptive, since it distinguishes benign from malignant thymoma only on the basis of encapsulated versus invasive or metastasizing tumour, and accords little prognostic value to the histological aspect.

Under these conditions the histological typing of a thymic tumour is still controversial. As a practical approach the following procedure may be recommended. First, the tumour should be classified into non-invasive thymoma (presumed benign), invasive thymoma (presumed malignant), and thymic carcinoma (with obvious architectural and cytological atypia). Invasion is best evaluated at the time of surgery, but careful histological control is necessary in the case of fibrous adhesion. Second, the major histological characteristics of the tumour should be evaluated. These include the size and shape of the epithelial cells, the degree of differentiation of the tumour (lobular pattern, delimitation of the lobules, perivascular spaces), and the lymphocyte–epithelial cell ratio. Hereafter, concluding remarks should indicate if the tumour is *clinically* benign or malignant, i.e. non-invasive or invasive, and if it is *histologically* benign or potentially malignant, i.e. composed of small (round or spindle) epithelial cells of medullary type, or composed of large well-differentiated epithelial cells of cortical type. In the case of thymic carcinoma the histological type should be specified, and the tumour classified into low- or high-grade histology categories.

Thymoma and associated diseases

A major feature of thymoma is the association with a number of autoimmune diseases or haematological disorders, among which the most common is myasthenia gravis (MG). The incidence of MG in patients with thymoma ranges from 7% to 54% in various series, with a mean of approximately 35%. Conversely, 10–15% of patients with MG are found to have a thymoma. Patients with MG tend to be younger at diagnosis of their thymoma, due to improved methods in the management of myasthenic patients and earlier detection of the tumour. Associated diseases other than MG occur in approximately 10% of patients with thymoma and are not exceptionally coincident with MG. Table 2.4 indicates the decreasing frequency of the different associated disorders.

Red-cell hypoplasia occurs in about 5% of thymoma patients and over half of the patients with red-cell hypoplasia harbour a thymoma. Thus, although red-cell hypoplasia is a rarer disease than MG, the relation between red-cell hypoplasia and thymoma is closer than that between MG and thymoma. The disease is either isolated or associated with MG or hypogammaglobulinaemia (Masaoka *et al.*, 1989).

The association of thymoma and hypogammaglobulinaemia is less frequent but seems to be underestimated. Approximately 10% of patients with hypogammaglobulinaemia have a thymoma and 12% of patients with thymoma would have hypogammaglobulinaemia (Waldmann *et al.*, 1975).

Table 2.4 Thymoma and associated diseases

Myasthenia gravis	Rheumatoid arthritis
Red-cell hypoplasia	Scleroderma
Hypogammaglobulinaemia	Kaposi's sarcoma
Polymyositis	Hashimoto's disease
Myocarditis	Peripheral neuropathy
Systemic lupus erythematosus	Erythrocytosis
Pemphigus vulgaris	Megakaryocytopenia
Myeloma, acute leukaemia	Others
Sjögren's disease	

Clinical features

Thymomas are the most common neoplasms of the anterosuperior mediastinum in adults, representing 25–47% of the tumours in this compartment. They are primarily tumours of middle to later life with a mean age at diagnosis of approximately 50 years, without any sex predilection. Thymic carcinomas occur in younger

Table 2.3 Tentative correspondence between the classifications of thymoma and thymic carcinoma

Degree of malignancy	*Levine and Rosai (1978)*	*Verley and Hollmann (1985)*	*Marino and Müller-Hermelink (1989)*
Benign	Non-invasive thymoma	Spindle-cell and lymphocyte-rich thymoma	Medullary type Mixed type
Malignant	Invasive thymoma	Differentiated epithelial thymoma	Predominant cortical type Cortical type
	Thymic carcinoma	Undifferentiated thymoma = thymic carcinoma	Well-differentiated thymic carcinoma
			Epidermoid carcinoma Endocrine carcinoma Undifferentiated carcinoma

patients with a median of 40 years, and a male predominance is noted in most series. In children, primary thymic epithelial neoplasms are extremely rare and display unusual morphological features (Cajal and Suster, 1991).

Approximately half of the thymomas are incidentally discovered at routine chest radiography, especially in myasthenic patients. Other patients are symptomatic with signs due to compression or invasion of mediastinal structures. The most common symptoms are cough, dyspnoea, chest pain or superior vena cava syndrome. Only exceptionally is thymoma revealed by lymphogenous or haematogenous metastasis, or diagnosed at autopsy. Sometimes the tumour is discovered at therapeutic thymectomy in myasthenic patients.

On chest roentgenogram, thymoma typically presents as a lobulated anterior or anterosuperior mediastinal mass, usually sharply demarcated and asymmetrically placed (Fig. 2.1). Ectopic location in the superior, middle or inferior (Fig. 2.2), or more exceptionally in the posterior mediastinum have been reported. Some cases may develop in the neck from a thymus that has failed to descend (Chan and Rosai, 1991). A very exceptional intrapulmonary occurrence has also been described. Small tumours may escape observation on anteroposterior radiographs. In such cases CT scans or MRI are helpful (Figs 2.3 and 2.4). Adversely, large invasive thymomas and thymic carcinomas project beyond the mediastinal boundaries into the surrounding structures (Figs 2.5 and 2.6). Again CT scans are useful to delineate the extent of the tumour, and can reveal small tumorous grafts on the pleura and/or pulmonary metastases.

Calcifications are present in about 20% of cases but are without diagnostic value. Thymic epithelial tumours have no radiographic signs distinguishing them from other mediastinal tumours. Nevertheless, if the patient suffers from MG, red-cell hypoplasia or hypogammaglobulinaemia, in the presence of a mediastinal mass the diagnosis of thymoma is virtually assumed.

Gross pathology

The majority of thymomas present as lobulated, well-circumscribed and encapsulated masses (Figs 2.7–2.13). The size varies greatly, with the majority between 5 and 10 cm in diameter. The tumour develops inside a thymic horn (Fig. 2.7) or occupies the whole gland, or sometimes appears distant from the gland and appended to a horn. In about 30% of the cases, thymomas are incompletely encapsulated and are locally invasive. These invasive thymomas tend to encroach the mediastinal fat tissue and the adjacent structures (Figs 2.14–2.17). On section, the tumours are either firm, pinkish to grey (Figs 2.9, 2.11, 2.12, 2.15), or soft, white, of fish-flesh appearance (Fig. 2.10). They are usually lobulated by large fibrous septa (Figs 2.9, 2.12, 2.15, 2.16). Many tumours show foci of cystic degeneration or true cysts, whereas haemorrhagic or necrotic areas are less common (Figs 2.11, 2.13, 2.16). Calcifications are frequently present in the capsule or the internal fibrous bands. Intrathoracic tumorous grafts may be present (Fig. 2.18). Thymic carcinomas are not encapsulated tumours that usually largely invade the surrounding tissues. The cut section is firm, white to yellow, with large areas of necrosis (Fig. 2.17) and hyaline fibrosis.

Based on the gross inspection at surgery four clinical stages have been described by Masaoka *et al.* (1981). This clinical staging is now extensively in use, sometimes with minor modifications (Table 2.5).

Histology

The various histological patterns of thymomas depend on two factors:the shape and size of the epithelial cells, and the number, degree of maturation and distribution of the accompanying lymphocytes. Other features, such as the presence of large fibrous septa lobulating the tumour, enlarged perivascular spaces, and Hassall's corpuscle differentiation, are characteristic of certain types of tumour. The fibrous septa characteristically intersect at sharp acute angles and divide the tumour into irregular angular lobules (Fig. 2.19) that differ from the rounded aspect observed in Hodgkin's disease (see Fig. 3.11).

Table 2.5 Thymoma and thymic carcinoma, clinical stages

Stage I	Macroscopically completely encapsulated and microscopically no capsular invasion
Stage II	1. Macroscopic invasion into surrounding fatty tissue or mediastinal pleura, or 2. Microscopic invasion into capsule
Stage III	Macroscopic invasion into neighbouring organs, i.e. pericardium, great vessels, or lung
Stage IVa	Pleural or pericardial dissemination
Stage IVb	Lymphogenous or haematogenous metastasis

According to Masaoka *et al.* (1981)

Benign thymomas are well-encapsulated, non-invasive, stage I tumours. When fibrous adherence to adjacent structures occurs, a thorough histological examination must be performed to indicate whether microscopic capsular invasion exists.

Many thymomas are composed of large epithelial cells, corresponding to the *predominantly epithelial* and *lymphoepithelial* types of Levine and Rosai (1978), *the cortical* and *predominant cortical* variants of Marino and Müller-Hermelink (1985), and the *differentiated epithelial* thymoma of Verley and Hollmann (1985) (Figs 2.19–2.29). The epithelial cells are round or star-like in areas rich in lymphocytes, and more polygonal and epidermoid-like in predominantly epithelial regions. The cytoplasm is clear and abundant and the nuclei are large, vesicular and clear or homogeneous. Nucleoli are small or large, usually prominent. Nuclear abnormalities are at times present, but without hyperchromasia, and the nucleocytoplasmic ratio remains low, less than 0.5–1. There is no anaplasia. Araldite-embedded half-thin sections show the large epithelial cells, with abundant cytoplasm and well-defined outlines, linked to adjacent cells by numerous desmosomes (Figs 2.22 and 2.27). In most instances the tumours are sharply lobulated by large fibrous septa, without penetration of the tumour cell into the capsule or the septa (Fig. 2.19). Enlarged vascular spaces, and peripheral palisading of epithelial cells around the blood vessels are frequent characteristic features (Figs 2.23, 2.25 and 2.26). The enlarged vascular spaces are empty, penetrated by lymphocytes or foamy cells, or hyalinized. Focal medullary differentiation is another typical aspect. It consists of paler zones, due to a higher epithelial–lymphocyte ratio than the surrounding thymoma, and resembles the medulla of normal thymus. Hassall's corpuscles and microcalcifications may be present. Necrosis occurs occasionally. Lymphocytes are usually blastic in appearance and their number varies from area to area and from one tumour to another.

Spindle-cell thymomas are composed of small to medium-sized, oval or spindle-shaped epithelial cells with scant eosinophilic cytoplasm, and thin cellular processes. The nuclei are oval to fusiform, with coarser chromatin structure and inconspicuous nucleoli. The tumours exhibit a diversity of architectural aspects (Figs 2.31–2.45). Some tumours are composed of spindle epithelial cells arranged in interlacing fascicles (Fig. 2.38). Other

[*continued on p. 23*]

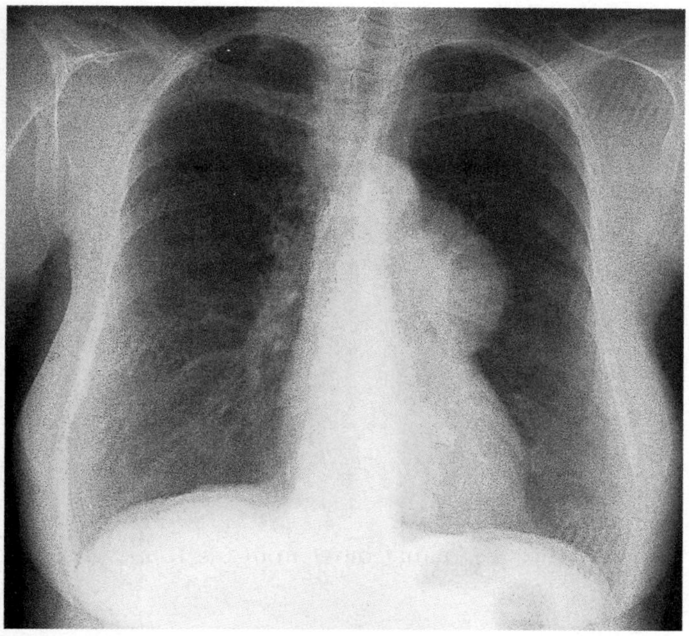

Figure 2.1 Thymoma. Chest X-ray shows a well-circumscribed mass of the antero-superior mediastinum

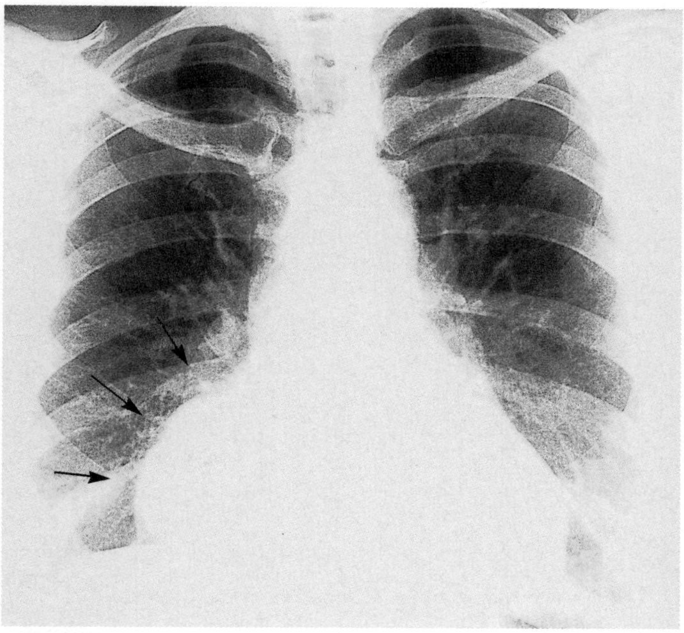

Figure 2.2 Ectopic thymoma presenting as a well-limited mass situated in the right cardiophrenic angle and simulating a pericardial cyst

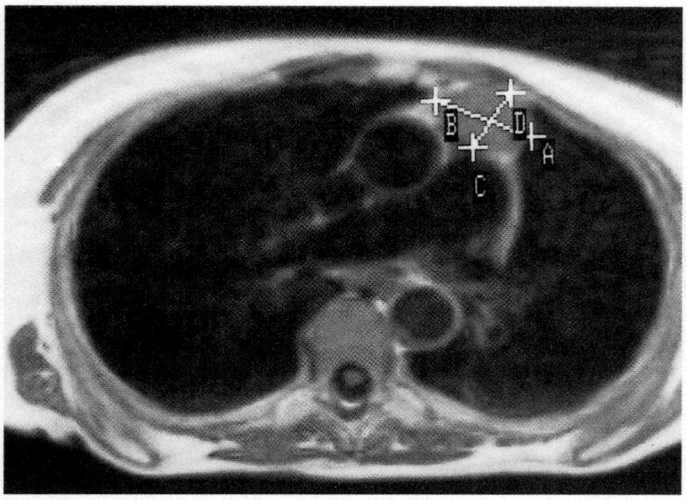

Figures 2.3 and 2.4 Thymoma. MR imaging delineates a small tumour situated in the anterior mediastinum. **Fig. 2.3**: transaxial view; **Fig. 2.4**: sagittal view

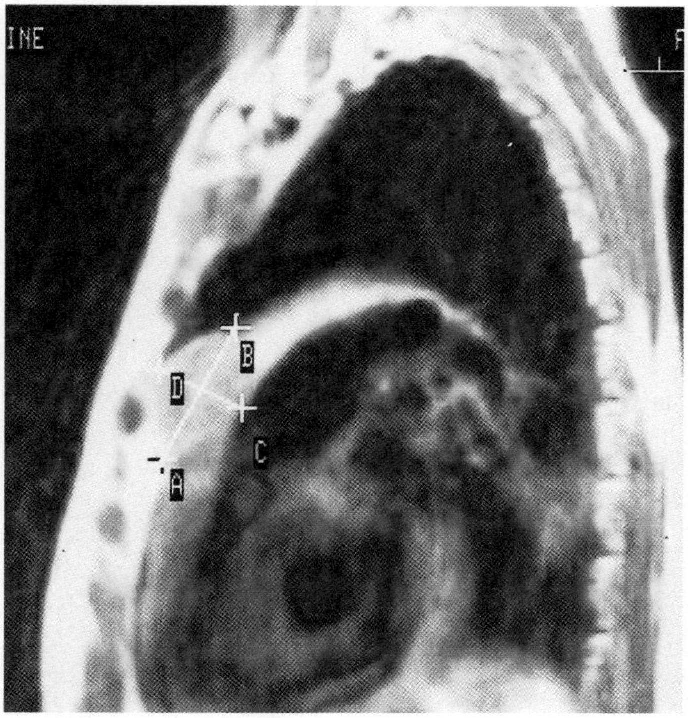

Figure 2.4

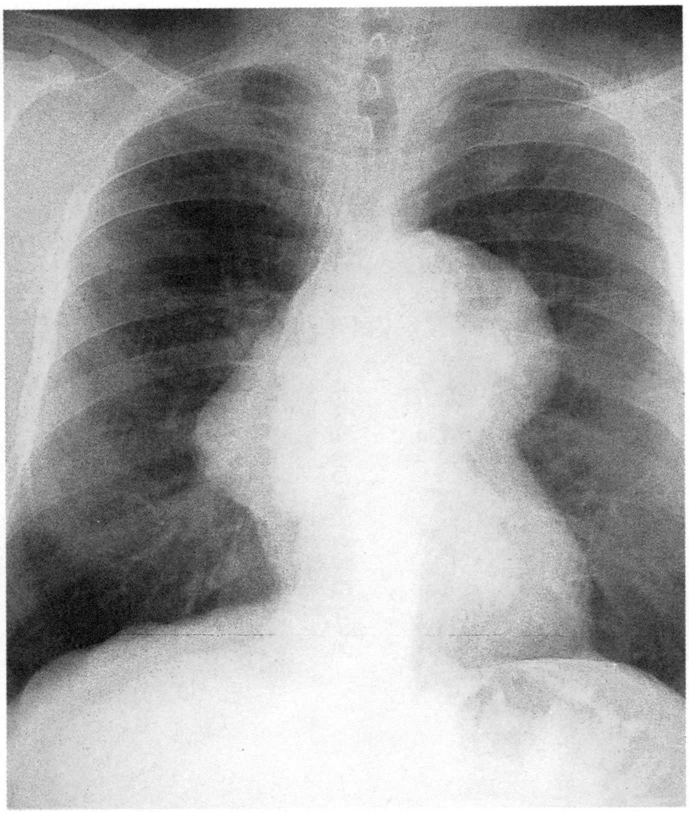

Figures 2.5 and 2.6 Invasive thymoma. Chest X-ray shows a large anterior mediastinal mass compressing the trachea. **Fig. 2.5**: posteroanterior view; **Fig. 2.6**: lateral view

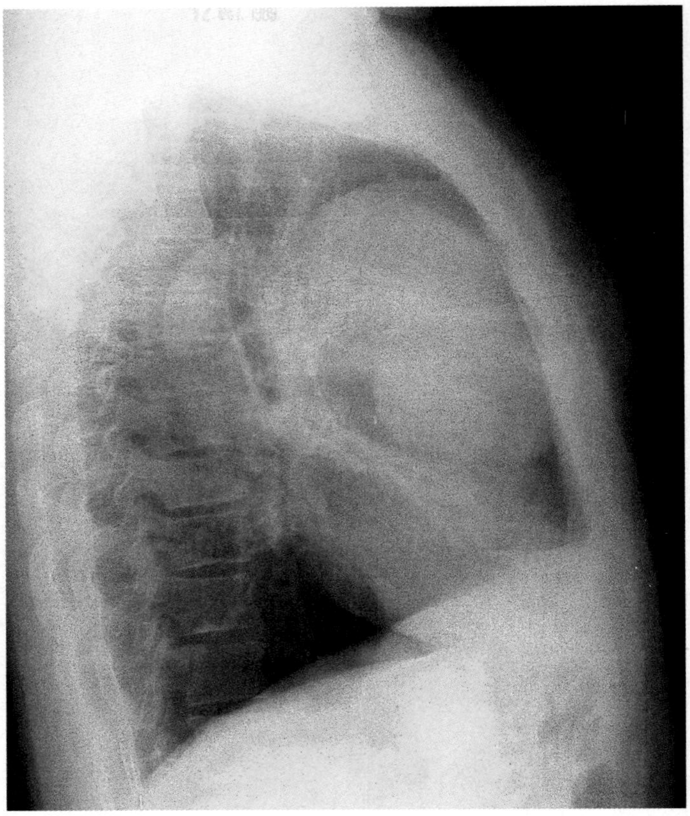

Figure 2.6

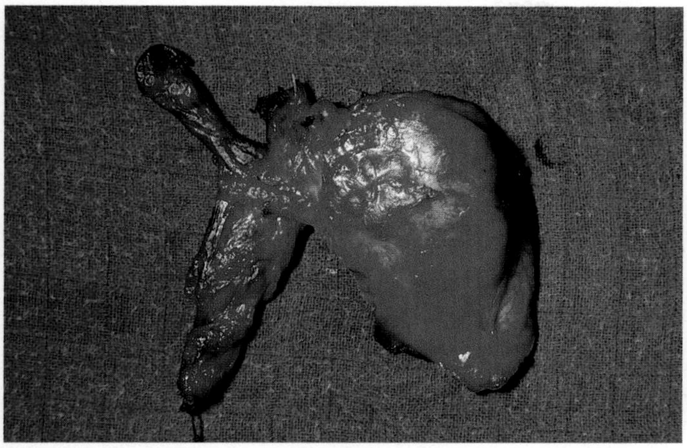

Figure 2.7 Benign thymoma. The tumour develops inside the left thymic horn

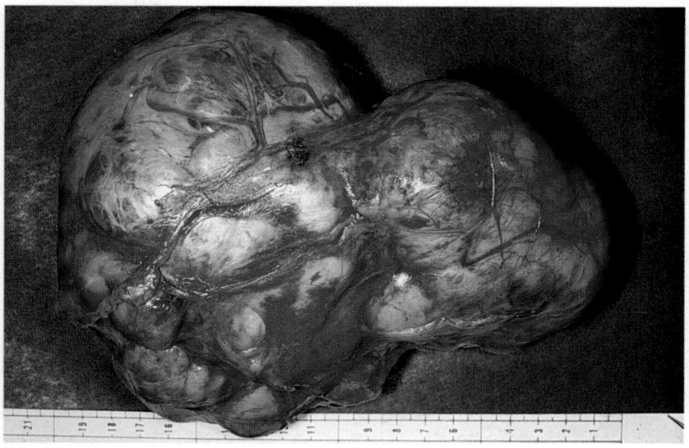

Figure 2.8 Benign thymoma, spindle-cell type. Large lobulated, well-encapsulated tumour

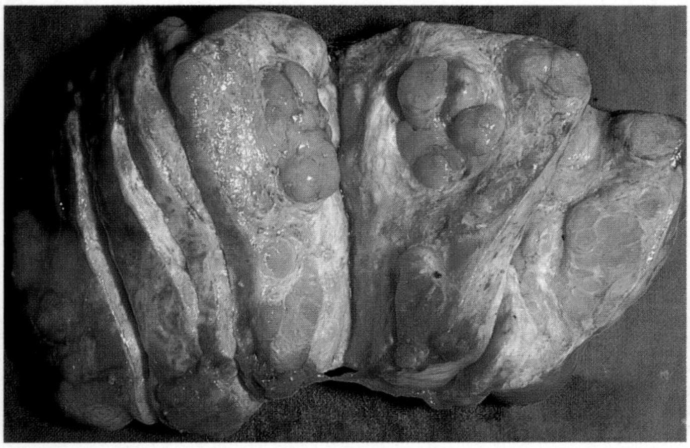

Figure 2.9 Benign thymoma, same tumour. On section the tumour is lobulated by large fibrous septa

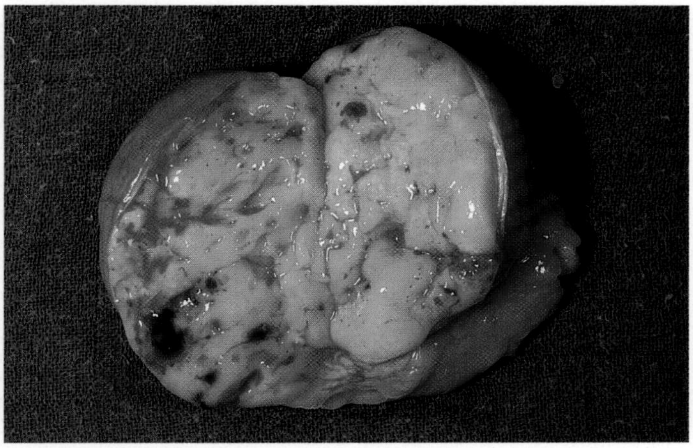

Figure 2.10 Benign thymoma, lymphocyte-rich. The tumour has a fish-flesh appearance that evokes a lymphoma

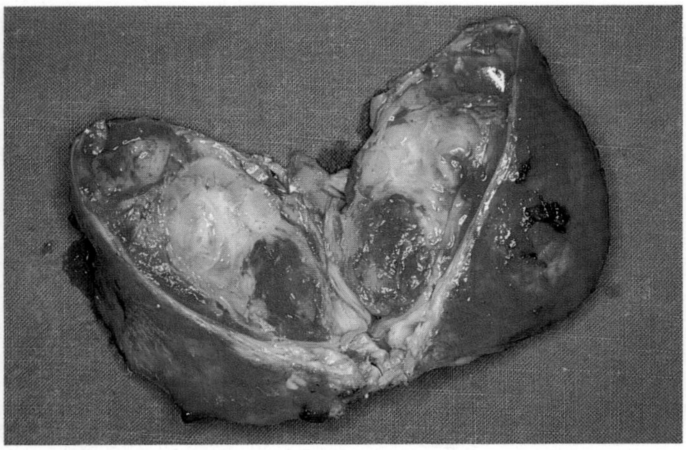

Figure 2.11 Benign thymoma, lymphoepithelial type. The tumour is well-encapsulated and shows haemorrhagic and necrotic areas

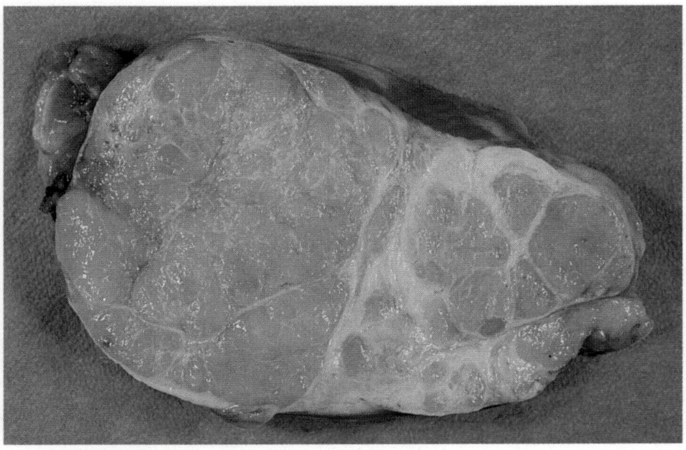

Figure 2.12 Benign thymoma, spindle-cell type. Lobulation by thin fibrous septa simulates Hodgkin's disease

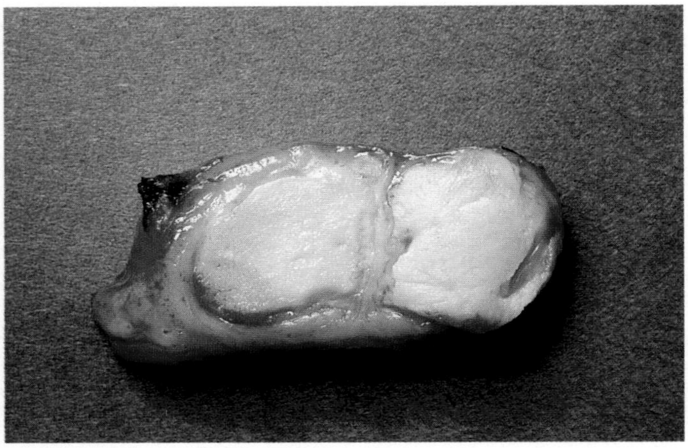

Figure 2.13 Benign thymoma. The tumour shows massive necrotic changes

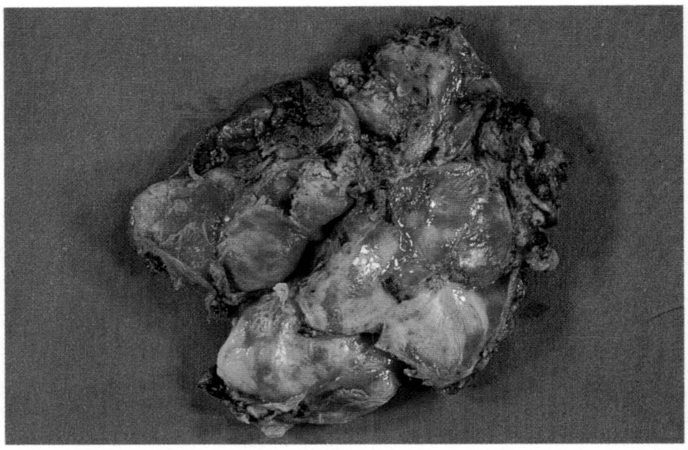

Figure 2.14 Invasive thymoma. Nodular, irregular tumour with capsular invasion

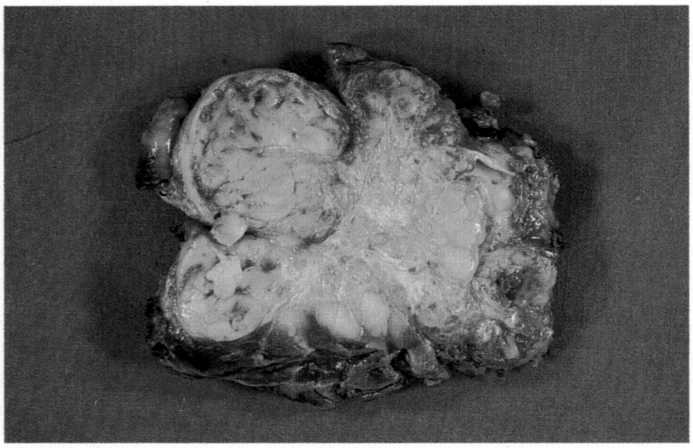

Figure 2.15 Invasive thymoma. The cut section of the same tumour shows a typical aspect with fibrous bands and lobulation

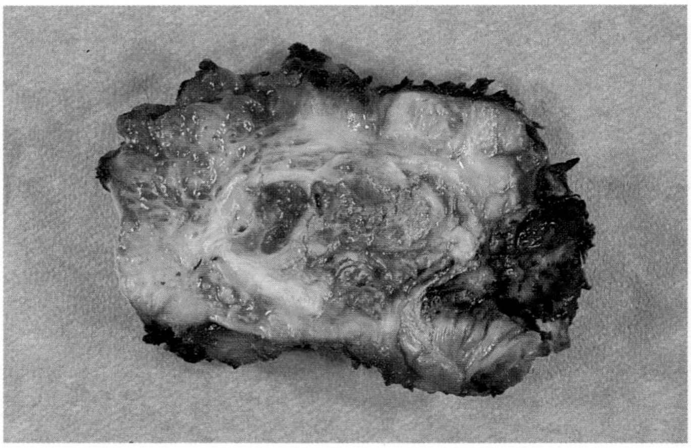

Figure 2.16 Invasive thymoma. The non-encapsulated tumour has a large central area of cystic degeneration and fibrosis

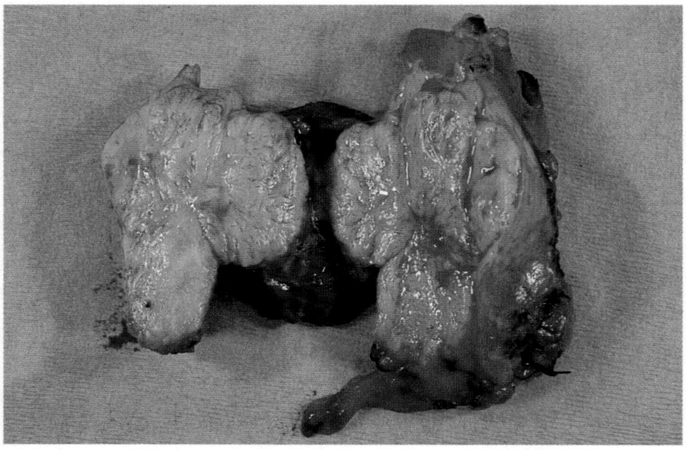

Figure 2.17 Thymic carcinoma. Large, bosselated and fleshy tumour invading a lung

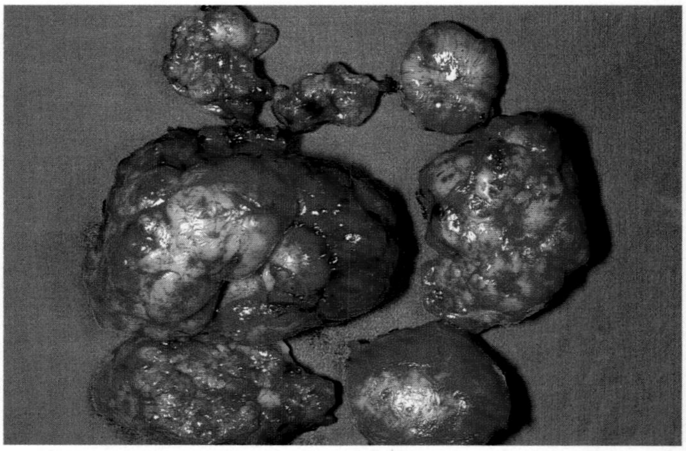

Figure 2.18 Thymic carcinoma. Multiple tumorous grafts resected from the pleura

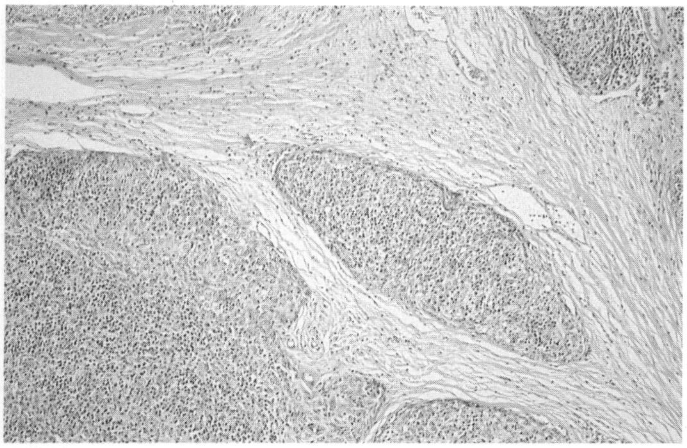

Figure 2.19 The tumour is lobulated by large fibrous septa that characteristically intersect at sharp acute angles and divide the tumour into irregular angular lobules.

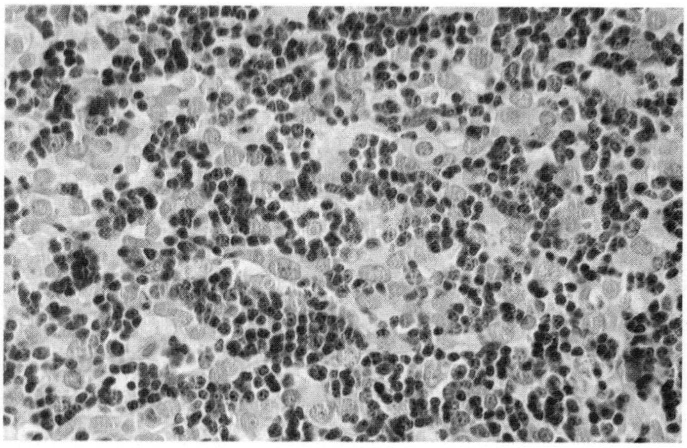

Figures 2.20 and 2.21 Benign thymoma, mixed lymphoepithelial type. The figures show the typical aspect of a thymoma from a myasthenic patient and illustrate the variable admixture of epithelial cells and lymphocytes. The epithelial cells are large, with an abundant clear cytoplasm, and round homogeneous nuclei. Note the continuous row of epithelial cells at the periphery of the lobules

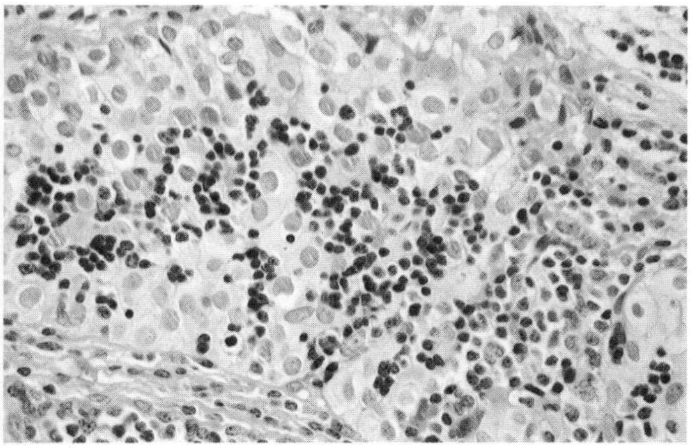

Figure 2.21

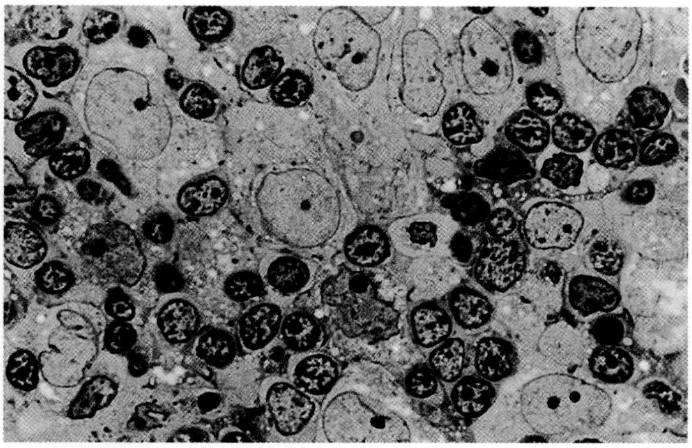

Figure 2.22 Benign thymoma, mixed lymphoepithelial type. A half-thin section of the same tumour depicts the large well-defined epithelial cells contrasting with the smaller dense lymphocytes

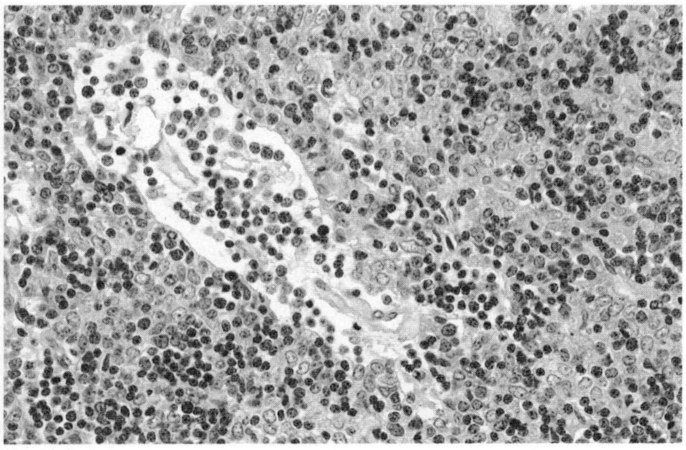

Figure 2.23 Benign thymoma, mixed lymphoepithelial type. The figure displays the characteristic aspect of an enlarged vascular space with central vessel. The space contains lymphocytes and is surrounded by epithelial cells

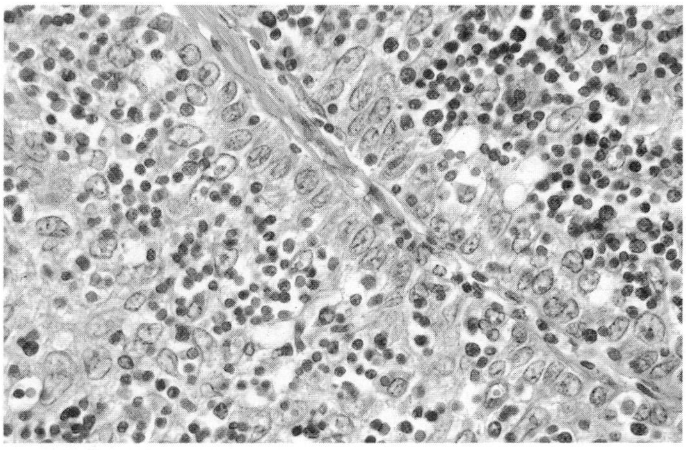

Figure 2.24 Benign thymoma, mixed lymphoepithelial type. Epithelial cells along the septa are higher and arranged in palisade

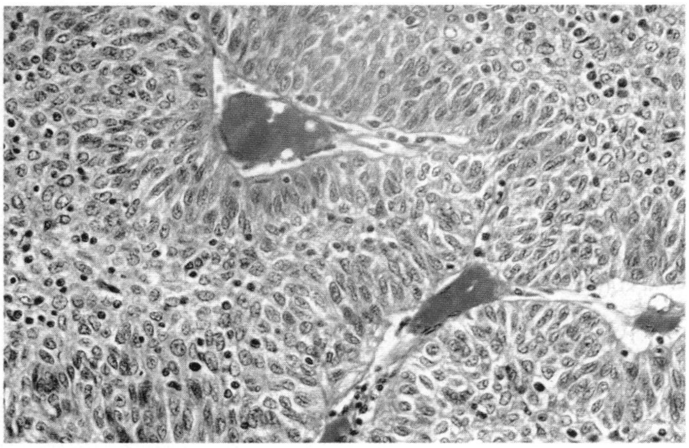

Figures 2.25 and 2.26 Benign thymoma, epithelial-predominant. The epithelial cells are large and polygonal and show a peripheral palisading around vascular spaces. The enlarged spaces contain lymphocytes

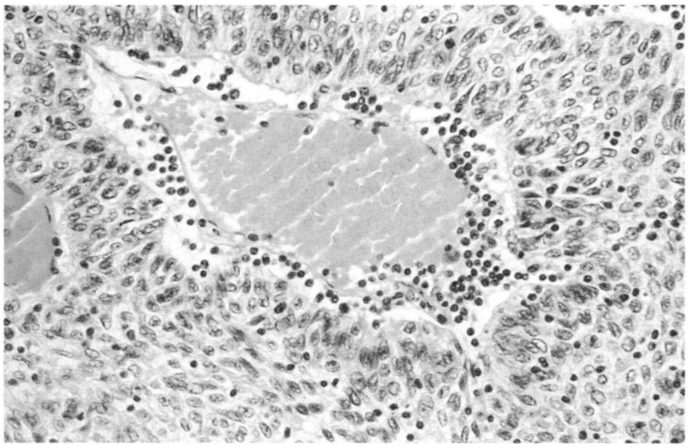

Figure 2.26

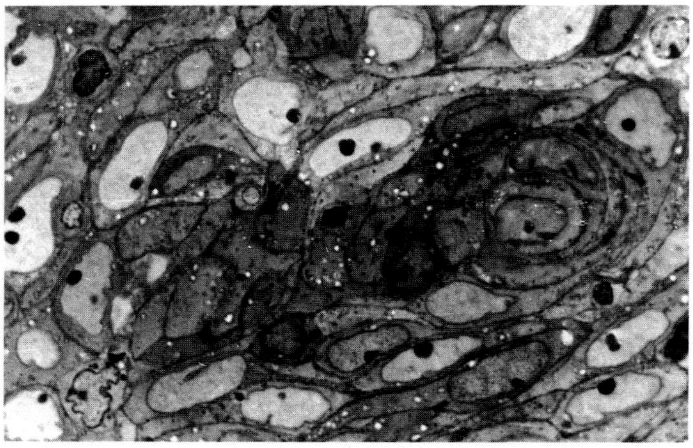

Figure 2.27 Benign thymoma, epithelial-predominant. The half-thin section emphasizes the epidermoid-like arrangement of the tumour cells. The cytoplasmic borders are well-defined, and linked togther with numerous desmosomes. The nuclei are large and homogeneous, and contain conspicuous nucleoli

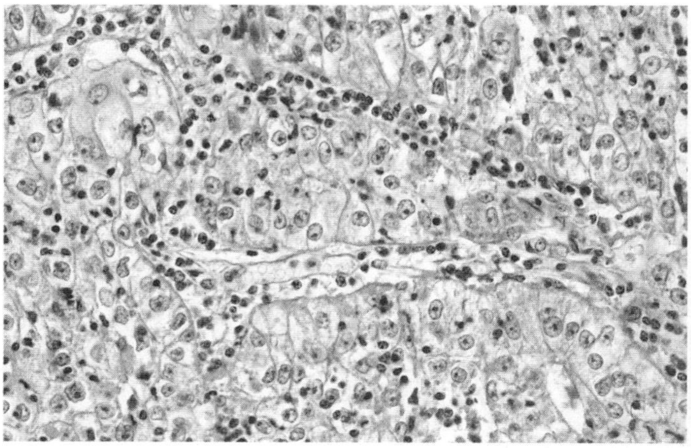

Figure 2.28 Benign thymoma, epithelial-predominant. The tumour is composed of large clear epithelial cells interspersed with few lymphocytes

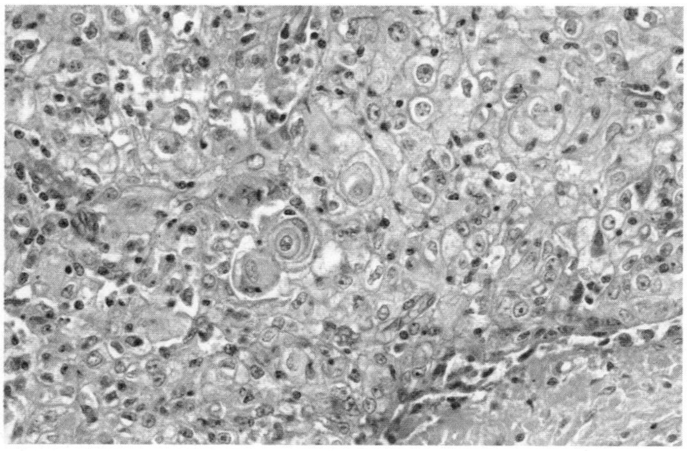

Figure 2.29 Benign thymoma, epithelial-predominant. The whorled arrangement of the epithelial cells evokes a Hassall's corpuscle differentiation

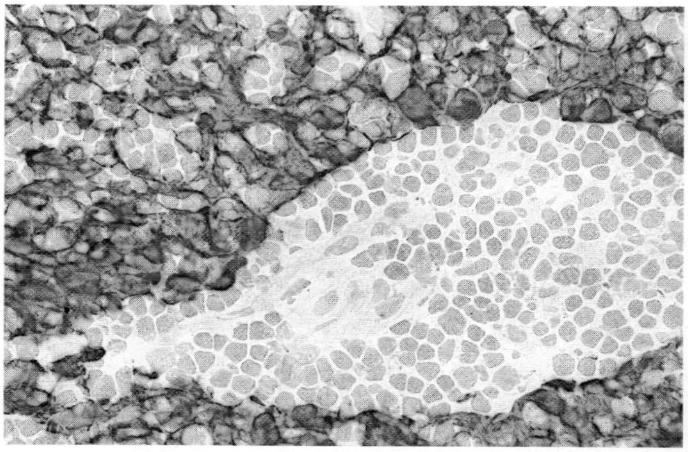

Figure 2.30 Benign thymoma, epithelial-predominant. Immunostaining with cytokeratin highlights the closely connected epithelial cells, which stain brown. The lymphocytes scattered among the epithelial cells, or filling the enlarged vascular lake, are not stained

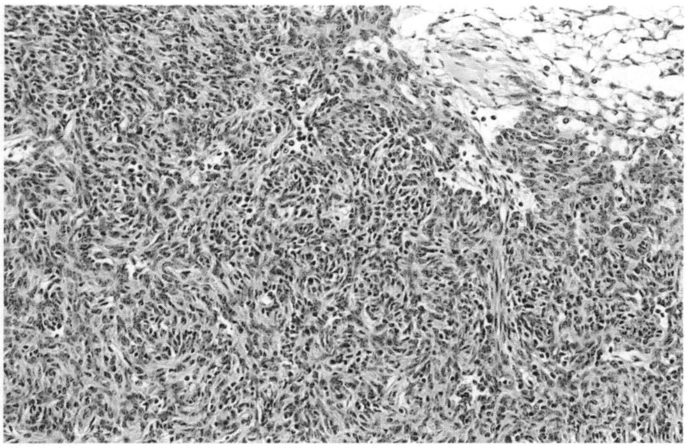

Figure 2.31 Benign thymoma, spindle-cell type. The tumour is composed of thin elongated epithelial cells. The lobular pattern is indistinct

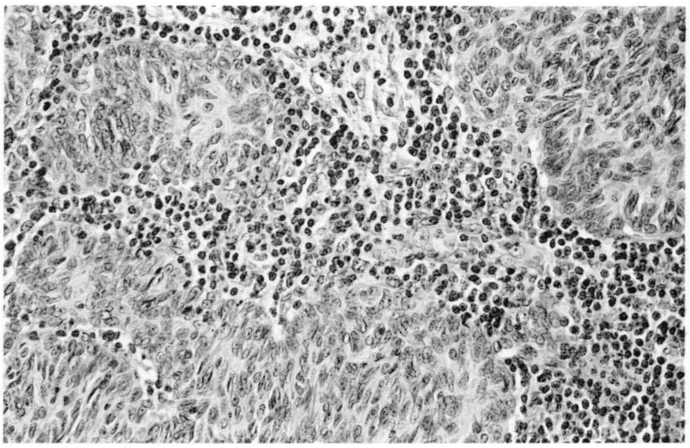

Figure 2.32 Benign thymoma, spindle-cell type. In this tumour there is a sharp separation, between the ovoid epithelial cells exhibiting a whorled arrangement, and the lymphocytes

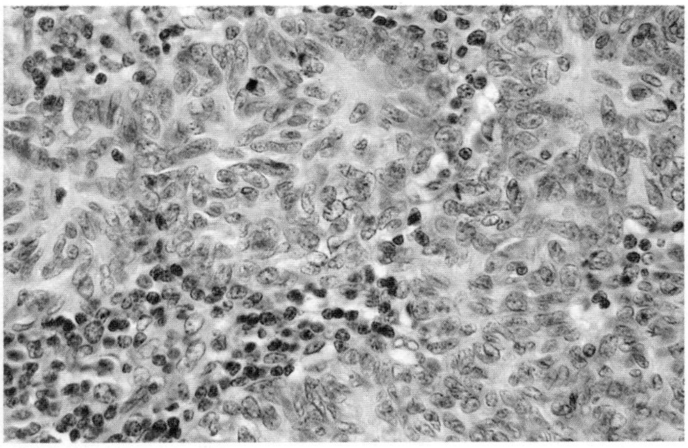

Figure 2.33 Benign thymoma, spindle-cell type. Higher magnification of the same tumour

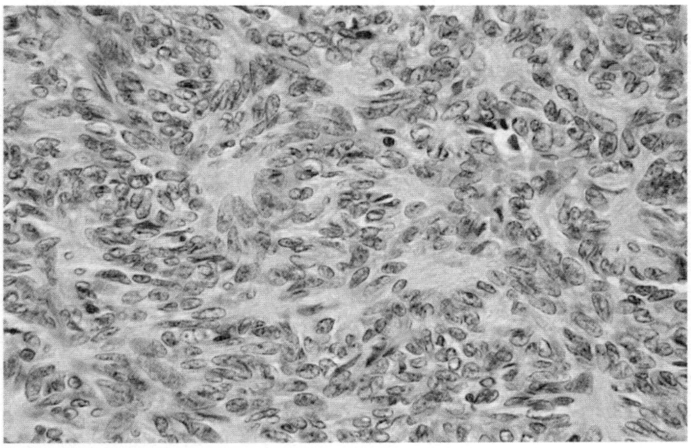

Figure 2.34 Benign thymoma, spindle-cell type. Rosette pattern reminiscent of that seen in neuroblastoma

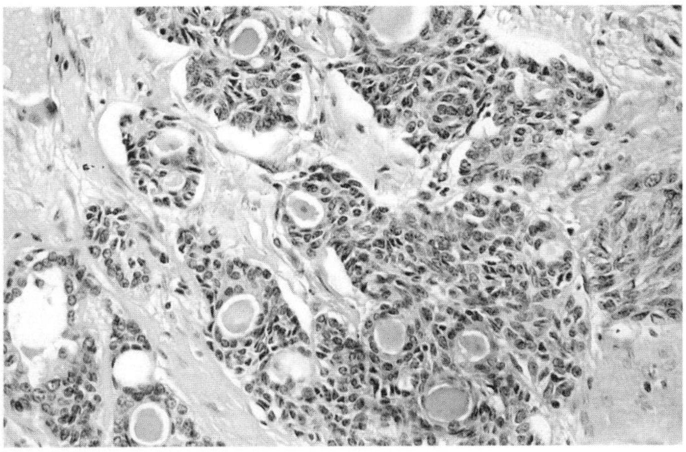

Figure 2.35 Benign thymoma, spindle-cell type. The tumour displays a cylindroma-like configuration

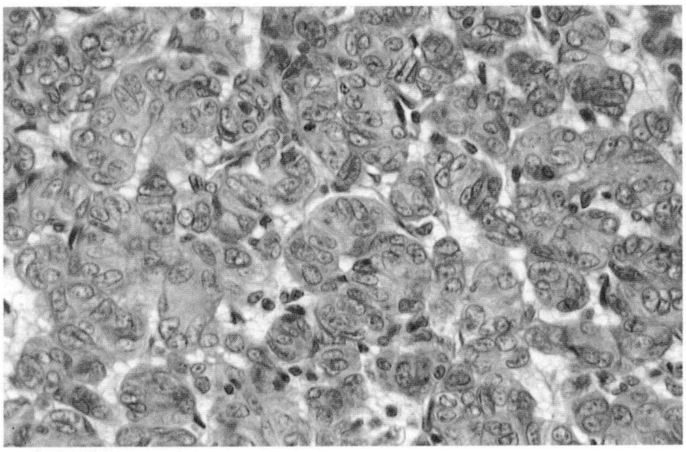

Figure 2.36 Benign thymoma, spindle-cell type. Nesting pattern resembling that in carcinoid or paraganglion tumours

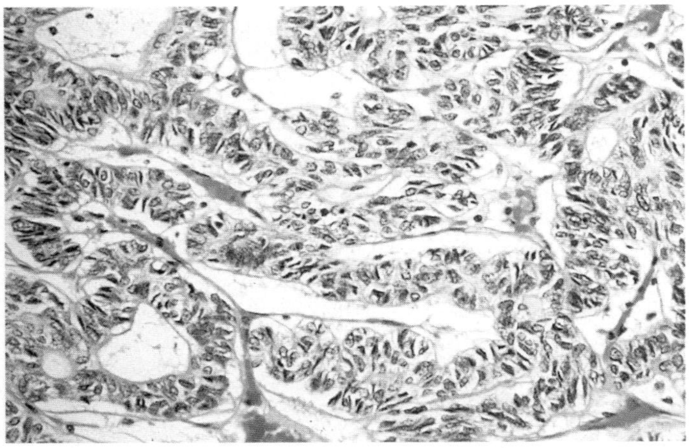

Figure 2.37 Benign thymoma, spindle-cell type. The trabecular arrangement and the rich vascularization evoke a carcinoid tumour

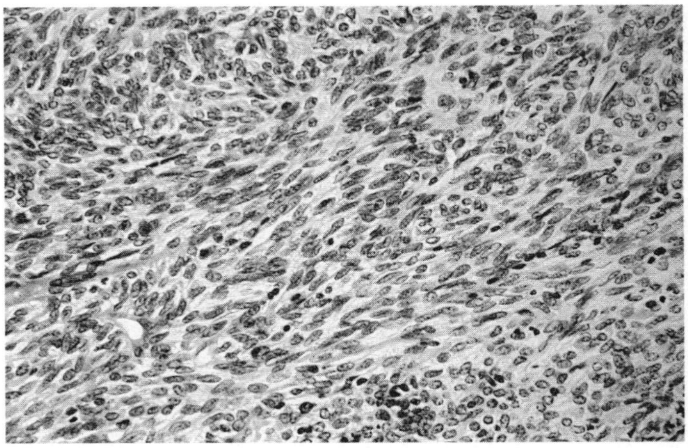

Figure 2.38 Benign thymoma, spindle-cell type. This figure illustrates a storiform pattern

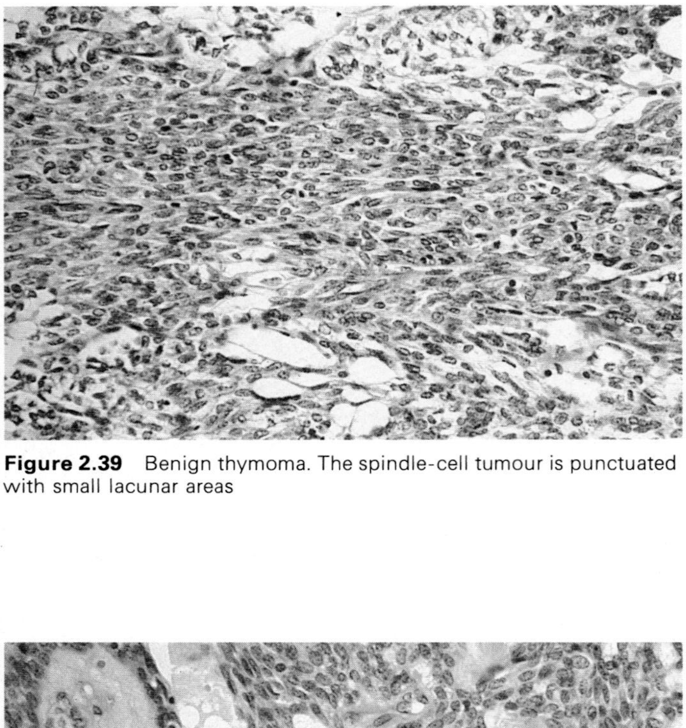

Figure 2.39 Benign thymoma. The spindle-cell tumour is punctuated with small lacunar areas

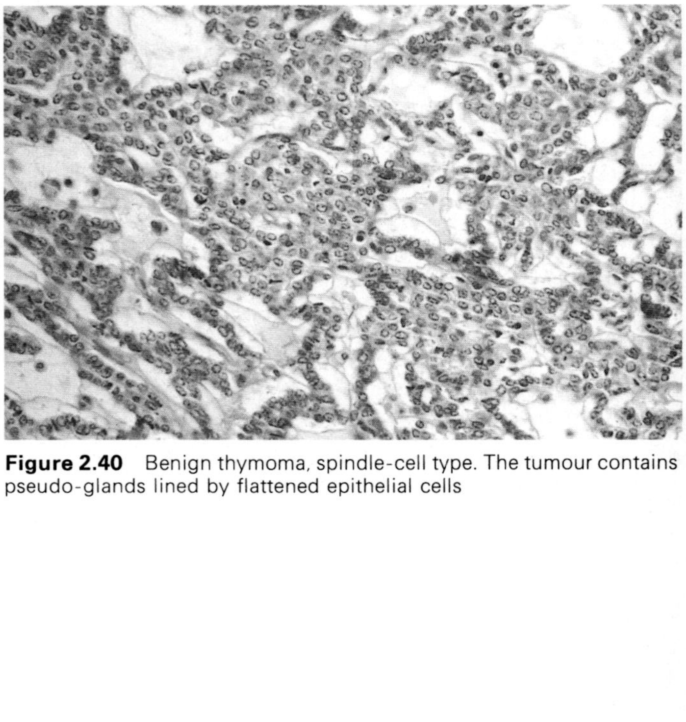

Figure 2.40 Benign thymoma, spindle-cell type. The tumour contains pseudo-glands lined by flattened epithelial cells

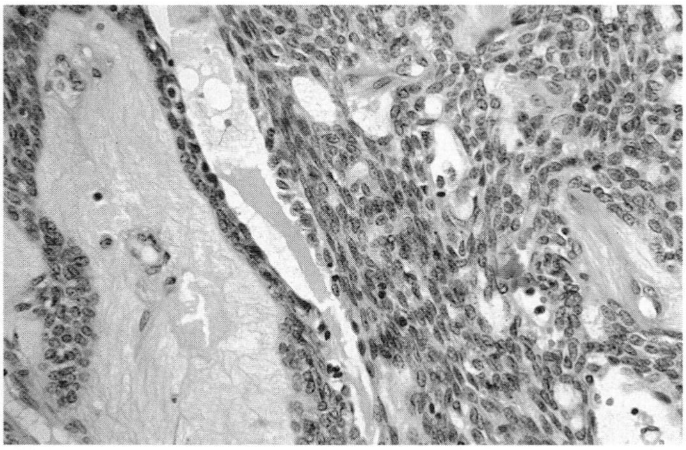

Figure 2.41 Benign thymoma, spindle-cell type. The abundant pale material separating the tumour cells probably corresponds to the hyalinization of vascular spaces

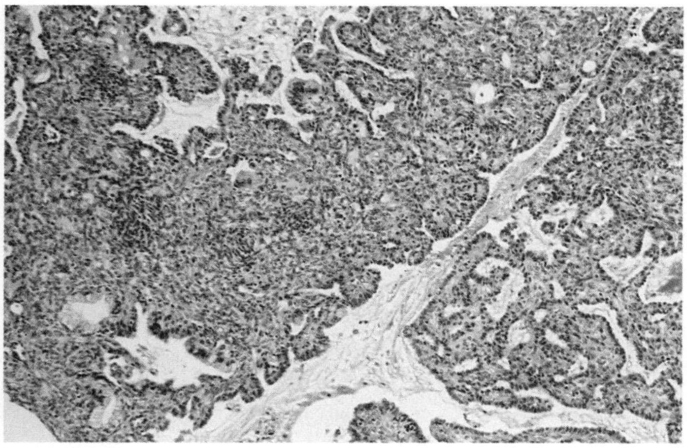

Figure 2.42 Benign thymoma, spindle-cell type. The tumour shows pseudo-glandular and true glandular differentiation

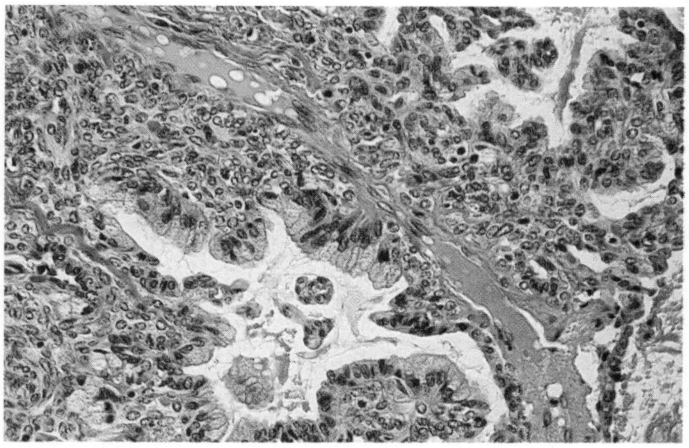

Figure 2.43 Benign thymoma, spindle-cell type. Higher magnification of the same tumour. The glandular formations are lined with mucus-secreting goblet cells

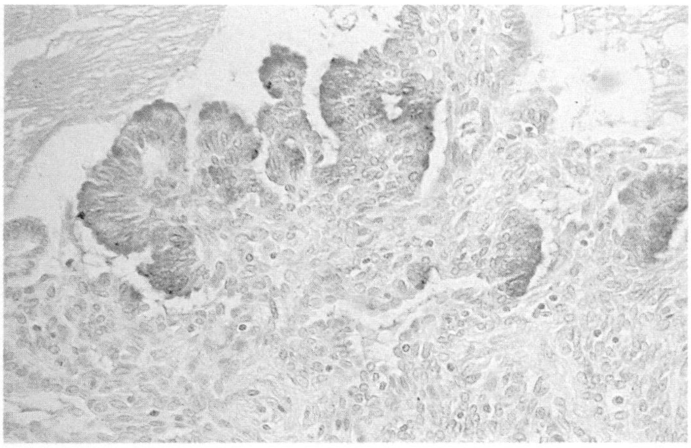

Figure 2.44 Benign thymoma, spindle-cell type. Same tumour. The mucus is stained with alcian blue. (Figures 2.42–2.44 are from the same tumour.) Courtesy of Dr J.J. Adnet, Reims, France

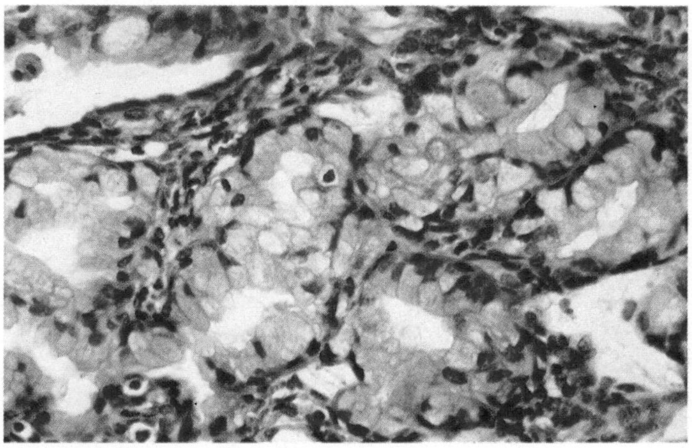

Figure 2.45 Benign thymoma, spindle-cell type. Focal glandular differentiation in another tumour

tumours are predominantly made of small oval cells showing a variable tendency to a whorled arrangement (Figs 2.32 and 2.33), pseudoglandular (Fig. 2.40) or rosette formation (Fig. 2.34), and cribriform or microcystic areas. True glandular formations are occasionally encountered (Figs 2.42–2.45). In these tumours the typical lobular pattern is indistinct and the perivascular spaces are ill-defined. Necrosis, Hassall's corpuscles, and microcalcifications are uncommon. Reticulin is usually abundant, outlining the epithelial cell individually. Lymphocytes, generally present in small numbers, are of the mature thymocyte type. Occasionally lymphocytes and epithelial cells accumulated in different areas (Figs 2.32 and 2.33).

In *lymphocyte-rich thymoma* the epithelial cells appear isolated or in clusters of two or three among numerous lymphocytes. The epithelial cells are small to medium-sized, round, polygonal or star-like. Their nuclei are rounded, clear and vesicular, and regular in outline, with small indistinct nucleoli. In lymphocyte-rich thymomas, epithelial cells are often difficult to identify on paraffin sections (Fig. 2.46) and half-thin Araldite sections are particularly useful in demonstrating the characteristic features of larger, pale epithelial cells among the small lymphocytes (Fig. 2.47). In these tumours, Hassall's corpuscles and medullary differentiation are frequent, occurring in approximately 40% of the cases (Figs 2.48 and 2.49). Microcalcifications are also encountered (Fig. 2.50). The perivascular spaces are well-defined, but not enlarged. Reticulin is sparse, and only localized around the vessels. A strong lobulation by fibrous trabeculae is present, without invasion of epithelial cells into the capsule or the septa. Lymphocyte-rich thymoma not infrequently combines with thymoma of spindle-cell type (Fig. 2.51).

Occasionally, lymphocyte-rich thymomas are composed of large epithelial cells, thus corresponding to the cortical-type thymoma of Marino and Müller-Hermelink. Pescarmona *et al.* (1991) describe an *'organoid' variant of thymoma*, characterized by the presence of several areas of medullary differentiation, surrounded by a predominant cortical-type neoplastic tissue. Normal-appearing Hassall's corpuscles are present in areas of medullary differentiation. This well-differentiated variant of thymoma has a distinct clinicopathological profile, with low-grade aggressiveness.

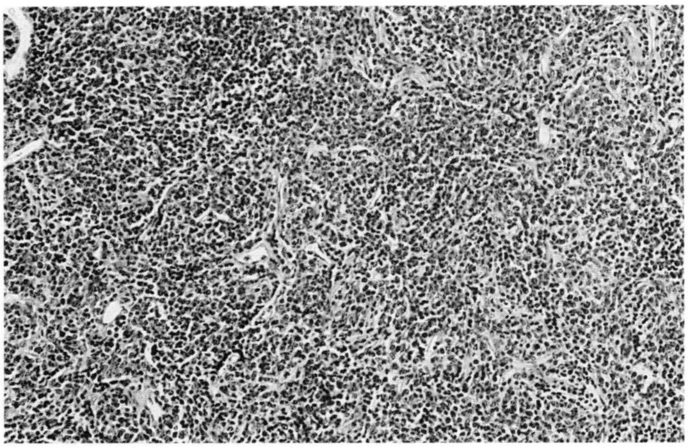

Figure 2.46 Benign thymoma, lymphocyte-predominant. The tumour is composed of a sheet of lymphocytes, interspersed with few, nearly indistinct epithelial cells

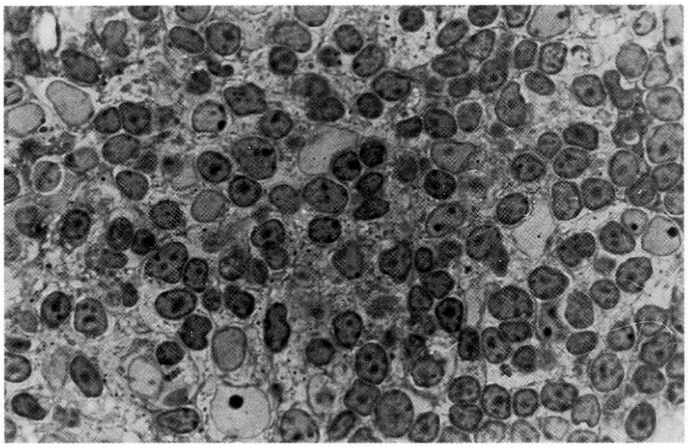

Figure 2.47 Benign thymoma, lymphocyte-predominant. Half-thin Araldite section demonstrates the characteristic feature of the pale epithelial cells scattered among lymphocytes

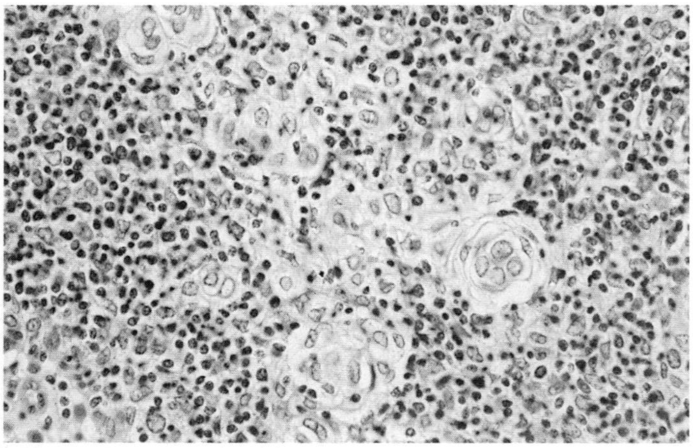

Figure 2.48 Benign thymoma, lymphocyte-predominant. The epithelial cells are small and display focal Hassall-like whorled arrangement

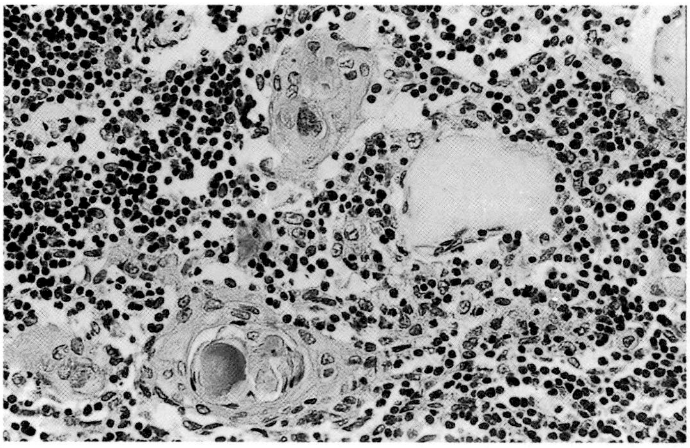

Figure 2.49 Benign thymoma, lymphocyte-predominant. The figure illustrates the predominant lymphocytic population, a hyalin vascular space, well-developed Hassall's corpuscles, and few, small, indistinct epithelial cells

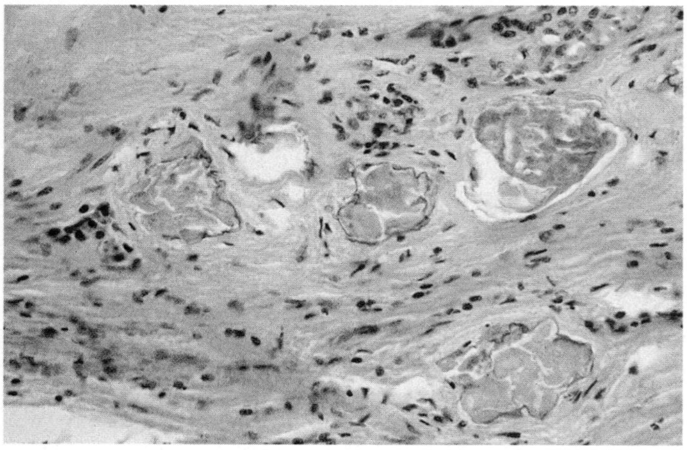

Figure 2.50 Benign thymoma, lymphocyte-predominant. Cluster of calcifications within a fibrous septum

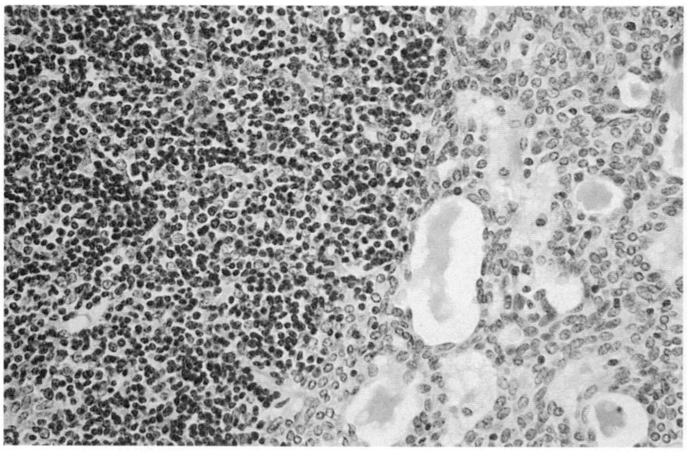

Figure 2.51 Benign thymoma. Sharply demarcated spindle cell (right) and lymphocyte-predominant areas (left)

Invasive thymomas have the same histological aspect as non-invasive tumours. However, they are mostly of the lymphoepithelial or of the predominantly epithelial types, and frequently present a certain degree of architectural and cytologic atypia (Figs 2.52–2.68). The borders of the lobules are no longer sharply circumscribed and the epithelial tumour cells show an invasive pattern in the fibrous septa and the capsule (Figs 2.53, 2.54, 2.57, 2.60). The epithelial cells exhibit some nuclear abnormalities, an increase of the nucleocytoplasmic ratio, and mitoses may be observed (Figs 2.62, 2.67, 2.68). Spindle cell thymomas and lymphocyte-rich thymomas are rarely invasive.

Thymic carcinomas have gained recognition during the past decade and are now well documented (Kuo *et al.*, 1990; Truong *et al.*, 1990; Suster and Rosai, 1991). They are defined as primary thymic epithelial neoplasms exhibiting obvious malignant cytological features and are characterized by their potential to differentiate into various histological types. Thus, several variants are described. Levine and Rosai (1978) distinguish five variants: squamous-cell, lymphoepithelioma-like, clear-cell, sarcomatoid, and undifferentiated carcinoma. Wick *et al.* (1982) additionally recognize a small-cell neuroendocrine carcinoma type. Müller-Hermelink and Kirchner (1989) separate the well-differentiated thymic carcinoma as a low-grade variant, and the more aggressive epidermoid carcinoma, endocrine carcinoma and undifferentiated carcinoma. Snover *et al.* (1982) report two additional variants: mucoepidermoid and basaloid carcinoma. Kuo *et al.* (1990) emphasize the variety in histological types and the frequency of mixed epithelial features, with a frequent neuroendocrine component presenting as small-cell carcinoma. In a number of cases the thymic carcinoma is seen in transition from a thymoma. Suster and Rosai (1991) emphasize that thymic carcinomas constitute a heterogeneous group of tumours, and group the various tumour types into low- and high-grade histology categories. Tumours included in the low-grade histology group are well-differentiated (keratinizing) squamous-cell carcinoma, well-differentiated mucoepidermoid carcinoma, and basaloid carcinoma. Tumours in the high-grade histology group include lymphoepithelioma-like (large-cell non-keratinizing) carcinoma, small-cell neuroendocrine carcinoma, sarcomatoid carcinoma, clear-cell carcinoma, and undifferentiated/anaplastic carcinoma.

Squamous-cell carcinomas of varying degrees of keratinization are the most common type, the keratinization varies from individual cell keratinization to large keratinized areas (Figs 2.69 to 2.71). Resemblance to Hassall's corpuscles is observed when keratinization is focal and abrupt (Figs 2.72–2.74). Pure squamous-cell carcinomas seem to indicate a better prognosis than the other subtypes.

Undifferentiated carcinomas of lymphoepithelioma, sarcomatoid or spindling types are also frequent and often associated (Figs 2.75–2.82). They are characterized by the loss of cellular and architectural differentiation. The typical lobular pattern is either absent or upset by numerous invading epithelial tumour cells, and the perivascular spaces are indistinct. Unless a characteristic feature of tumour cells with large vesicular nuclei and prominent nucleoli, or the association of areas of thymoma, their diagnosis remains questionable.

Pure small-cell neuroendocrine carcinomas of the thymus are described by Wick *et al.* (1982), Müller-Hermelink and Kirchner (1989), and Suster and Rosai (1991). Association of areas of small-cell carcinoma with squamous-cell carcinomas or adenosquamous carcinoma is also reported by Kuo *et al.* (1990). The classification of neuroendocrine carcinomas with the epithelial thymic tumours is nevertheless a matter of debate. In this book, these tumours are described in Chapter 5.

Clear-cell carcinomas, mucoepidermoid carcinomas (Figs 2.83–2.86), and basaloid carcinomas are exceedingly rare and are only reported as isolated cases.

Thymic carcinomas lack the characteristic angular lobular pattern seen in thymomas. The neoplastic cells proliferate predominantly, with minimal or no admixture of lymphocytes. They are anaplastic, with nuclear hyperchromasia and an increased nucleocytoplasmic ratio. The nuclei are often pleomorphic, the nucleoli prominent, and mitoses are frequent. Extended tumour necrosis is invariably found, whereas typical features such as enlarged vascular spaces or Hassall's corpuscles are not present.

The presence of *myoid cells* in thymic tumour has been occasionally reported and is distinctly unusual. Myoid cells are large cells with an abundant eosinophilic cytoplasm and large nuclei with prominent nucleoli (Fig. 2.87). Staining with Masson's trichrome (Fig. 2.88) or phosphotungstic acid haematoxylin (PTAH), half-thin section (Fig. 2.89) or electron microscopic study reveal the characteristic intracytoplasmic fibrillary pattern. Myoid cells are a component of aggressive thymic tumours, and may be responsible for some primary spindle-cell sarcomas of the mediastinum.

Distribution of histopathological types

Spindle-cell, lymphocyte-rich, and differentiated epithelial thymomas roughly occur with the same frequency, with a predominance for the differentiated epithelial type (i.e. the lymphoepithelial or predominantly epithelial thymoma of Levine and Rosai, and the cortical or cortical predominant variant of Marino and Müller-Hermelink). Thymic carcinomas (undifferentiated epithelial type) are much rarer, and occur in less than 10% of patients (Verley and Hollmann, 1985; Table 2.6).

In patients with MG, differentiated epithelial thymomas largely predominate, and represent nearly 50% of the cases. Spindle-cell thymomas occur in only 15%, but are more frequent (86%) in patients with other autoimmune diseases. In patients without any autoimmune disorder, differentiated thymoma is less frequent than in MG patients, whereas undifferentiated tumours, i.e. thymic carcinomas, are more frequent.

Table 2.6 Histological types and associated disease in 200 patients with thymoma

	Histological types				
	1	*2*	*3*	*4*	*Total*
Myasthenia gravis	17 (15.5%)	34 (33.1%)	50 (47.6%)	4 (3.8%)	105
Erythrocyte hypoplasia	4		1		5
Hypogamma-globulinaemia	4				4
Systemic lupus erythematosus	3				3
Pemphigus vulgaris	1				1
Sjögren's disease			1		1
Without disease	31 (38.5%)	25 (30.9%)	15 (18.5%)	10 (12.3%)	81
Total	60 (30%)	59 (29.5%)	67 (33.5%)	14 (7%)	200

Type 1: Spindle-cell thymoma; type 2: lymphocyte-rich thymoma; type 3: differentiated epithelial thymoma; type 4: undifferentiated epithelial thymoma or thymic carcinoma. From Verley and Hollmann, 1985

[*continued on p. 32*]

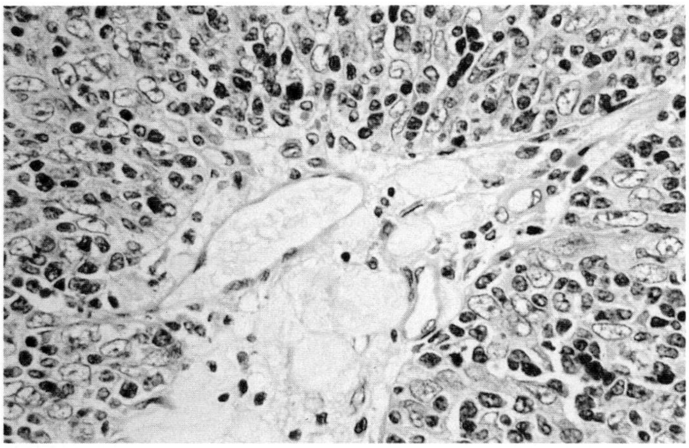

Figure 2.52 Invasive thymoma. Mixed lymphoepithelial thymoma showing a typical enlarged vascular space. Note the nuclear pleomorphism, with increase of the nucleocytoplasmic ratio

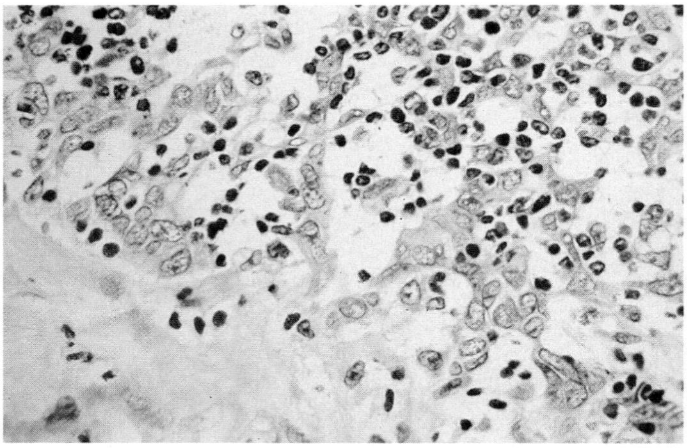

Figure 2.53 Invasive thymoma. The border of the lobule is no longer well-circumscribed and the epithelial cells show a tendency to invade the fibrous septa

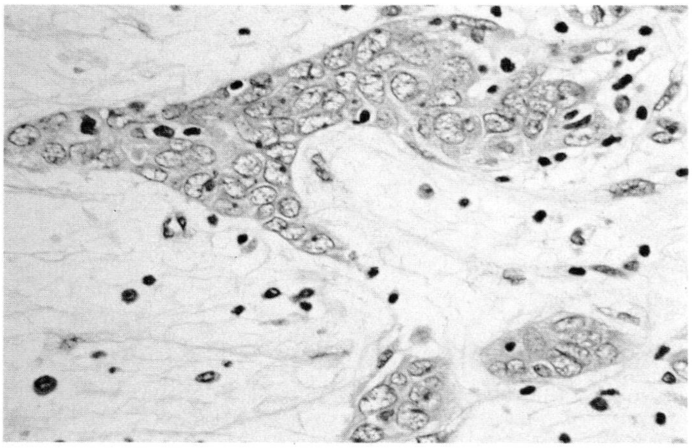

Figure 2.54 Invasive thymoma. The epithelial cells infiltrate the septa

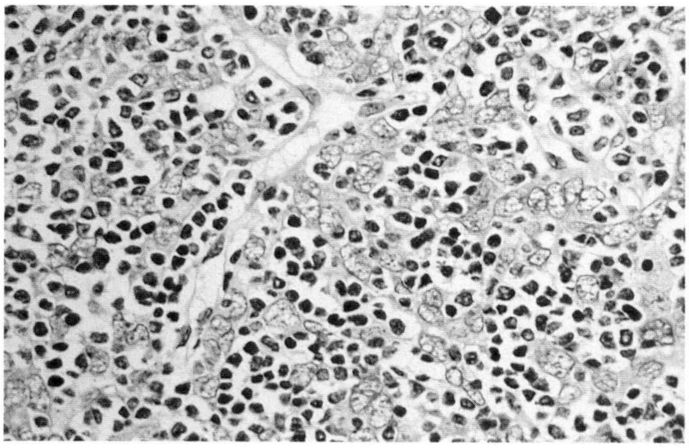

Figure 2.55 Invasive thymoma. There is a lack of cohesion of the epithelial cells, with disorganization of the lobular architecture (Figures 2.52–2.55 are from the same tumour.)

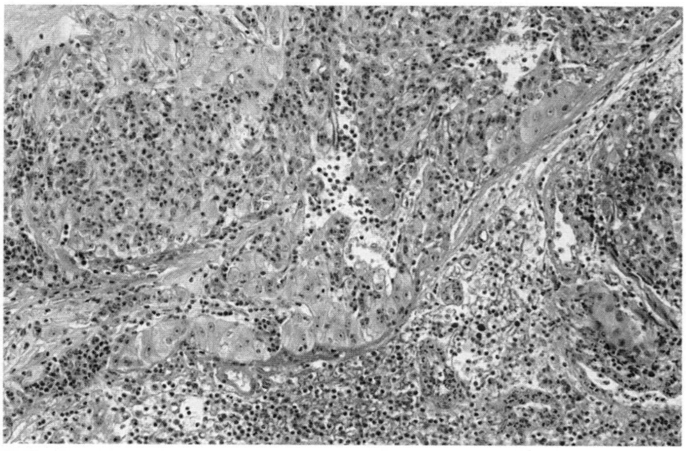

Figure 2.56 Invasive thymoma. This mostly epithelial tumour displays extensive area of necrosis

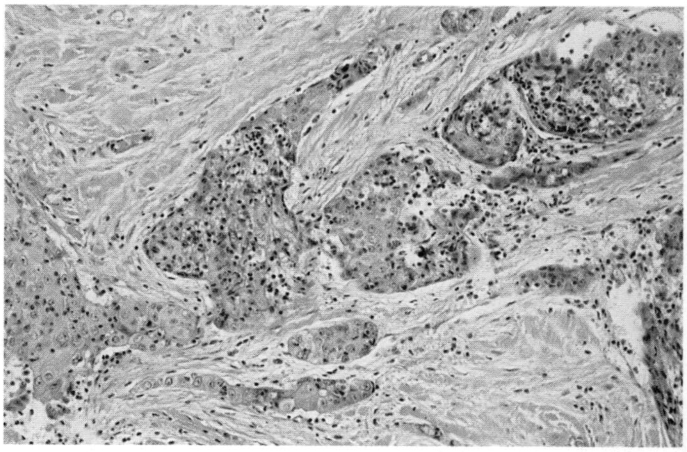

Figure 2.57 Invasive thymoma. The same tumour largely invades the surrounding fibrous tissue

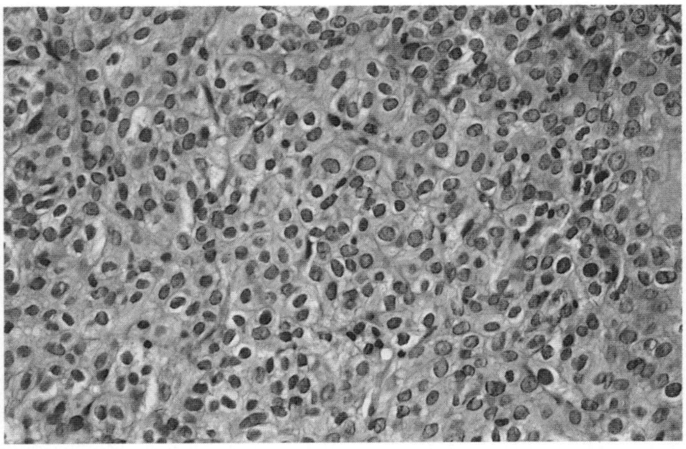

Figure 2.58 Invasive thymoma. Pure epithelial tumour composed of medium-sized cells with increased nucleocytoplasmic ratio. The nuclei are homogeneous, without obvious atypia. The tumour is suggestive of a carcinoid

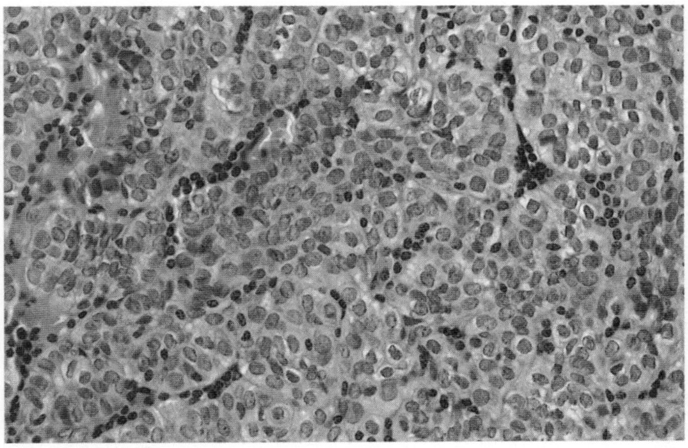

Figure 2.59 Invasive thymoma. In another area the presence of lymphocytes along the vessels gives to the tumour the typical appearance of a thymoma

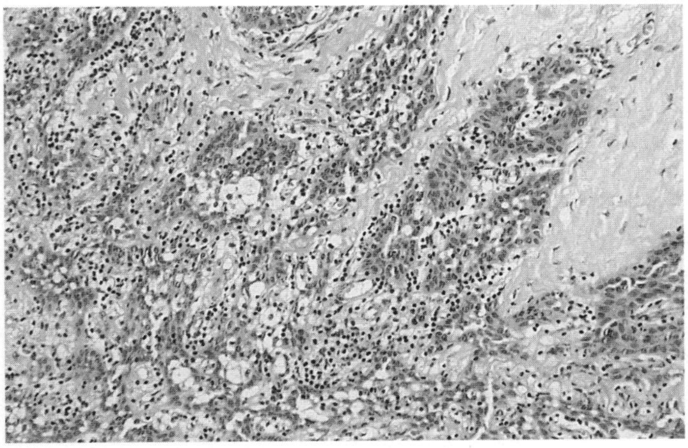

Figure 2.60 Invasive thymoma. Elsewhere the tumour infiltrates the surrounding tissue. (Figures 2.58–2.60 are from the same tumour.)

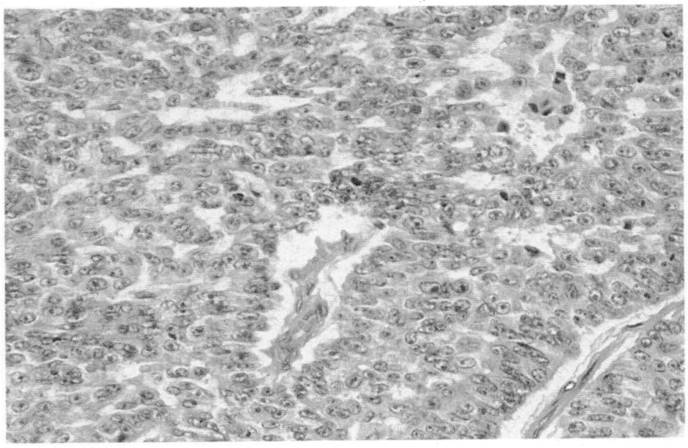

Figure 2.61 Invasive thymoma. Pure epithelial tumour composed of strands and trabeculae of cells with large open nuclei and prominent nucleoli, resembling a carcinoid tumour

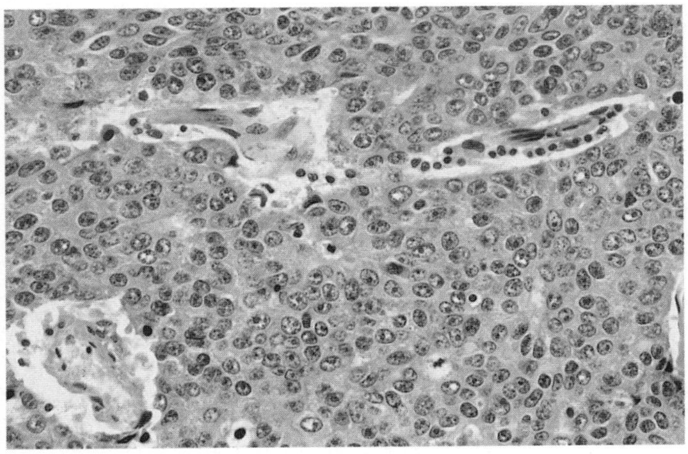

Figure 2.62 Invasive thymoma. Pure epithelial tumour with typical vascular feature of thymoma. Slight nuclear atypia and mitoses are present

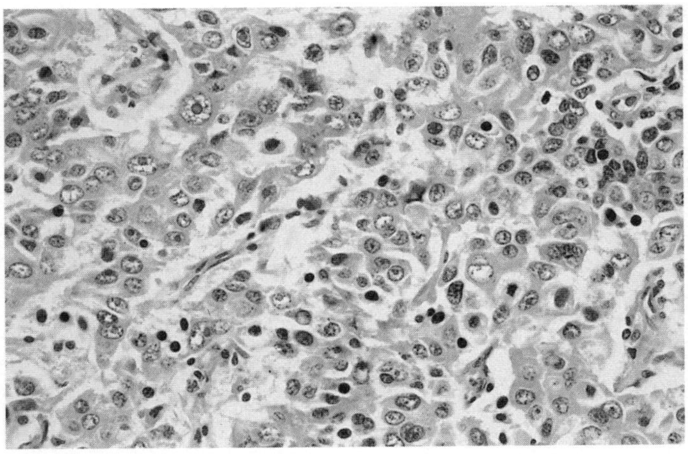

Figure 2.63 Invasive thymoma. In another area strands of epithelial cells are growing in a disorganized fashion

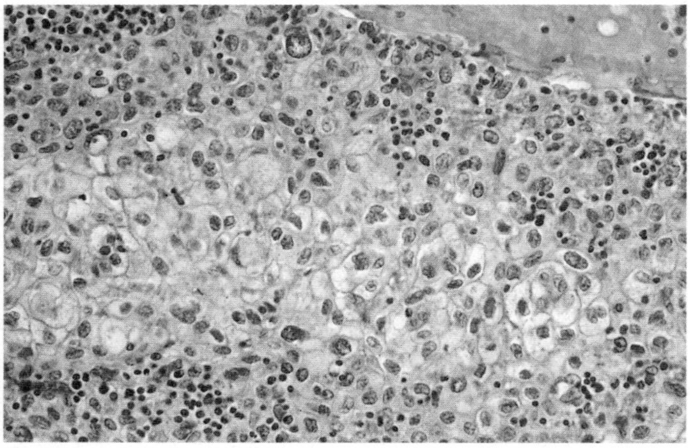

Figure 2.64 Invasive thymoma. Predominantly epithelial tumour with numerous cytonuclear atypia

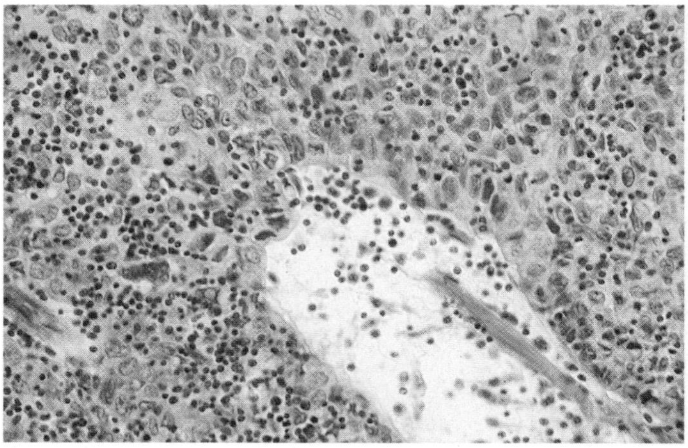

Figure 2.65 Invasive thymoma. Another area of the same tumour with a typical enlarged vascular space

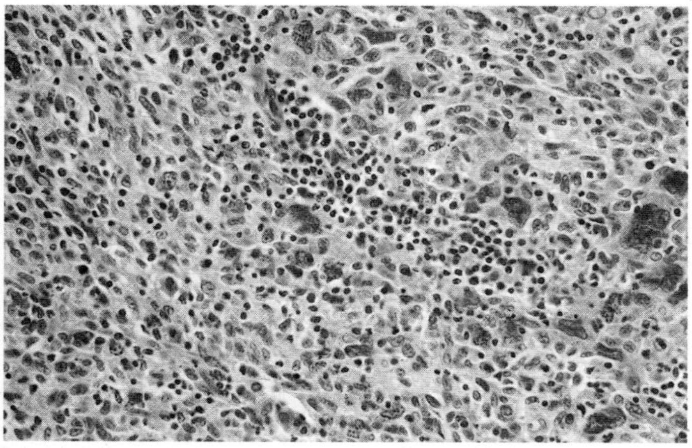

Figure 2.66 Invasive thymoma. In this area nuclear atypia are obvious. (Figures 2.64–2.66 are from the same tumour.) The patient was myasthenic. He was alive and well, without evidence of tumour, 15 years 6 months after surgery

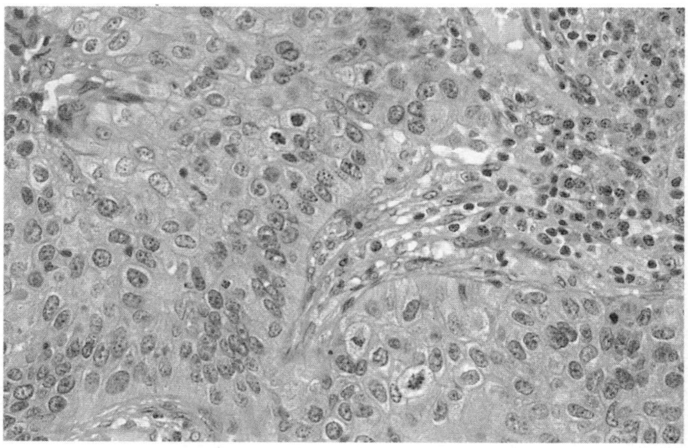

Figure 2.67 Invasive thymoma. Numerous mitoses in an otherwise typical pure epithelial thymoma

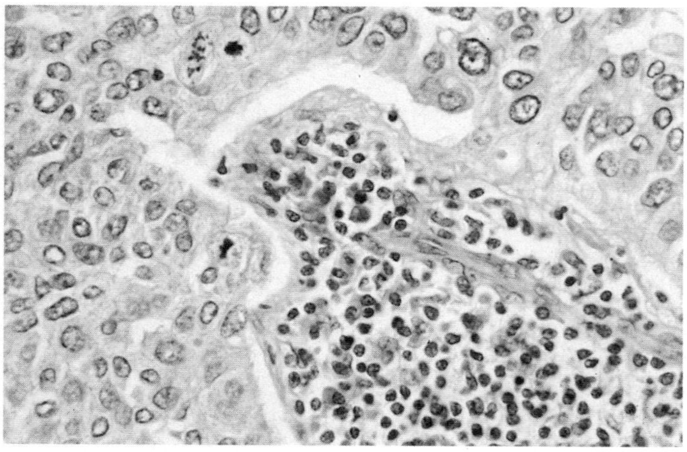

Figure 2.68 Invasive thymoma. Obvious mitoses around a vascular space

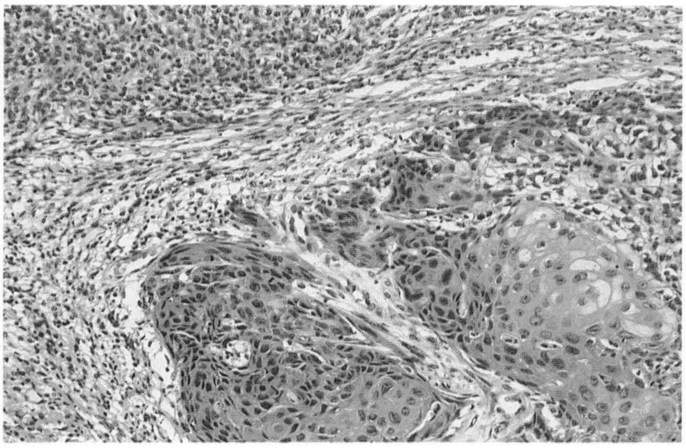

Figure 2.69 Thymic carcinoma. The tumour displays both squamous (right) and undifferentiated areas (upper left)

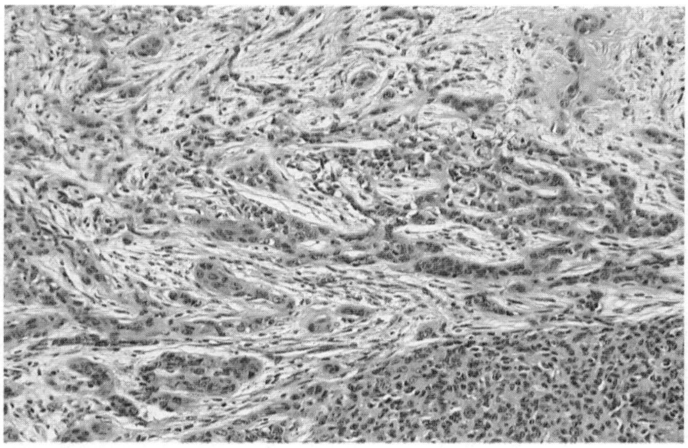

Figure 2.70 Thymic carcinoma. The undifferentiated component largely invades the surrounding fibrous tissue

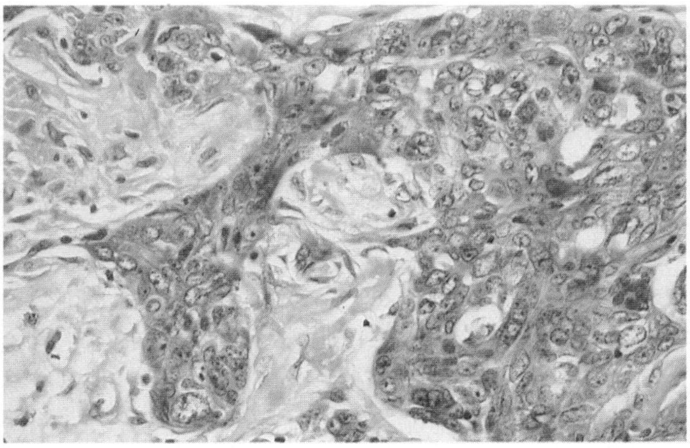

Figure 2.71 Thymic carcinoma. Sarcomatoid changes also occur. (Figures 2.69–2.71 are from the same tumour.) Thymic carcinomas are characterized by their potential to differentiate into various histological types

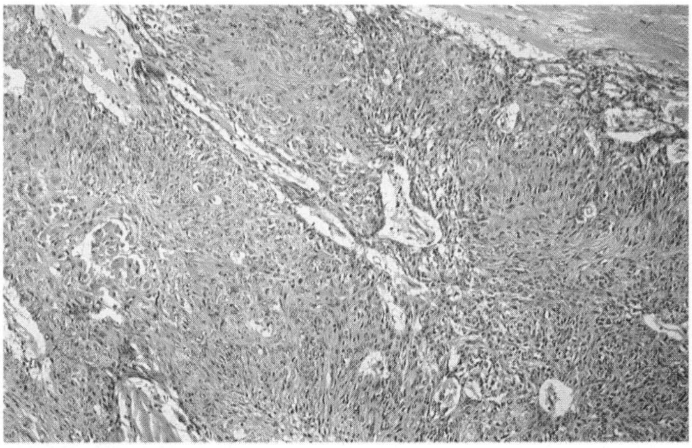

Figure 2.72 Thymic carcinoma. Undifferentiated epithelial tumour, without distinguishing features to indicate its thymic origin

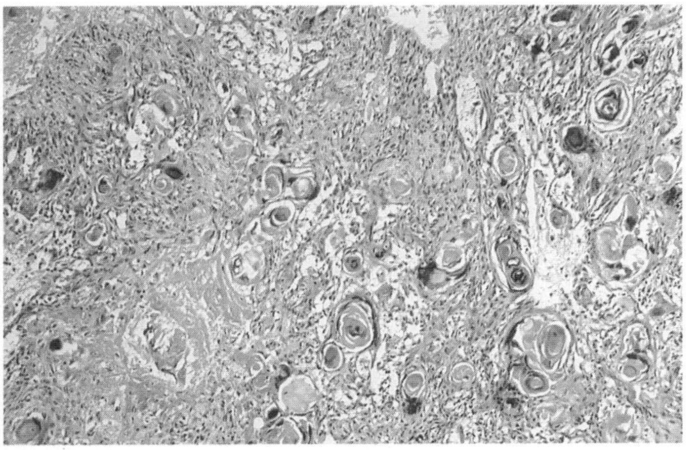

Figure 2.73 Thymic carcinoma, squamous-cell variant, With Hassall's corpuscle formation. Focal keratinization gives the tumour a squamous-cell carcinoma appearance

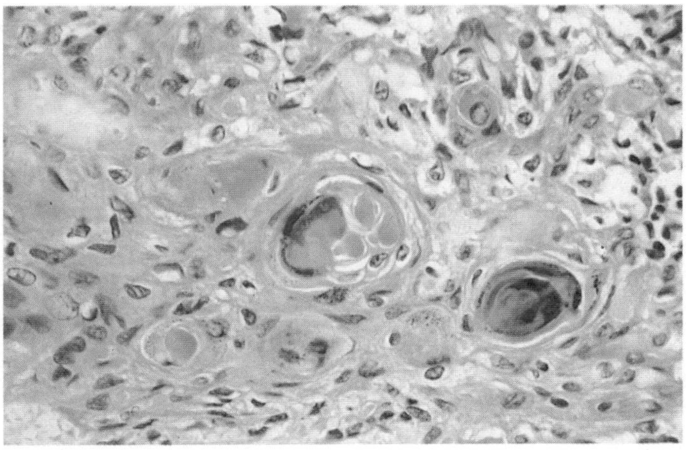

Figure 2.74 Thymic carcinoma, squamous-cell variant, with Hassall's corpuscle formation. At higher magnification keratinization is abrupt, as seen in Hassall's corpuscles. (Figures 2.72–2.74 are from the same tumour.)

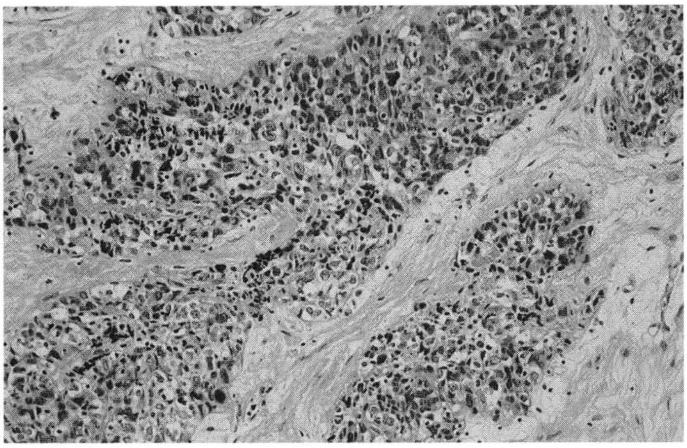

Figure 2.75 Thymic carcinoma, undifferentiated variant. The tumour is massive, and strongly lobulated by fibrous septa

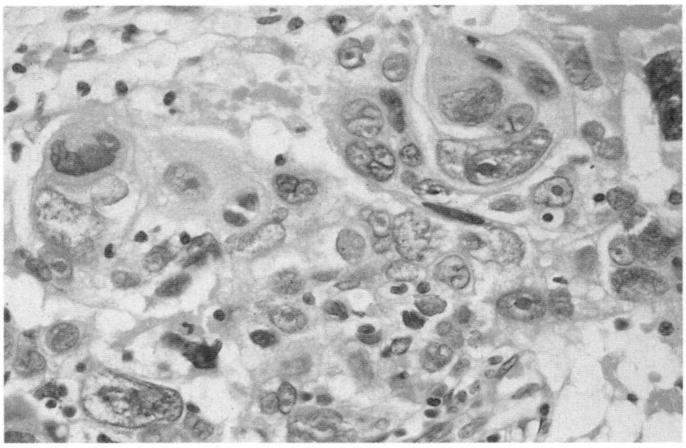

Figure 2.76 Thymic carcinoma, undifferentiated variant. Marked cellular pleomorphism and atypia are present

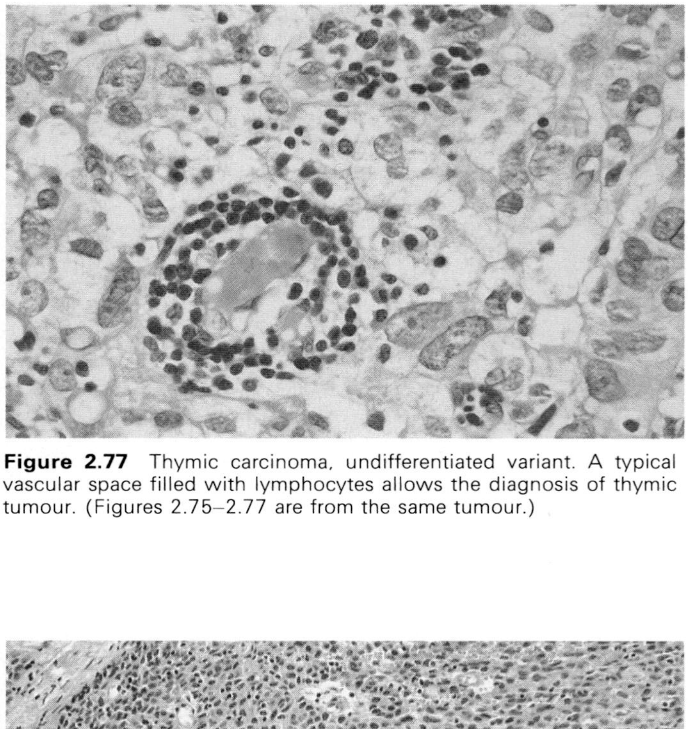

Figure 2.77 Thymic carcinoma, undifferentiated variant. A typical vascular space filled with lymphocytes allows the diagnosis of thymic tumour. (Figures 2.75–2.77 are from the same tumour.)

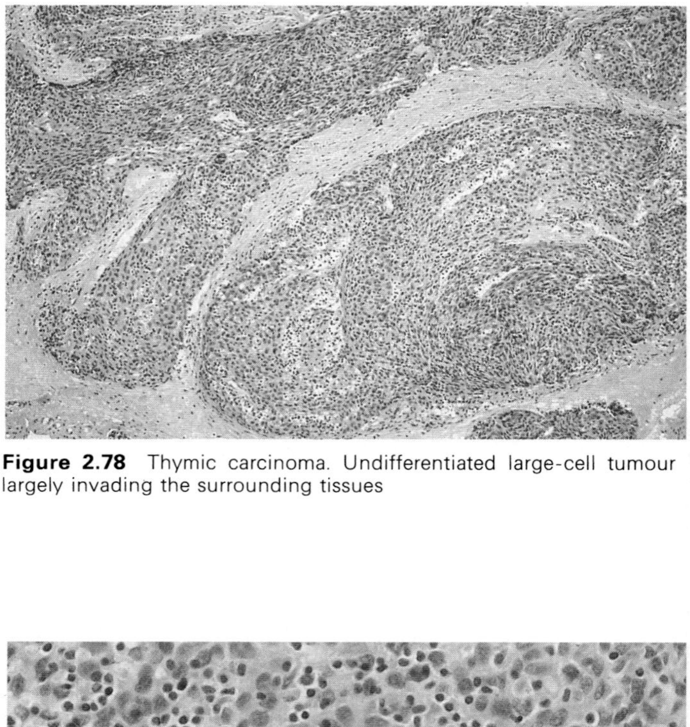

Figure 2.78 Thymic carcinoma. Undifferentiated large-cell tumour largely invading the surrounding tissues

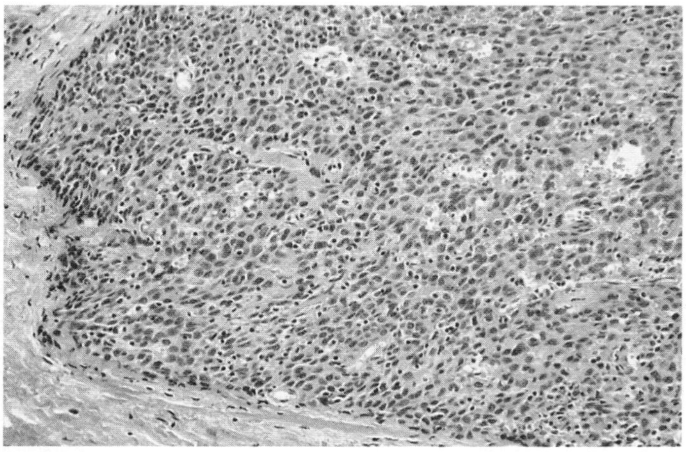

Figure 2.79 Thymic carcinoma. The tumour has no distinctive feature and is undifferentiated

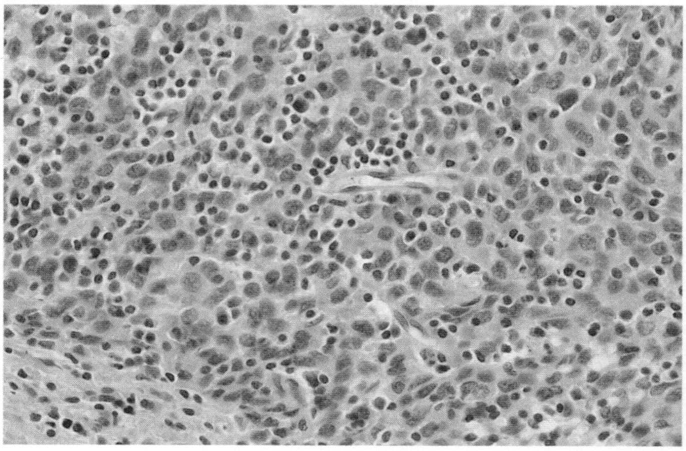

Figure 2.80 Thymic carcinoma. The tumour cells are anaplastic, with nuclear hyperchromasia and increased nucleocytoplasmic ratio. The presence of some lymphocytes within the tumour is indicative of the thymic origin. (Figures 2.78–2.80 are from the same tumour.)

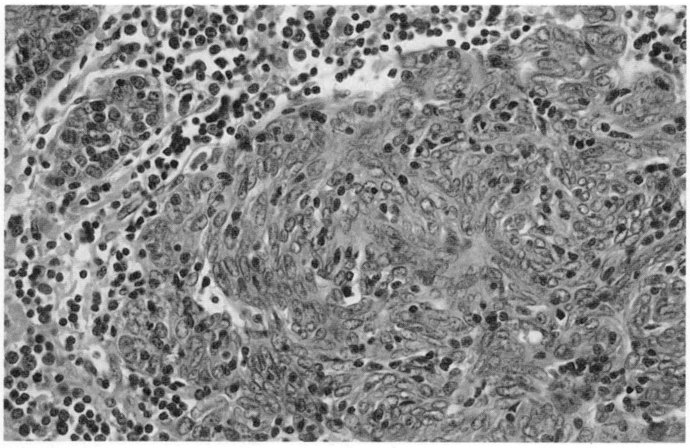

Figure 2.81 Thymic carcinoma. The tumour is poorly differentiated. Cells are oval to spindle-shaped and cytologically malignant

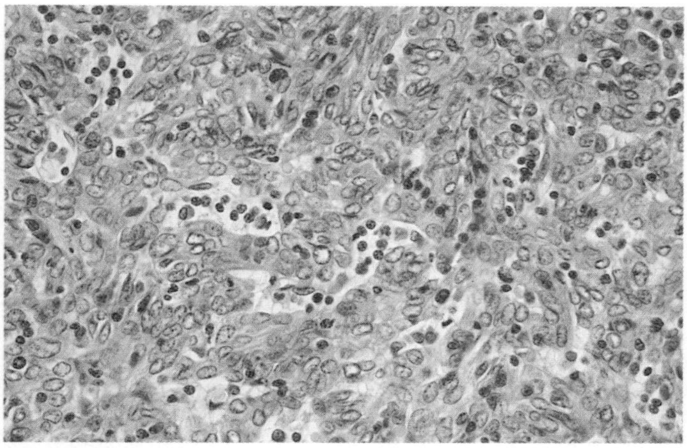

Figure 2.82 Thymic carcinoma. The vascular pattern may suggest hemangiopericytoma. (Figures 2.81–2.82 are from the same tumour.)

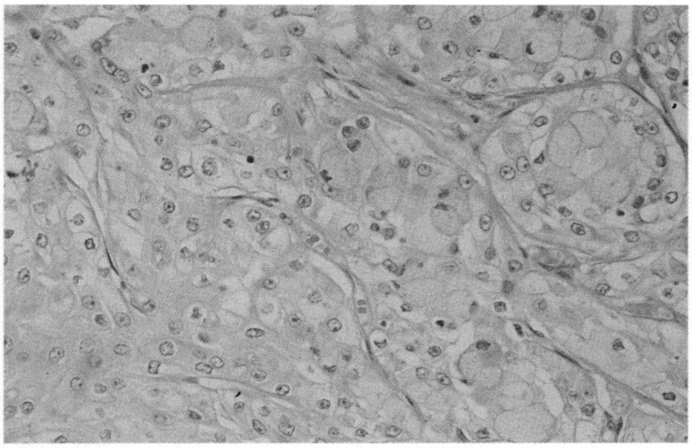

Figure 2.83 Thymic carcinoma, mucoepidermoid variant. The tumour is lobulated by thin fibrous septa and is composed of large cells with an abundant clear cytoplasm

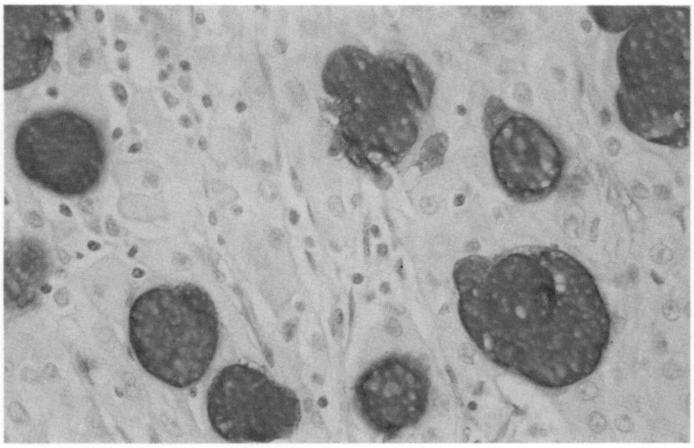

Figure 2.84 Thymic carcinoma, mucoepidermoid variant. Some cells stain positively with Alcian blue

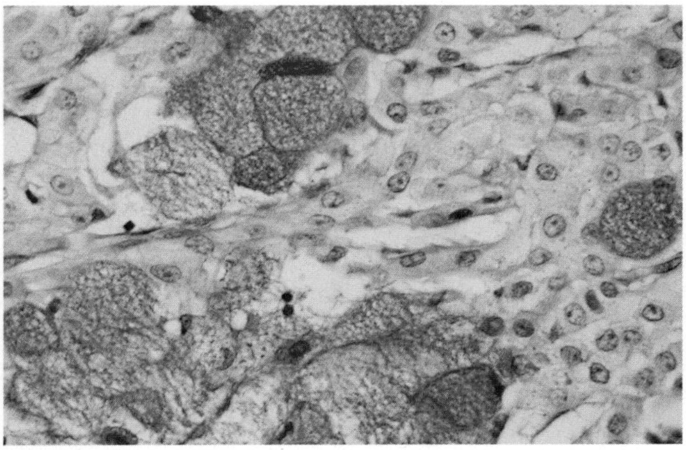

Figure 2.85 Thymic carcinoma, mucoepidermoid variant. Mucus-secreting cells are also stained with PAS

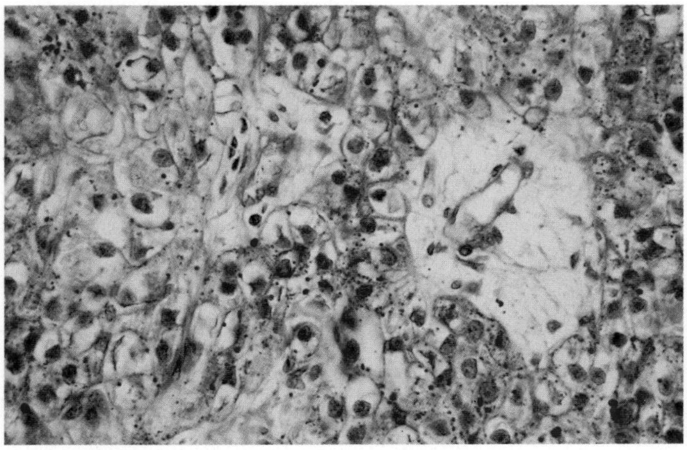

Figure 2.86 Thymic carcinoma, mucoepidermoid variant. In this area the cells contain only small intracytoplasmic droplets, PAS-positive. (Figures 2.83–2.86 are from the same case.) Courtesy of Dr R.H. Laeng-Danner, Bern, Switzerland

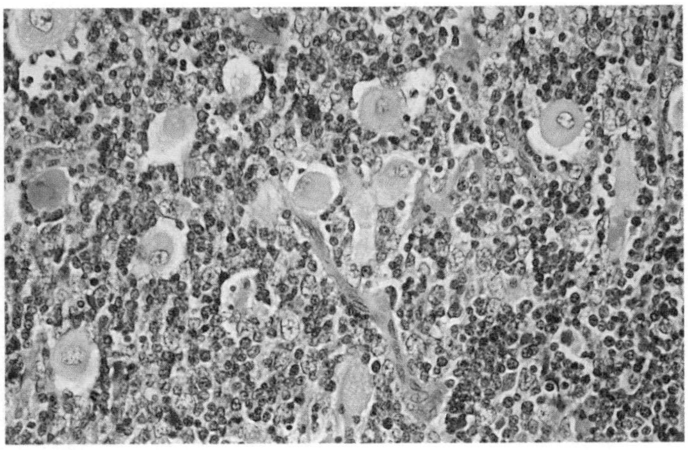

Figure 2.87 Thymoma with myoid cells. Scattered large acidophilic cells are present within the tumour

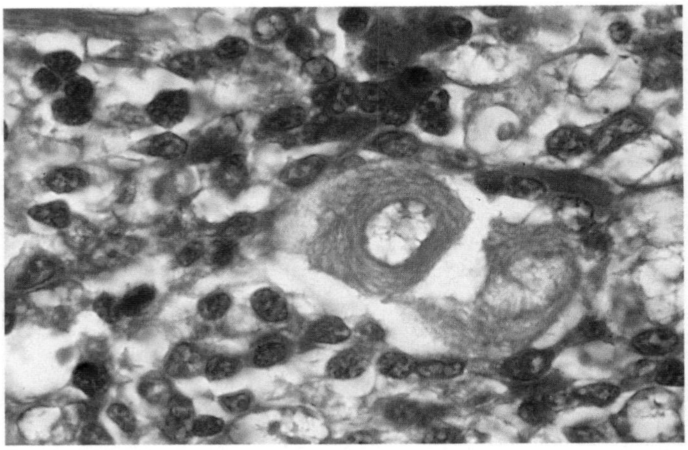

Figure 2.88 Thymoma with myoid cells. At higher magnification Masson's trichrome reveals a circular fibrillary pattern in the cytoplasm, characteristic of myoid cells

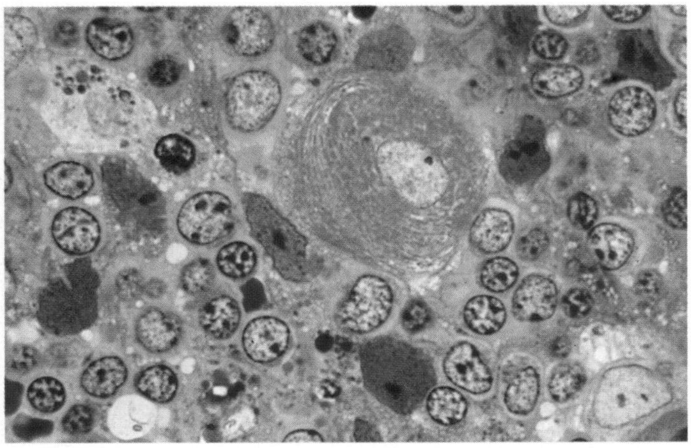

Figure 2.89 Thymoma with myoid cells. A toluidine blue-stained half-thin section emphasizes the fibrillary pattern

Thymoma and Epstein–Barr virus

To date there is evidence for the specific association of EBV and nasopharyngeal carcinoma with the histological features of lymphoepithelioma. Such an association has also been reported in cases of lymphoepithelioma of the thymus (Leyvraz *et al.*, 1985; Rosai, 1985; Dimery *et al.*, 1988; Weiss *et al.*, 1989; Perronne *et al.*, 1990) and the salivary glands, but not with lymphoepithelioma of other origin, or other types of tumour. The association is demonstrated by the presence of antibodies to the virus in sera of patients, and by the incorporation of the EBV genome into the tumour DNA, as detected by molecular hybridation analysis *in situ* or according to the Southern blot technique. This suggests that lymphoepitheliomas arising in sites derived from the primitive pharynx may often be associated with EBV. Nevertheless, more studies are needed to clarify the role of the virus in the pathogenesis of these tumours.

Immunohistochemistry and functional activity

The epithelial cells in thymomas and thymic carcinomas, like other epithelial cells, possess keratins which can be labelled by antikeratin antibodies. Unfortunately, whereas the different patterns of keratin subunit expression have been accurately described in normal thymic epithelial cells, studies concerning cytokeratin expression in the different types of thymic epithelial tumours remain sparse and limited. According to Savino *et al.* (1988), all thymomas react with the T2/30 antibody which recognizes a 64 kD cytokeratin. The thymic carcinomas positively stain with antikeratin antibodies AE1 (40, 50, 56.5 kD), and AE3 (46, 52, 58, 65–67 kD), but not with antibody AE2 (56.5, 65–67 kD), suggesting a lack of differentiation towards keratinized epidermal cell type in these tumours (Kuo *et al.*, 1990). Thus, the use of antikeratin antibodies indicates the epithelial nature of the tumour, but does not allow the distinction between a thymic epithelial tumour and an epithelial tumour of other origin.

Epithelial membrane antigen (EMA) is positive on epithelial cells, but is not specific. Neuron-specific enolase (NSE) antibody is useful for the identification of small-cell carcinoma components. Scattered S-100 protein-positive dendritic cells are also detected in all tumours.

The lymphocytes are not stained by keratin, EMA, NSE and S-100 protein antibodies, but react with leukocyte common antigen. The immature cortical thymocytes are terminal deoxynucleotidyl transferase (Tdt) positive, $CD1^+$, $T10^+$, and $CD3^-$, whereas mature thymocytes of peripheral lymphocyte type are Tdt^-, $CD1^-$, $T10^-$ and $CD3^+$.

Studies on the functional capacity of thymoma epithelial cells provide promising tools for the diagnostic and the determination of the degree of differentiation of thymomas. The thymic epithelial antigen, defined by the anti-p19 monoclonal antibody (initially raised against a protein isolated from the human T cell leukaemia virus), is normally acquired during the ontogenesis of the human thymic epithelium. In thymoma epithelial cells its expression is strongly altered: in benign thymomas a variable number of epithelial cells express the antigen, whereas in malignant cases no anti-p19 is found (Savino *et al.*, 1984). In another study, HLA-DR antigens, which are normally present on the majority of thymic epithelial cells, are not detected in thymomas (Savino *et al.*, 1985). These results suggest a possible change in antigen expression following neoplastic transformation. The production of thymic hormones, known to play an important role in T cell differentiation, is, however, preserved in thymomas. The thymoma epithelial cells contain thymic hormones (thymulin and thymosin a1), detected by immunohistochemistry (Savino *et al.*, 1985; Figs 2.90 and 2.91), a finding corroborated by the observation of elevated thymulin serum levels in patients with thymoma

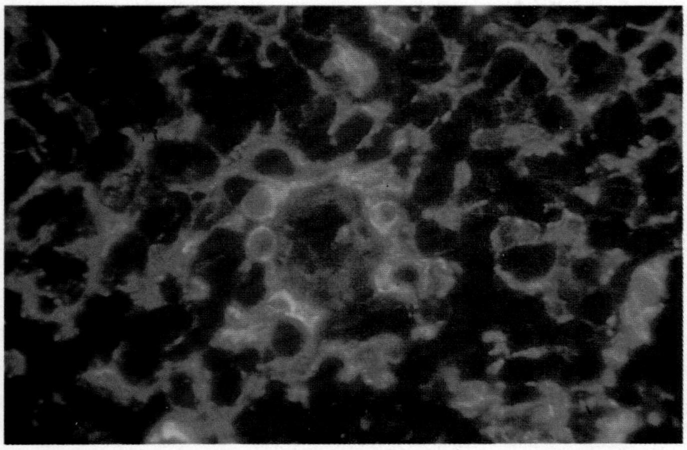

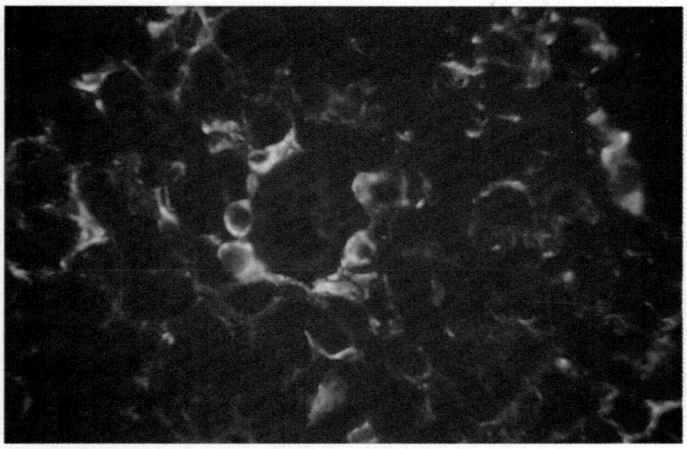

Figures 2.90 and 2.91 Thymoma frozen section immunolabelled by the antithymulin MAB (revealed by GAMIgG2b/FITC in **Fig. 2.90**) and the antikeratin antiserum (revealed by the GAR/TRITC in **Fig. 2.91**). Thymoma epithelial cells are sharply labelled by both antithymic hormone and antikeratin antibodies

Figure 2.91

(Kirkpatrick *et al.*, 1978; Chollet *et al.*, 1981). These data open the possibility of using antithymic hormone antibodies as specific markers of thymoma, but these antibodies are not easily available for routine pathology.

Electron microscopy

The ultrastructural features of thymomas are now well documented and electron microscopy is a valuable aid in the identification of difficult cases (Toker, 1968; Levine and Bensch, 1972; Levine *et al.*, 1975; Pascoe and Miner, 1976; Rosai and Levine, 1976; Cossman *et al.*, 1978).

Despite the histological varieties in thymomas, the fine structure of the tumours resembles that of the normal thymus and the complex anatomical interrelationships between epithelial cells, lymphocytes and blood vessels tend to be preserved.

The basic structure of thymomas consists of a network of epithelial cells showing complex interdigitations between adjacent cells and elongated cytoplasmic processes which are connected by well-developed desmosomes (Figs 2.92 and 2.93). The epithelial cells or their processes completely surround the capillaries and segregate lymphocytes either isolated or in small groups. The epithelial cells are rounded or spindle-shaped, with round to elongated nuclei and a finely dispersed chromatin. The nucleoli are either small or large, with a compact filamentous nucleolonema. The cytoplasm contains scattered ribosomes, a moderate number of lysosomes and small rounded mitochondria. The ergastoplasm and Golgi apparatus are usually well developed.

The two most characteristic features in thymomas are the presence of tonofilaments in the epithelial cells and the relationship between epithelial cells and vessels. In all cases tonofilaments are present at least in some cells (Fig. 2.94) and they are particularly abundant in spindle-cell thymomas. They form bundles of varying width which branch and interconnect. The filaments insert into desmosomes of maculae adherentes type. The capillary–epithelial relationships recall those of the normal thymus, but the perivascular space is frequently dilated. Both the vessels and epithelial cells possess a well-defined basal lamina. The laminae delineate the perivascular space which may be empty, hyalinized or packed with lymphocytes intermingled with various numbers of red cells, plasma cells, or histiocytes.

Differential diagnosis

The remarkable morphological varieties of thymomas and thymic carcinomas account for the well-known difficulty of diagnosing these tumours accurately.

In poorly preserved lymphocytic-rich thymoma the abundance of lymphocytes may obscure the epithelial nature of the tumour and the blastic immature appearance of the lymphocytes, together with numerous mitotic figures, may suggest a lymphoma of lymphoblastic type. Histological characteristics of a thymona, such as the fibrous capsule and the large fibrous bands lobulating the tumour, the enlarged perivascular spaces, and the absence of diffuse infiltration of lymphoid cells in the surrounding mediastinal fat tissue are distinctive features from a lymphoma. Isolated epithelial cells, difficult to identify in paraffin-embedded routine sections, become obvious in half-thin Araldite sections or after immunostaining with cytokeratin.

In spindle-cell thymomas the epithelial cells may grow in intercrossing or storiform pattern reminiscent of a mesenchymal tumour. Thymomas composed of ovoid cells show a variety of features simulating a haemangiopericytoma, a neuroendocrine tumour or a neuroepithelioma when a rosette pattern is prominent. The pathologist must be advised of these various features and has to search for the presence of interspersed lymphocytes and other characteristic patterns of thymomas. In doubtful cases immunocytochemical characterization of cytokeratin in the tumour cells or electron microscopic study will definitely determine the epithelial nature of the lesion.

There are no difficulties in the recognition of mixed lymphocytic and epithelial thymomas which possess a very characteristic histological appearance, but predominant or pure epithelial thymomas are more confusing. They may mimic a Hodgkin's disease of the thymus that associates fibrosis, lymphocytes and large Hodgkin's or Sternberg's cells simulating epithelial cells, sometimes intermingled with involuting thymic epithelial structures. The clinical features, the pleomorphism of the small infiltrating cells, the typical aspect of Sternberg's cells in Hodgkin's disease, and the different pattern of the sclerosis are helpful in differential diagnosis. Immunohistochemistry allows the identification of the Hodgkin's or Sternberg's cells and distinguishes them from residual thymic epithelial cells. Other predominant epithelial cells thymomas may simulate a germ-cell tumour, namely a seminoma composed of nests of large rounded cells

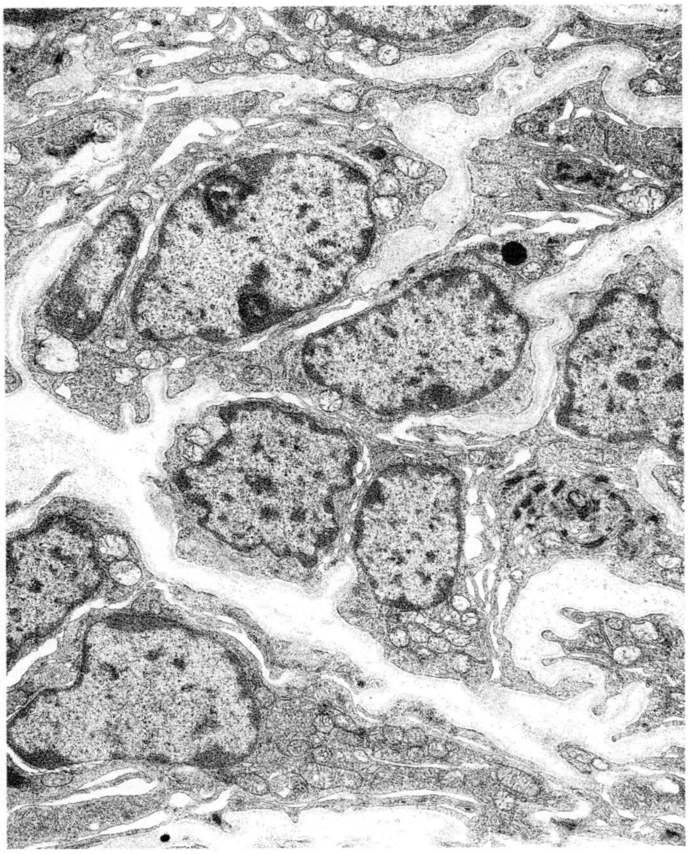

Figure 2.92 Spindle-cell thymoma. Electron micrograph illustrates the network of epithelial cells with elongated cytoplasmic processes connected by desmosomes. The cells are surrounded by a well-defined basal lamina

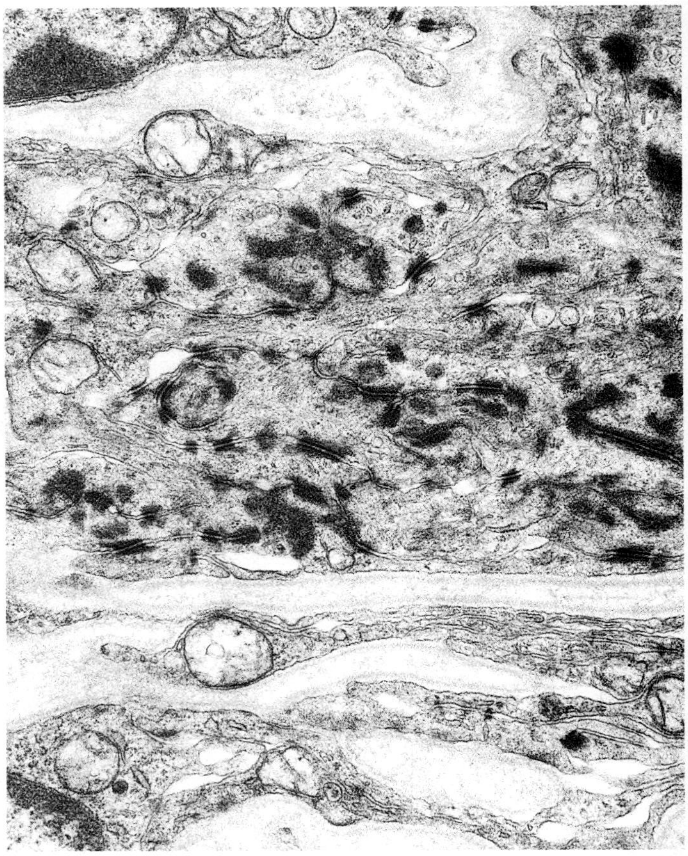

Figure 2.93 Spindle-cell thymoma. Electron micrograph shows the complex interdigitation between cell processes and the numerous desmosomes

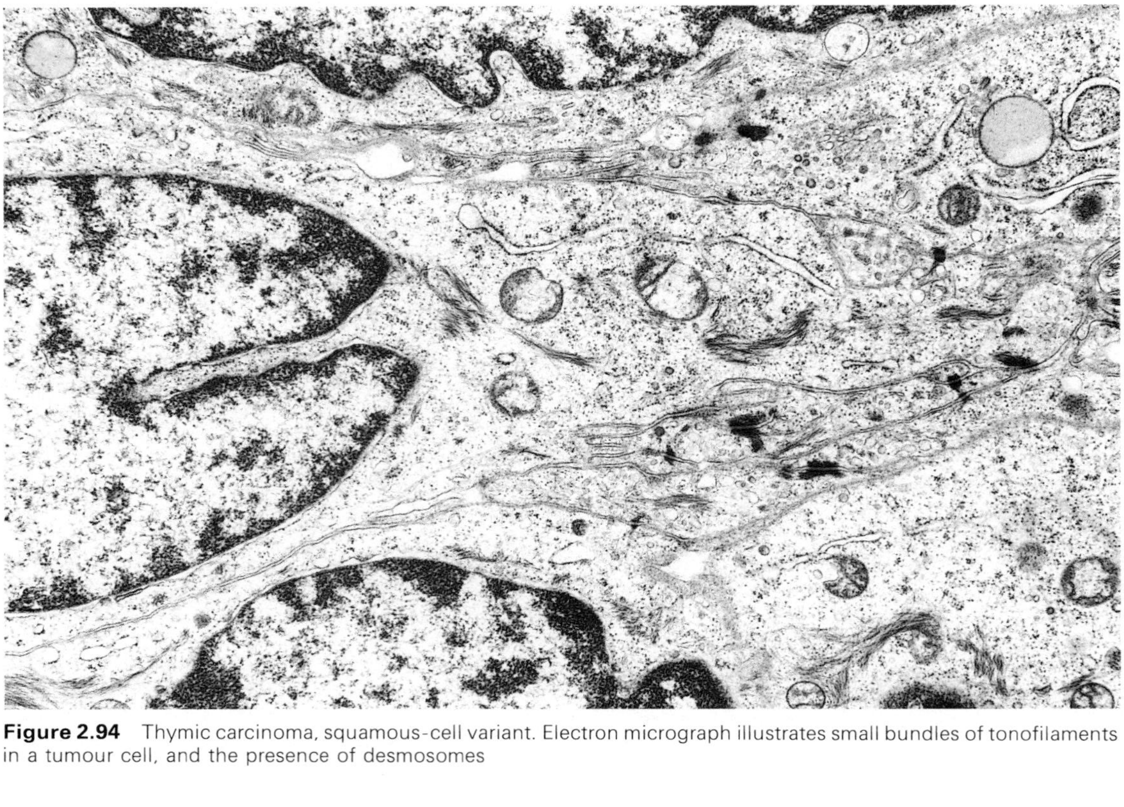

Figure 2.94 Thymic carcinoma, squamous-cell variant. Electron micrograph illustrates small bundles of tonofilaments in a tumour cell, and the presence of desmosomes

separated by strands of connective tissues heavily infiltrated by lymphocytes. The younger age and male sex of the patient, the abundance of glycogen in the cytoplasm, the characteristic feature of the large eosinophilic nucleoli, and the frequent granulomatous response with multinucleated Langhans cells are in favour of a seminoma. Immunohistochemistry is helpful since seminomatous cells are negative for cytokeratin and EMA, and positive for neuron-specific enolase and vimentin.

Thymic carcinomas always pose diagnostic problems because they simulate both lymphomas, either of the anaplastic Ki-1 type or of the large-cell B-type, and carcinomas of other origin.

In the presence of an undifferentiated, anaplastic tumour of the mediastinum, only immunochemistry enables a definite diagnosis, and is strongly recommended. It permits determination of the lymphoid or epithelial nature of the tumour, and in cases of lymphoma it allows immunophenotype characterization of the tumour.

When the epithelial character of the tumour is determinate, the marked stromal fibrosis, the increased mitotic activity, and the extensive central necrosis are important differential pathological features from bronchogenic carcinoma invading the mediastinum (Kuo *et al.*, 1990). Half-thin sections are useful in demonstrating poorly distinct perivascular spaces, the characteristic feature of the nuclei of thymic tumours, and the presence of lymphocytes penetrating inside the epithelial lobules. But the final diagnosis of thymic carcinoma can be made with certainty only when metastasis to the mediastinum is excluded.

Clinical course and prognosis

The majority of thymomas are composed of cytologically bland elements and are slow-growing tumours with a benign clinical course. They show a propensity for local invasion and intrathoracic recurrence (Figs 2.95–2.98), but rarely metastasize outside the thorax. On the other hand, thymic carcinomas show a marked tendency for rapid invasion and widespread extrathoracic metastases.

Invasiveness and the possibility of complete resection are considered by most authors as the most important factors influencing long-term survival of patients (Rosai and Levine, 1976; Wilkins and Castleman, 1979; Masaoka *et al.*, 1981; Salyer and Eggleston, 1976; Bergh *et al.*, 1978; Cohen *et al.*, 1984; Nakahara *et al.*, 1988). Well-encapsulated thymomas are almost always cured by surgical excision alone, and show a 5-year survival rate of about 83% and a 10-year survival of 80%. Invasive thymoma patients who receive radical surgery survive at 80% after 5 years compared to 59% and 45% of patients who had a subtotal resection or biopsy only. Thus, the radicality of the operation is the determining factor in the equal survival statistics for both invasive and non-invasive cases (Maggi *et al.*, 1986, 1991). Nevertheless, even after complete resection of non-invasive thymoma, 2–10% of tumours recur, sometimes months or years following surgery (Fechner, 1969; Monden *et al.*, 1985; Verley and Hollmann, 1985). In incompletely resected invasive thymomas the survival rate decreases to about 50% at 5 years and 35% at 10 years. Recurrences are observed in 20–30% of cases. They present as local mediastinal recurrences or as pleural grafts, or exceptionally as distant metastases to the supraclavicular or axillary lymph nodes, lung, liver, brain or bone (Wilkins *et al.*, 1966; Bernatz *et al.*, 1973; Rosai and Levine, 1976; Chahinian *et al.*, 1981; Monden *et al.*, 1985, Verley and Hollmann, 1985; Lewis *et al.*, 1987). Thymic carcinomas are always largely invasive with metastases frequently present at diagnosis, and their prognosis is considered as very poor (Wick *et al.*, 1982; Marino and Müller-Hermelink, 1985; Verley and Hollmann, 1985; Kuo *et al.*, 1990). Invasiveness usually correlates with presence of symptoms, size of the tumour, histological type and extent of surgical excision. But the relationship between these different variables is still debated. From statistical analysis, Lewis *et al.* (1987) found four independent variables of poor prognosis: the presence of invasion or metastasis (most heavily weighted), the presence of symptoms, age under 30 years, and lack of total surgical excision.

The predictive value of histological features as an individual variable remains controversial. Many authors state that histology is valueless in establishing a prognosis (Bernatz *et al.*, 1973; Levine and Rosai, 1978; Masaoka *et al.*, 1981). Paradoxically, they agree that spindle-cell and lymphocyte-rich thymomas tend to be well encapsulated and are benign in behaviour, and that the predominantly epithelial tumours tend to be more invasive and follow a more aggressive course. In the study of Marino and Müller-Hermelink (1985) the three major histological subtypes correlate with the surgical stage of the tumours and long-term prognosis: the medullary type and mixed type are essentially benign in nature. The cortical and predominant cortical types are often invasive and of poorer prognosis. Ricci *et al.* (1989) observe a 5-, 10-, 15-, and 20-year survival of 100% for medullary thymoma; 85%, 76%, 65%, and 65% respectively for mixed thymoma; and 52%, 45%, 45%, and 45% for cortical thymoma. Verley and Hollmann (1985) also observe a clear concordance between histological type of thymomas and survival rate of patients (Fig. 2.99). In thymic carcinomas the morphological features of the tumours correlate with the clinical behaviour, and the histological type constitutes the most reliable and important predictor of prognosis (Suster and Rosai, 1991).

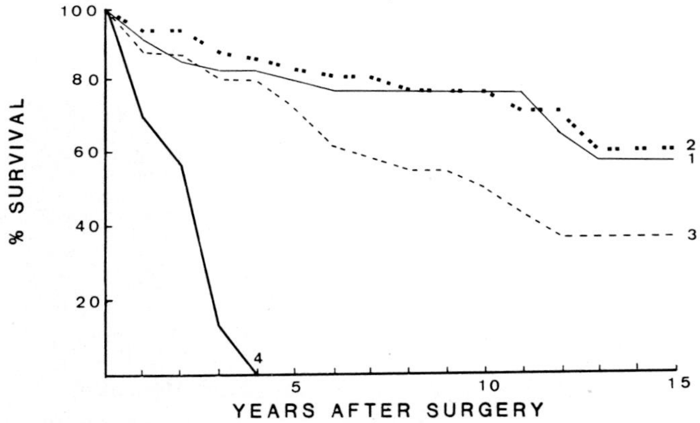

Figure 2.99 Survival rates of 181 patients with thymomas according to the histological types of the tumours. Type 1: Spindle-cell thymoma (54 patients); type 2: lymphocyte-rich thymoma (53 patients); type 3: differentiated epithelial thymoma (63 patients); type 4: undifferentiated epithelial thymoma or thymic carcinoma (11 patients). From Verley and Hollmann, 1985)

The presence of nuclear atypia is another factor whose significance is discussed. A number of authors have emphasized a lack of correlation between the clinical course of the tumour and the cytological features of thymomas. Conversely, other authors found the presence of epithelial atypia to be significantly associated with local or regional recurrences. Furthermore, thymic carcinomas are characterized by the presence of malignant cytological abnormalities and a poor prognosis. Thus, thymic epithelial neoplasms may be viewed as a spectrum encompassing both thymomas and thymic carcinomas (Lewis *et al.*, 1987). A careful cytological examination is needed to assess the presence, importance and number of atypia. Even slight cytological atypia warrant closer follow-up. Obvious malignant cytological features lead to the diagnosis of thymic carcinoma of very poor prognosis.

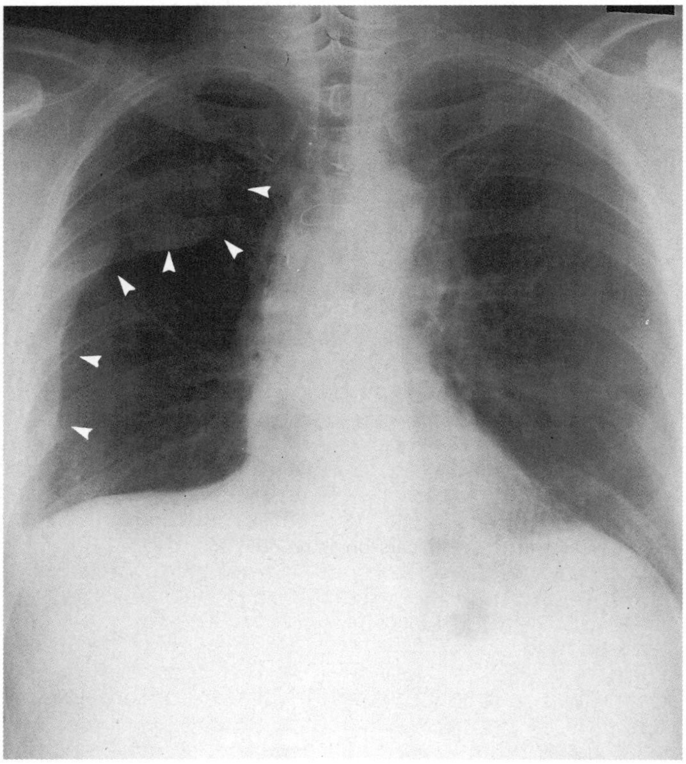

Figures 2.95–2.97 Recurrent thymoma. Pleural recurrence in the right hemithorax. There is no recurrence in the anterior mediastinum. **Fig. 2.95**: roentgenogram, posteroanterior view; **Fig. 2.96**: roentgenogram, lateral view; **Fig. 2.97**: CT scan

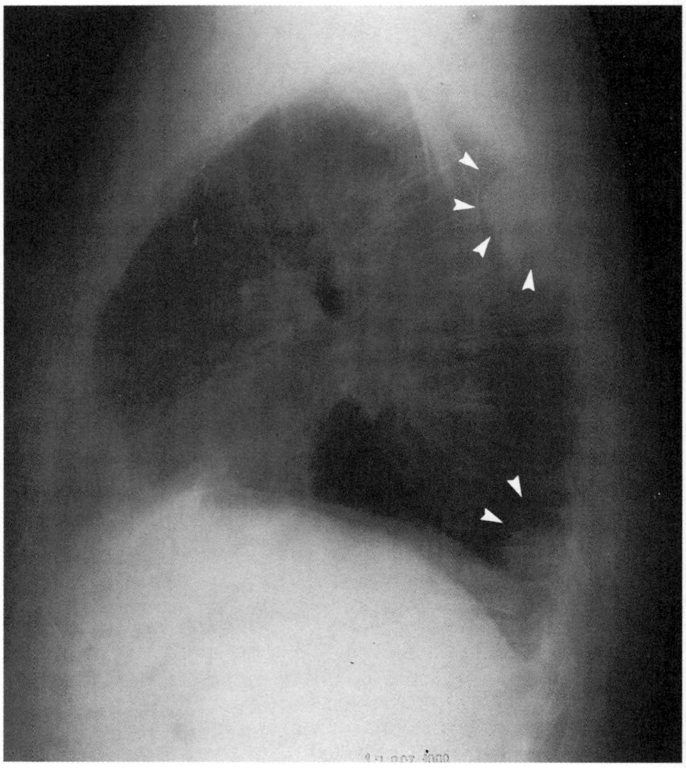

Figure 2.96

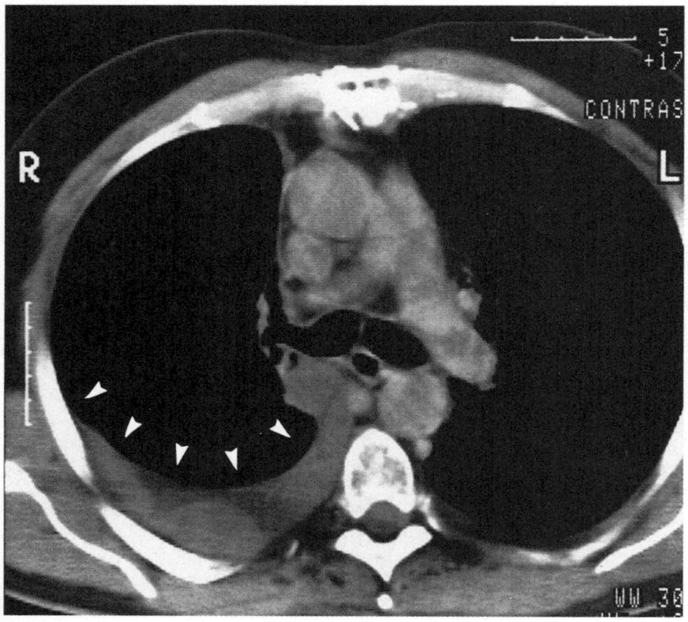

Figure 2.97

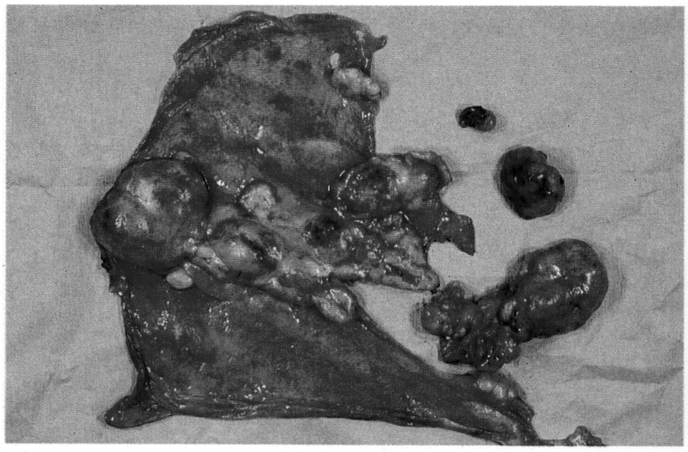

Figure 2.98 Recurrent thymoma. The recurrence occurs as numerous grafts on the pleural surface of the lung. (Figures 2.95–2.98 are from the same patient.)

Occasional cases with a high proportion of epithelial cells demonstrating variable degrees of cytological atypia may be difficult to classify, and would be expected to behave in an intermediate manner.

The association with autoimmune disease has long been reported as an indicator of poor prognosis, the mortality rate related to associated syndrome being equal or superior to that due to tumour. More recent studies, however, have recognized that associated diseases are no longer an adverse factor affecting survival, due to the earlier detection of the thymoma and improved methods in management of patients (Wilkins and Castleman, 1979; Masaoka *et al.*, 1981; Verley and Hollmann, 1985; Lewis *et al.*, 1987; Maggi *et al.*, 1991).

Treatment

Surgery, radiotherapy, and chemotherapy are the main therapeutic modalities in thymomas and thymic carcinomas.

Surgery, with an attempt at complete resection, is the basic treatment of tumours. Surgery permits the histopathological diagnosis and determination of the extent of the disease. It allows a complete thymectomy to be performed, avoiding recurrences or a second primary thymoma. Surgery is capable of resecting completely 100% of the non-invasive thymomas, and about 60% of invasive cases. In very largely invasive thymoma and thymic carcinoma an aggressive surgical approach, such as resection of the superior vena caval system followed by reconstruction and/or complete pleuropneumonectomy, has been proposed (Bergh *et al.*, 1978; Nakahara *et al.*, 1988), but the long-term result of such extended operation is unresolved and controversial. With improvements in modern radiotherapy there seems to be no difference between patients having partial excision and those having biopsy only (Cohen *et al.*, 1984; Verley and Hollmann, 1985). These data imply that there is no value in so-called 'debulking procedures'. A second thoracotomy for local relapse, with an attempt at curative resection of pleural grafts or localized metastases, may be recommended, since the results of radiotherapy remain poor in cases of recurrent disease after surgery.

All authors agree that radiotherapy is effective for treatment of thymomas, and numerous authors advocate postoperative irradiation in all cases of invasive thymoma. Postoperative radiation therapy is always indicated when the tumour is incompletely removed (Arriagada *et al.*, 1981; Fujimura *et al.*, 1987). For the majority of authors this is also advised in completely resected invasive tumours (Rosai and Levine, 1976; Chahinian *et al.*, 1981; Nakahara *et al.*, 1988).

The indication of postoperative radiotherapy in well-encapsulated totally resected tumours is more debated. Most of the authors report that radiotherapy is not necessary in the management of these non-invasive thymomas (Rosai and Levine, 1976; Cohen *et al.*, 1984; Maggi *et al.*, 1986, 1991; Fujimura *et al.*, 1987). On the other hand, based on the evidence that (1) all thymomas have malignant potential, (2) even completely excised thymomas can recur, and (3) non-invasive thymomas can also recur after operation, more recent studies recommend postoperative irradiation of all patients with thymoma regardless of the stage, extent of surgery, and histological type (Monden *et al.*, 1985; Nakahara *et al.*, 1988).

The volume to be treated should be the mediastinum, the supraclavicular nodes and all the thoracic extensions found at operation. When the tumour is completely removed postoperative irradiation should deliver 40–50 Gy. When the resection is incomplete, or the tumour unresectable, 50–55 Gy may be delivered to the anterior mediastinum. Irradiation alone of inoperable tumours should be carried out with high doses (55–60 Gy) to decrease the risk of local recurrence (Arriagada *et al.*, 1981; Chahinian *et al.*, 1981).

Information regarding the effect of chemotherapy on thymoma is limited, but all reports indicate that combination chemotherapy is an effective treatment in invasive thymoma and also in the treatment of local or metastatic relapses after radiotherapy (Chahinian *et al.*, 1981; Giaccone *et al.*, 1985; Kosmidis *et al.*, 1988; Dy *et al.*, 1988; Göldel *et al.*, 1989). Some authors have even suggested the use of combination chemotherapy in incompletely resectable thymoma before radiotherapy (Evans *et al.*, 1980; Göldel *et al.*, 1989). The more effective combined regimens are not established definitely, but cisplatin-containing regimens seem of interest.

References

Arriagada, R., Gerard-Marchant, R., Tubiana, M., Amiel, J. L. and Hajj, L. (1981). Radiation therapy in the management of malignant thymic tumors. *Acta Radiol. Oncol.*, **20**, 167–172

Bergh, N. P., Gatzinsky, P., Larsson, S., Lundin, P. and Ridell, B. (1978). Tumors of the thymus and thymic region: I. Clinicopathological studies on thymomas. *Ann. Thorac. Surg.*, **25**, 91–98

Bernatz, P. E., Khonsari, S., Harrison, E. G. and Taylor, W. F. (1973). Thymoma: factors influencing prognosis. *Surg. Clin. N. Am.*, **53**, 885–892

Cajal, S. R. and Suster, S. (1991). Primary thymic epithelial neoplasms in children. *Am. J. Surg. Pathol.*, **15**, 466–474

Chahinian, P., Bhardwaj, S., Meyer, R. J., Jaffrey, I. S., Kirschner, P. A. and Holland, J. F. (1981). Treatment of invasive or metastatic thymoma: Report of eleven cases. *Cancer*, **47**, 1752–1761

Chan, J. K. C. and Rosai, J. (1991). Tumors of the neck showing thymic or related branchial pouch differentiation: a unifying concept. *Hum. Pathol.*, **22**, 349–367

Chollet, P., Plagne, R., Fonck, Y. *et al.* (1981). Thymoma with hypersecretion of thymic hormone. *Thymus*, **3**, 321–334

Cohen, D. J., Ronnigen, L. D., Graeber, G. M. *et al.* (1984). Management of patients with malignant thymoma. *J. Thorac. Cardiovasc. Surg.*, **87**, 301–307

Cossman, J., Deegan, M. J. and Schnitzer, B. (1978). Thymoma: an immunologic and electron microscopic study. *Cancer*, **41**, 2183–2191

Dimery, I. W., Lee, J. S., Blick, M., Pearson, G., Spitzer, G. and Hong, W. K. (1988). Association of the Epstein–Barr virus with lymphoepithelioma of the thymus. *Cancer*, **61**, 2475–2480

Dy, C., Calvo, F. A., Mindan, J. P. *et al.* (1988). Undifferentiated epithelial-rich invasive malignant thymoma: Complete response to cisplatin, vinblastine and bleomycin therapy. *J. Clin. Oncol.*, **6**, 536–542

Evans, W. K., Thompson, D. M., Simpson, W. J., Feld, R. and Phillips, M. J. (1980). Combination chemotherapy in invasive thymoma. *Cancer*, **46**, 1523–1527

Fechner, R. E. (1969). Recurrence of noninvasive thymomas: report of four cases and review of literature. *Cancer*, **23**, 246–254

Fujimura, S., Kondo, T., Handa, M., Shiraishi, Y., Tamahashi, N. and Nakada, T. (1987). Results of surgical treatment for thymoma based on 66 patients. *J. Thorac. Cardiovasc. Surg.*, **93**, 708–714

Giaccone, G., Musella, R., Bertetto, O. *et al.* (1985). Cis-platinum containing chemotherapy in the treatment of invasive thymoma: report of 11 cases. *Cancer Treat. Rep.*, **69**, 695–697

Göldel, N., Böning, L., Fredrik, A., Hölzel, D., Hartenstein, R. and Wilmanns, W. (1989). Chemotherapy of invasive thymoma. A retrospective study of 22 cases. *Cancer*, **63**, 1493–1500

Ito, M., Taki, T., Miyake, M. and Mitsuoka, A. (1988). Lymphocyte subsets in human thymoma studied with monoclonal antibodies. *Cancer*, **61**, 284–287

Kirkpatrick, H., Lynn, E. and Greenberg, S. (1978). Plasma thymic hormone activity in patients with chronic mucocutaneous candidiasis. *Clin. Exp. Immunol.*, **34**, 311–317

Kosmidis, P. A., Iliopoulos, E. and Penetea, S. (1988). Combination chemotherapy with cyclophosphamide, adriamycin and vincristine in malignant thymoma and myasthenia gravis. *Cancer*, **61**, 1736–1740

Kuo, T.-T., Chang, J.-P., Lin, F.-J., Wu, W.-C. and Chang, C.-H. (1990). Thymic carcinomas: histopathological varieties and immunohistochemical study. *Am. J. Surg. Pathol.*, **14**, 24–34

Levine, G. D. and Rosai, J. (1978). Thymic hyperplasia and neoplasia: A review of current concepts. *Hum. Pathol.*, **9**, 495–515

Levine, G. D. and Bensch, K. G. (1972). Epithelial nature of spindle-cell thymoma. An ultrastructural study. *Cancer*, **30**, 500–511
Levine, G. D., Rosai, J., Bearman, R. M. and Polliack, A. (1975). The fine structure of thymoma, with emphasis on its differential diagnosis: a study of ten cases. *Am. J. Pathol.*, **81**, 49–86
Lewis, J. E., Wick, M. R., Scheithauer, B. W., Bernatz, P. E. and Taylor, W. F. (1987). Thymoma. A clinicopathologic review. *Cancer*, **60**, 2727–2743
Leyvraz, S., Henle, W., Chahinian, A. P. *et al.* (1985). Association of Epstein–Barr virus with thymic carcinoma. *N. Engl. J. Med.*, **312**, 1296–1299
Maggi, M., Giaccone, G., Donadio, M. *et al.* (1986). Thymomas. A review of 169 cases, with particular reference to results of surgical treatment. *Cancer*, **58**, 765–776
Maggi, G., Casadio, C., Cavallo, A., Cianci, R., Molinatti, M. and Ruffini, E. (1991). Thymoma: results of 241 operated cases. *Ann. Thorac. Surg.*, **51**, 152–156
Marino, M. and Müller-Hermelink, H. K. (1985). Thymoma and thymic carcinoma: Relation of thymoma epithelial cells to the cortical and medullary differentiation of the thymus. *Virchows Arch. (A)*, **407**, 119–149
Masaoka, A., Monden, Y., Nakahara, K. and Tanioka, T. (1981). Follow-up study of thymomas with special reference to their clinical stages. *Cancer*, **48**, 2485–2492
Masaoka, A., Hashimoto, T., Shibata, K., Yamakawa, Y., Nakamae, K. and Iizuka, M. (1989). Thymomas associated with pure red cell aplasia. Histologic and follow-up studies. *Cancer*, **64**, 1872–1878
Monden, Y., Nakahara, K., Iioka, S. *et al.* (1985). Recurrence of thymoma: clinocopathological features, therapy and prognosis. *Ann. Thorac. Surg.*, **39**, 165–169
Müller-Hermelink, H. K. and Kirchner, T. (1989). The diagnosis of thymic epithelial tumors. In *Thymic Tumors*, Sarrazin, Vrousos and Vincent (eds), Karger, Basel, pp. 37–44
Nakahara, K., Ohno, K. and Hashimoto, J. (1988). Thymoma: results with complete resection and adjuvant postoperative irradiation in 141 consecutive patients. *J. Thorac. Cardiovasc. Surg.*, **95**, 1041–1047
Nomori, H., Horinouchi, H., Kaseda, S., Ishihara, T. and Torikata, C. (1988). Evaluation of the malignant grade of thymoma by morphometric analysis. *Cancer*, **61**, 982–988
Nomori, H., Ishihara, T. and Torikata, C. (1989). Malignant grading of cortical and medullary differentiated thymoma by morphometric analysis. *Cancer*, **64**, 1694–1699
Pascoe, H. R. and Miner, M. H. (1976). An ultrastructural study of nine thymomas. *Cancer*, **37**, 317–326
Perronne, C., Ooka, T., De Thé, G., Berrih-Aknin, S. and Verley, J. M. (1990). Antibodies to Epstein–Barr virus in 50 patients with thymic tumor. *J. Am. Med. Assoc.*, **264**, 570–571
Pescarmona, E., Pisacane, A., Rendina, E. A., Ricci, C., Ruco, L. P. and Baroni, C. D. (1991). 'Organoid' thymoma: a well-differentiated variant with distinctive clinicopathological features. *Histopathology*, **18**, 161–164
Ricci, C., Rendina, E. A., Pescarmona, E. O., Venuta, F., Di Tolla, R., Ruco, L. P. and Baroni, C. D. (1989). Correlations between histological type, clinical behaviour, and prognosis in thymoma. *Thorax*, **44**, 455–460
Rosai, J. (1985). 'Lymphoepithelioma-like' thymic carcinoma. Another tumor related to Epstein–Barr virus? *New Engl. J. Med.*, **312**, 1320–1322
Rosai, J. and Levine, G. D. (1976). Tumors of the thymus. In *Atlas of Tumor Pathology*, 2nd series, fascicle 13. Washington, DC: Armed Forces Institute of Pathology
Salyer, W. R. and Eggleston, J. C. (1976). Thymoma: A clinical and pathological study of 65 cases. *Cancer*, **37**, 229–249
Savino, W., Manganella, G., Verley, J. M., Wolff, A., Berrih, S., Levasseur, Ph., Binet, J.-P., Dardenne, M. and Bach, J.-F. (1985). Thymoma epithelial cells secrete thymic hormone but do not express class II antigens of the major histocompatibility complex. *J. Clin. Invest.*, **76**, 1140–1146
Savino, W., Berrih, S. and Dardenne, M. (1984). Thymic epithelial antigen, acquired during ontogeny and defined by the anti-p19 monoclonal antibody, is lost in thymomas. *Lab. Invest.*, **51**, 292
Savino, W., Takacs, L., Monostori, E. and Dardenne, M. (1988). Phenotypic changes of the subseptal thymic epithelium in myasthenia gravis. *Thymus*, **12**, 111–116
Snover, D. C., Levine, G. D. and Rosai, J. (1982). Thymic carcinoma. Five distinctive histological variants. *Am. J. Surg. Pathol.*, **6**, 451–470
Suster, S. and Rosai, J. (1991). Thymic carcinoma. A clinicopathologic study of 60 cases. *Cancer*, **67**, 1025–1032
Toker, C. (1968). Thymoma – an ultrastructural study. *Cancer*, **21**, 1157–1163
Truong, L. D., Mody, D. R., Cagle, P. T., Jackson-York, G. L., Schwartz, M. R. and Wheeler, T. M. (1990). Thymic carcinoma: a clinicopathologic study of 13 cases. *Am. J. Surg. Pathol.*, **14**, 151–166
Verley, J. M. and Hollmann, K. H. (1985). Thymoma: A comparative study of clinical stages, histologic features, and survival in 200 cases. *Cancer*, **55**, 1074–1086
Waldmann, T. A., Broder, S., Durm, M., Blackman, M., Krakauer, R. and Meade, B. (1975). Suppressor T cells in the pathogenesis of hypogammaglobulinemia associated with a thymoma. *Trans. Assoc. Am. Phys.*, **88**, 120–134
Weiss, L. M., Movahed, L. A., Butler, A. E. *et al.* (1989). Analysis of lymphoepithelioma and lymphoepithelioma-like carcinomas for Epstein–Barr viral genomes by in situ hybridization. *Am. J. Surg. Pathol.*, **13**, 625–631
Wick, M. R., Weiland, L. H., Scheithauer, B. W. and Bernatz, P. E. (1982). Primary thymic carcinoma. *Am. J. Surg. Pathol.*, **6**, 613–630
Wilkins, E. W., Jr and Castleman, B. (1979). Thymoma: A continuing survey at the Massachusetts General Hospital. *Ann. Thorac. Surg.*, **28**, 252–255
Wilkins, E., Edmunds, L. and Castleman, B. (1966). Cases of thymoma at the Massachusetts General Hospital. *J. Thorac. Cardiovasc. Surg.*, **52**, 322–330

THYMIC HYPERPLASIA

True thymic hyperplasia is defined as an increase in both size and weight of the thymus occurring during the first two decades of life, with retention of a normal microscopic appearance for age. The lesion ranges from borderline enlarged thymus to massive thymic hyperplasia (weight > 100 g). True thymic hyperplasia differs from the lymphoid hyperplasia, which is characterized by the presence of lymphoid follicles with germinal centres, regardless of the size or weight of the thymus: this is the type classically associated with myasthenia gravis and other autoimmune diseases (Levine and Rosai, 1978).

According to Mullen and Richardson (1986), 170 cases of thymic hyperplasia in children less than 15 years of age are reported in the literature over a 25-year period in whom 50 resections were performed. The lesion is usually detected on routine chest roentgenogram, and is seen on CT as homogeneous, diffuse, symmetric anterior mediastinal mass (Arliss *et al.*, 1988). The enlarged normal thymus does not appear as a forerunner of neoplastic change or immunological difficulty, and is not associated with haematological or metabolic disorders. However, several cases of myasthenia gravis associated with thymic hyperplasia are reported in children (LaFranchi and Fonkalsrud, 1973), and peripheral lymphocytosis is described in some cases (Lack, 1981; Arliss *et al.*, 1988).

Enlarged thymic shadow seems safe in asymptomatic infants up to 3 years of age, since involution can be expected in 98% of such enlargements. Respiratory complications or symptoms are reported only occasionally. In the older child, who is asymptomatic and who has typical roentgenographic features of thymic hyperplasia, surveillance with an annual chest X-ray also seems safe. Massive thymic hyperplasia can nevertheless simulate thymoma, and the development of symptoms or abnormal radiographic features should prompt removal of the mass.

References

Arliss, J., Scholes, J., Dickson, P. R. and Messina, J. J. (1988). Massive thymic hyperplasia in an adolescent. *Ann. Thorac. Surg.*, **45**, 220–222
Lack, E. E. (1981). Thymic hyperplasia with massive enlargement. Report of two cases with review of diagnostic criteria. *J. Thorac. Cardiovasc. Surg.*, **81**, 741–746
LaFranchi, J. and Fonkalsrud, E. W. (1973). Surgical treatment of lymphatic tumors of the mediastinum in children. *J. Thorac. Cardiovasc. Surg.*, **65**, 8–14
Levine, G. D. and Rosai, J. (1978). Thymic hyperplasia and neoplasia. A review of current concepts. *Hum. Pathol.*, **9**, 495–515
Mullen, B. and Richardson, J. D. (1986). Primary anterior mediastinal tumors in children and adults. *Ann. Thorac. Surg.*, **42**, 338–345

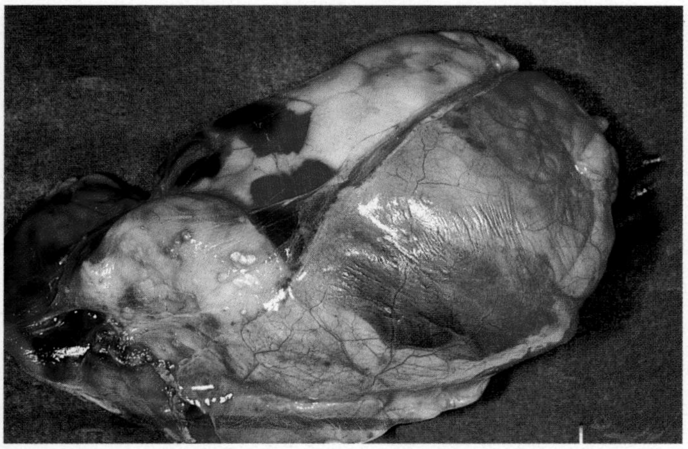

Figure 2.100 Thymolipoma. Large, well-encapsulated tumour of soft and yellow appearance

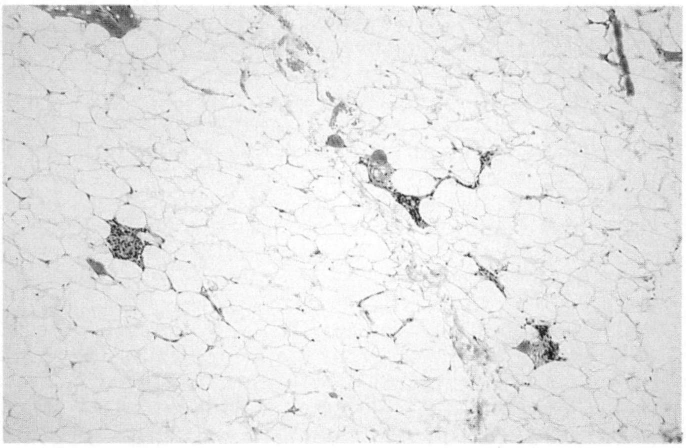

Figure 2.101 Thymolipoma. The tumour consists mainly of mature fat tissue

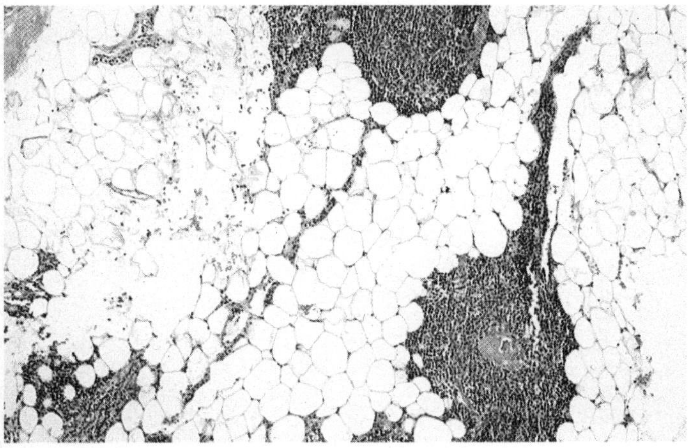

Figure 2.102 Thymolipoma. Foci of thymic tissue, containing a Hassall's corpuscle

THYMOLIPOMA

Thymolipoma is a rare, benign tumour composed of normal thymic tissue and mature adipose elements. It occurs with equal frequency in men and women, and shows a predilection for young adults (mean age 22 years). The tumour can attain a very large size and the weight of reported cases ranges from 22 to 16 000 g (Iseki *et al.*, 1990).

About 50% of thymolipomas are asymptomatic and are discovered incidentally on routine chest radiology. CT shows a mass of mixed density consistent with fat and soft-tissue component, and is of value in differentiating the tumour from a more homogeneous thymoma, or from a mediastinal lipoma displaying a characteristic low attenuation value (Winarso *et al.*, 1982). In rare instances a few systemic diseases, including Graves' disease, aplastic anaemia, and myasthenia gravis have been reported in association with thymolipoma (Otto *et al.*, 1982).

Grossly, the tumours are lobulated and well encapsulated, soft and yellow on section (Fig. 2.100). Histologically, they consist mainly of mature fatty tissue separated into distinct lobules by bands of fibrous tissues, with only few foci of thymic tissue containing Hassall's corpuscles but no germinal centres (Figs 2.101 and 2.102). The proportion of thymic tissue in the tumours varies from about 10% to 30%. Iseki *et al.* (1990) described a unique case of thymolipoma with striated myoid cells.

Thymolipoma may adhere to the pleura or pericardium and displace adjacent mediastinal organs, but invasion has never been documented. It is always cured by local excision.

References

Iseki, M., Tsuda, N., Kishikawa, M. *et al.* (1990). Thymolipoma with striated myoid cells. Histological, immunohistochemical, and ultrastructural study. *Am. J. Surg. Pathol.*, **14**, 395–398

Otto, H. F., Löning, Th., Lachenmayer, L. *et al.* (1982). Thymolipoma in association with myasthenia gravis. *Cancer*, **50**, 1623–1628

Winarso, P., Isherwood, I., Photiou, S. and Donnelly, R. J. (1982). Thymolipoma simulating cardiomegaly: use of computed tomography in diagnosis. *Thorax*, **37**, 941–942

THYMIC CYSTS

Mediastinal thymic cysts are uncommon, accounting for 1–2% of mediastinal cysts and tumours. Graeber *et al.* (1984) collected 46 patients with cystic lesion of the thymus, and Davis and Florendo (1988) record 44 further cases of mediastinal thymic cysts in the English-language literature from 1953.

Cysts of the thymus are classified as congenital, neoplastic, and degenerative. Congenital thymic cysts arise from a persistently patent thymopharyngeal duct. Usually this structure is obliterated by the seventh week of gestation. If not, accumulation of fluid or blood could result in formation of a cyst. This congenital aetiology is the most common. Degenerative cysts result from degeneration of Hassall's corpuscles. Neoplastic cysts occur within thymomas, benign or malignant (Figs 2.103–2.106), within Hodgkin's (Figs 2.107 and 2.108) or non-Hodgkin's lymphomas or, less commonly, within germ-cell tumours. Among the non-Hodgkin's lymphomas, the mediastinal lymphoma of B cell type with sclerosis, which develops from the thymus gland, is most likely to give rise to a cyst. In Hodgkin's disease of thymic origin, cysts are frequent and the tumour may occasionally present predominantly as a mediastinal cyst (Lewis and Manoharan, 1987). In these cases the cysts are either bordered by a well-preserved ciliated columnar epithelium, or result from cystic degeneration of Hassall's corpuscles and are then bordered by a stratified pseudo-squamous epithelium. All these neoplastic cysts may be grossly indistinguishable from a benign cyst of the thymus. Benign cystic lesions have also been recorded after successful chemotherapy or radiation therapy for Hodgkin's disease, raising the question of the recurrence of the disease.

Non-neoplastic thymic cysts are usually considered as asymptomatic, and are frequently either found incidentally at operation for unrelated cause or discovered on routine chest roentgenogram. Nevertheless, according to Davis and Florendo (1988) 39% have symptoms, the most common complaints being dyspnoea, shortness of breath, chest pain, and dysphagia. The cysts may also be found only on microscopic examination. No preoperative study is specifically diagnostic, and diagnosis requires surgical removal. However, a chest roentgenogram is of some help in delineating the size of the mass and the organs to which it is related. CT outlines the capsule of the mass, confirms the presence of central fluid and gives an accurate estimate of the size of the lesion and the organs it involves.

Mediastinal thymic cysts are round or ovoid, and are limited by a smooth, fibrous wall. They are solitary or multiple, sometimes multiloculated. The microscopic appearance of the cysts varies. A simple cyst is composed of a definite epithelial lining of cuboidal, squamous, or multilayered columnar cells, with thymic tissue present in the wall of the cyst (Figs 2.109–2.111). The cyst content is serous fluid. With degeneration from haemorrhage into the cyst, the epithelium lining is lost and is replaced with fibrous tissue. Cholesterol clefts are a typical degenerative change. With degeneration the content of the cyst modifies, consisting of blood and necrotic material with varied gross appearances. In this case the diagnosis depends on the presence of thymic tissue in the cyst wall.

Multilocular thymic cysts resulting from the cystic transformation of medullary duct epithelium-derived structures (including Hassall's corpuscles) induced by an acquired inflammatory process have been recently described as a distinctive entity (Suster and Rosai, 1991; Figs 2.112–2.114).

References

Davis, J. W. and Florendo, F. T. (1988). Symptomatic mediastinal thymic cysts. *Ann. Thorac. Surg.*, **46**, 693–694

Graeber, G. M., Thompson, L. D., Cohen, D. J. *et al.* (1984). Cystic lesion of the thymus. An occasionally malignant cervical and/or anterior mediastinal mass. *J. Thorac. Cardiovasc. Surg.*, **87**, 295–300

Lewis, C. R. and Manoharan, A. (1987). Benign thymic cysts in Hodgkin's disease: report of a case and review of published cases. *Thorax*, **42**, 633–634

Suster, S. and Rosai, J. (1991). Multilocular thymic cyst: an acquired reactive process. Study of 18 cases. *Am. J. Surg. Pathol.*, **15**, 388–398

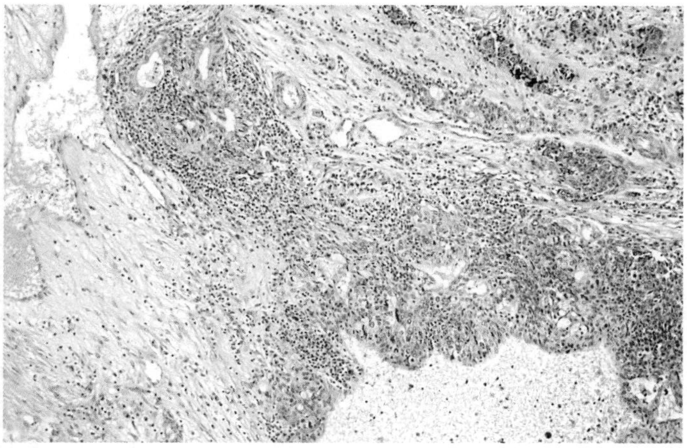

Figure 2.103 Thymic cysts within thymic carcinoma. Two large cysts and several smaller ones are surrounded by the neoplastic tissue

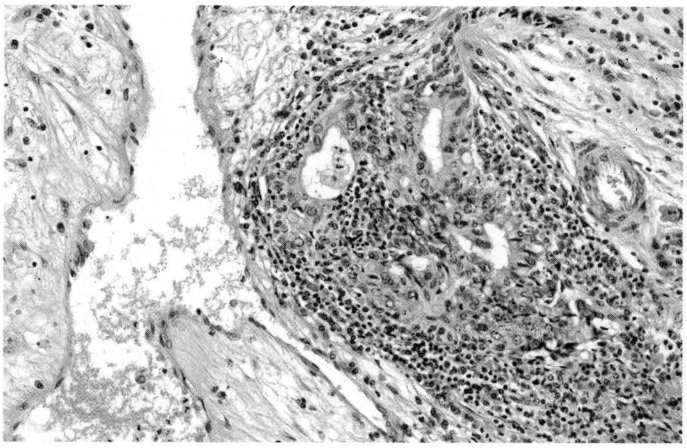

Figure 2.104 Thymic cysts within thymic carcinoma. The large cyst is lined by flattened epithelium, the small ones are bordered by ciliated columnar epithelium

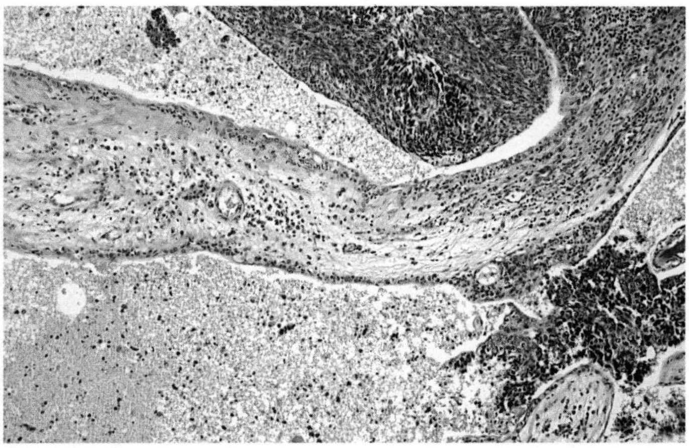

Figure 2.105 Thymic cysts within thymic carcinoma. The neoplastic tissue proliferates within the cysts

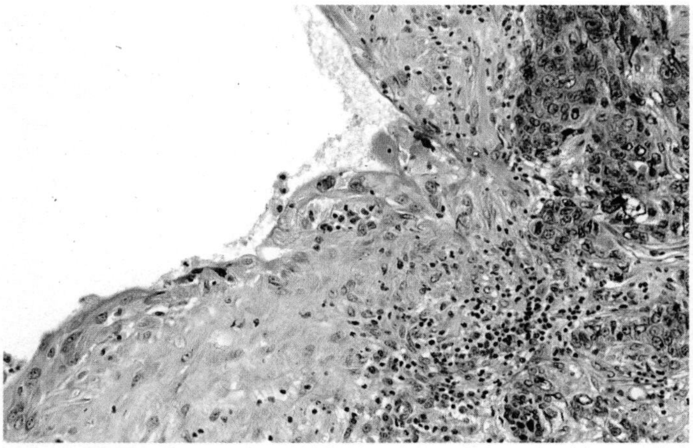

Figure 2.106 Thymic cyst within thymic carcinoma. In this area the cyst is lined by a flattened squamous epithelium

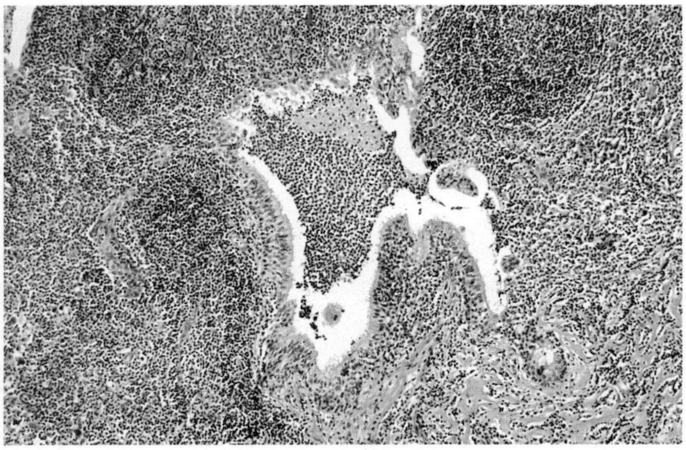

Figure 2.107 Thymic cyst within Hodgkin's disease. The cyst is lined by ciliated columnar epithelium, and is surrounded by Hodgkin's tissue

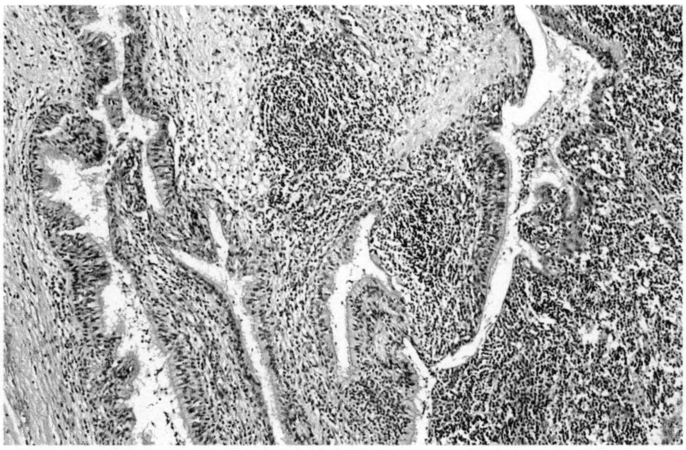

Figure 2.108 Thymic cysts within Hodgkin's disease. Another view of the same tumour gives a better illustration of the features of the cysts

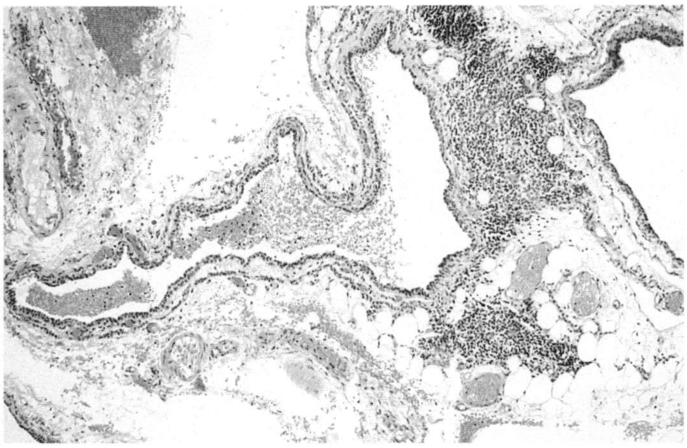

Figure 2.109 Congenital thymic cysts. The cysts are thin walled and contain serous to haemorrhagic fluid. Thymic tissue is present between the cysts

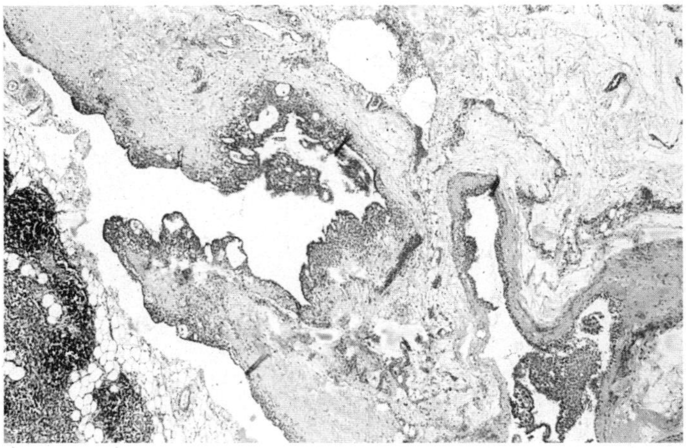

Figure 2.110 Congenital thymic cyst. The cyst develops in a loose connective tissue containing a thymic lobule (left) and atrophic thymic remnants (upper right)

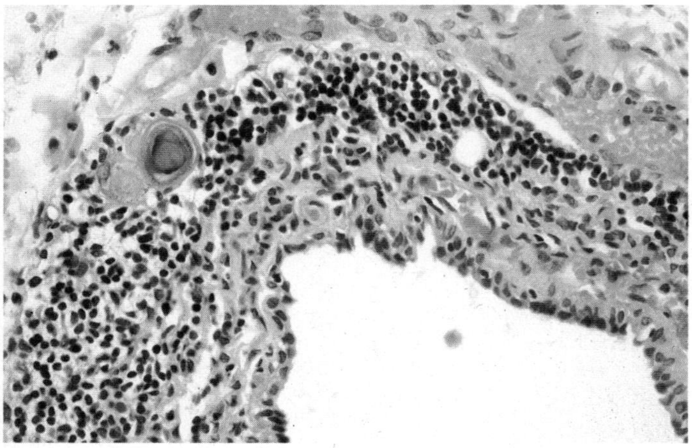

Figure 2.111 Congenital thymic cyst. The cyst is lined by a flat cuboidal epithelium, and is surrounded by atrophic thymic tissue with a Hassall's corpuscle (upper left)

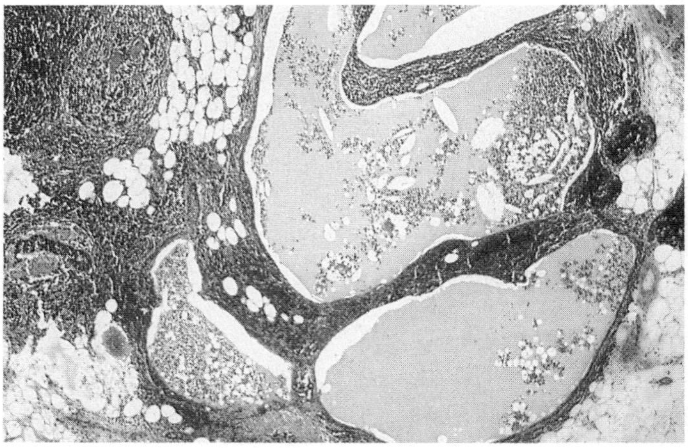

Figure 2.112 Multilocular thymic cysts. The cysts are surrounded by lymphocytes. On the left of the figure thymic tissue can be seen

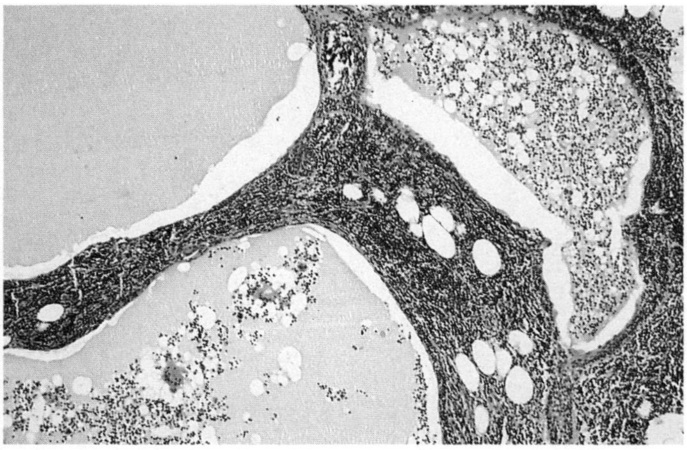

Figure 2.113 Multilocular thymic cysts. The cysts contain a serous fluid, lymphocytes, and necrotic debris. They are lined by a flattened squamous epithelium

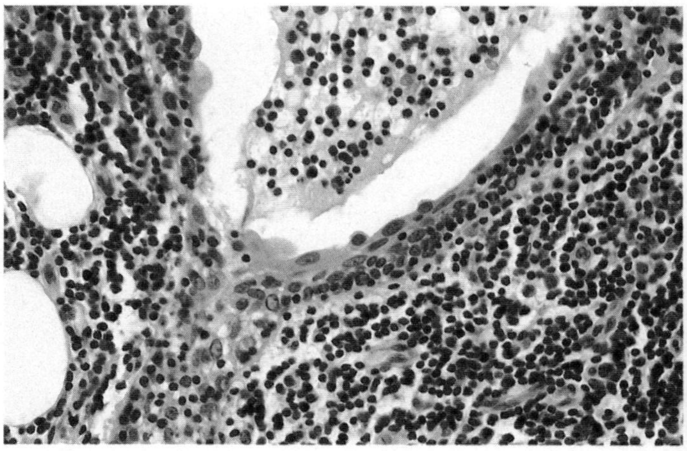

Figure 2.114 Multilocular thymic cyst. The figure illustrates inflammatory changes in the cyst wall

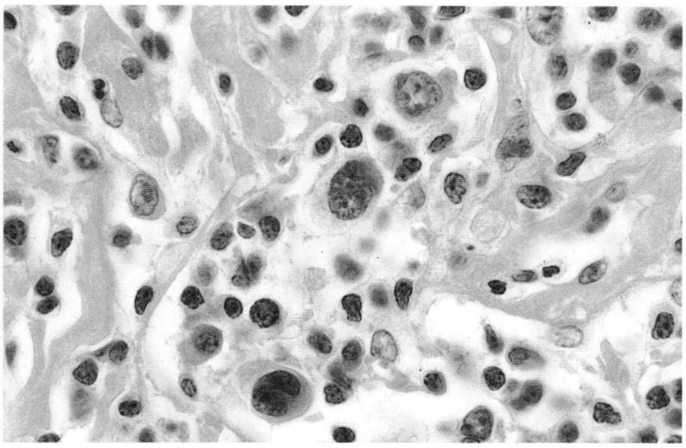

Figure 3.7 Hodgkin's disease. In this figure lacunar Reed–Sternberg cells have a small darkly stained cytoplasm shrunk away from the surrounding structures, leaving the cell in a clear lacuna. Nuclei are dense and pyknotic

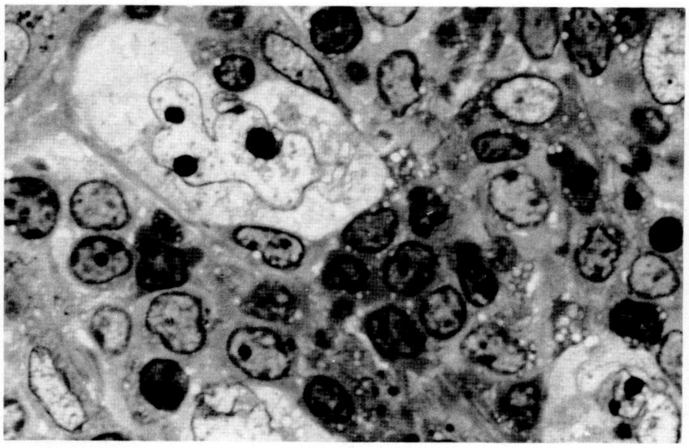

Figure 3.8 Hodgkin's disease. This half-thin section shows more clearly the feature of a Reed–Sternberg cell with the large well-delimited cytoplasm and the characteristic polylobated nucleus with prominent nucleoli

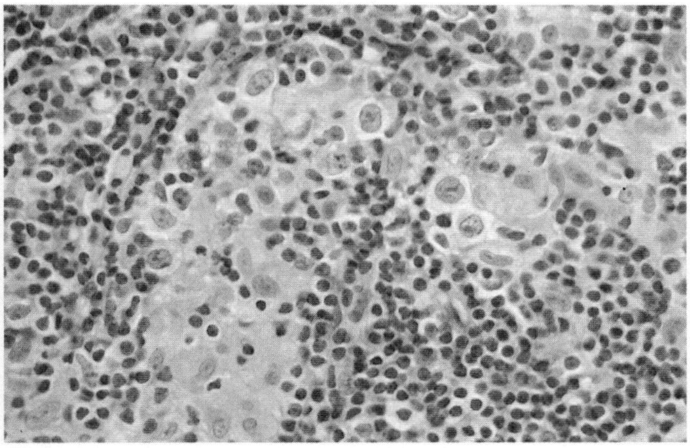

Figure 3.9 Hodgkin's disease, lymphocyte-predominant type. The tissue is composed of numerous lymphocytes, clusters of epithelioid histiocytes, and some scattered polylobated Reed–Sternberg cells

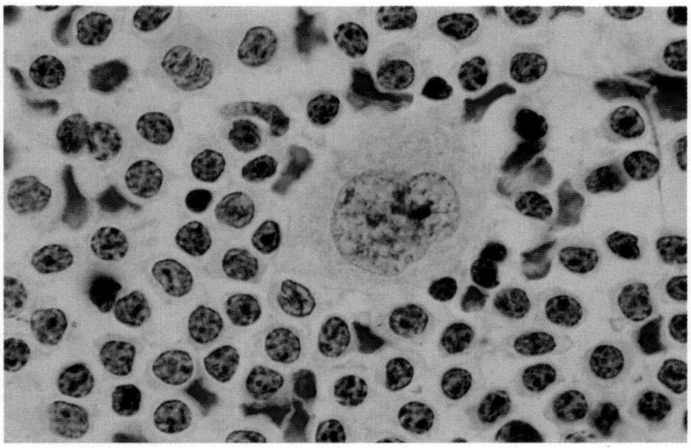

Figure 3.10 Hodgkin's disease, lymphocyte-predominant type. In the same case, imprint of the tumour shows a large polylobated Reed–Sternberg cell surrounded with lymphocytes. The nuclear chromatin is granular and the nucleolus is inconspicuous

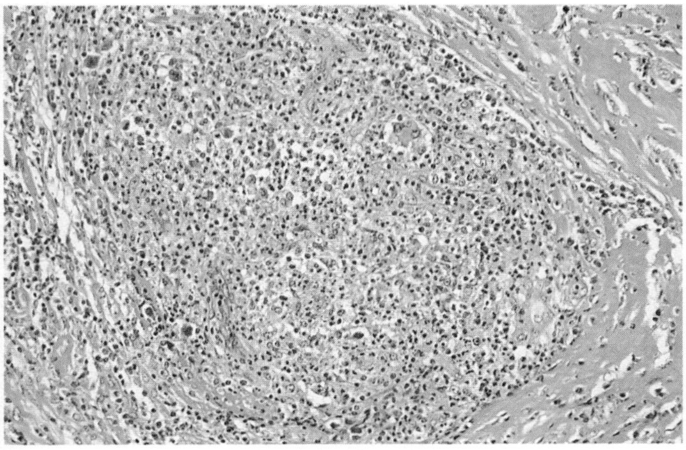

Figure 3.11 Hodgkin's disease. Low magnification of nodular sclerosing type. Bands of fibrous tissue surround a cellular tissue containing numerous lacunar Reed–Sternberg cells

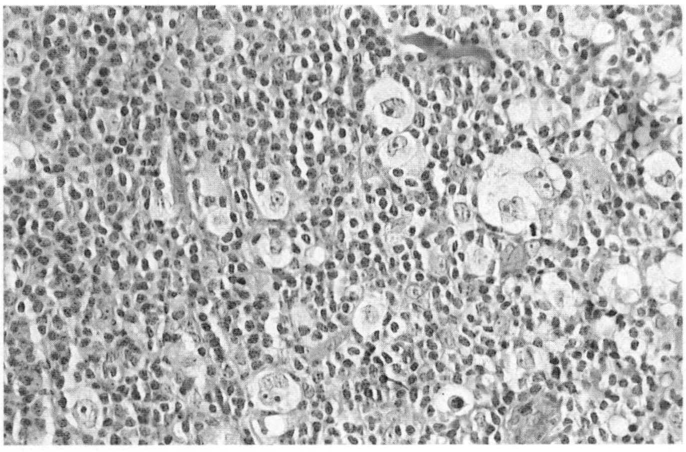

Figure 3.12 Hodgkin's disease. At higher magnification the cellular area consists mainly of lymphocytes and lacunar Reed–Sternberg cells

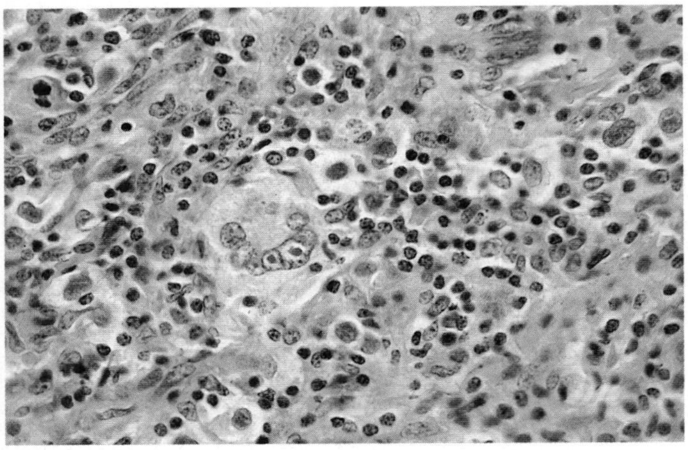

Figure 3.13 Hodkin's disease, nodular sclerosing type. Typical polymorphous aspect of Hodgkin's tissue with a Reed–Sternberg 'ring-cell'

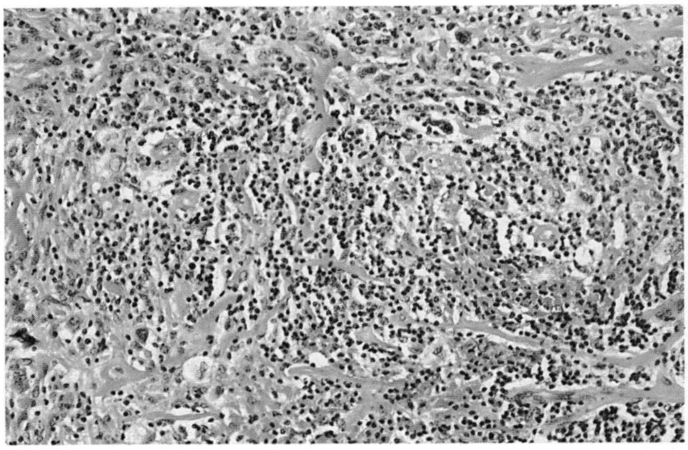

Figure 3.14 Hodgkin's disease, nodular sclerosing type, advanced fibrous phase. The fibrous tissue obliterates the Hodgkin's tissue, leaving only scattered lymphocytes and Reed–Sternberg cells

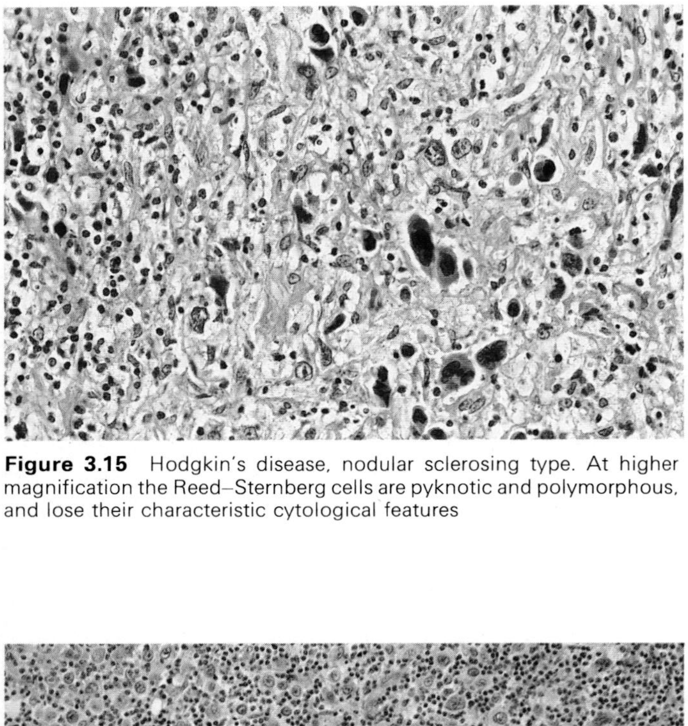

Figure 3.15 Hodgkin's disease, nodular sclerosing type. At higher magnification the Reed–Sternberg cells are pyknotic and polymorphous, and lose their characteristic cytological features

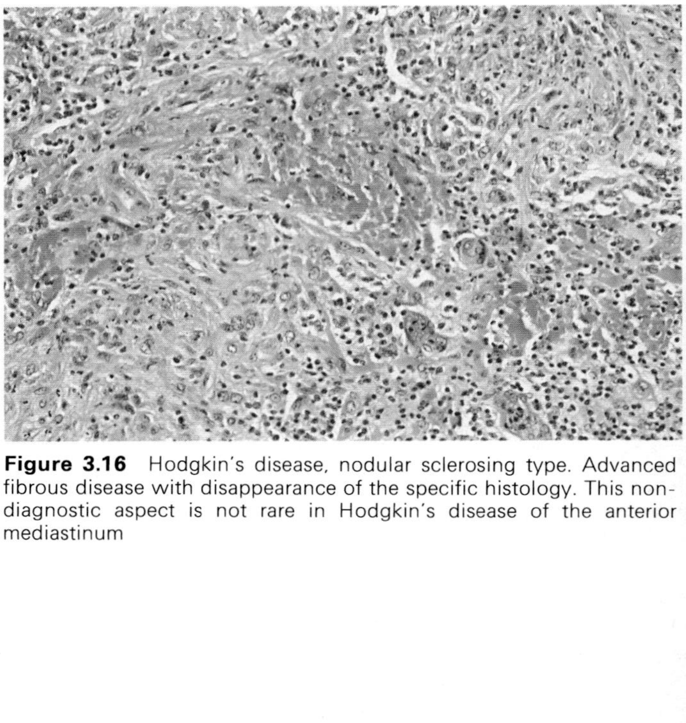

Figure 3.16 Hodgkin's disease, nodular sclerosing type. Advanced fibrous disease with disappearance of the specific histology. This non-diagnostic aspect is not rare in Hodgkin's disease of the anterior mediastinum

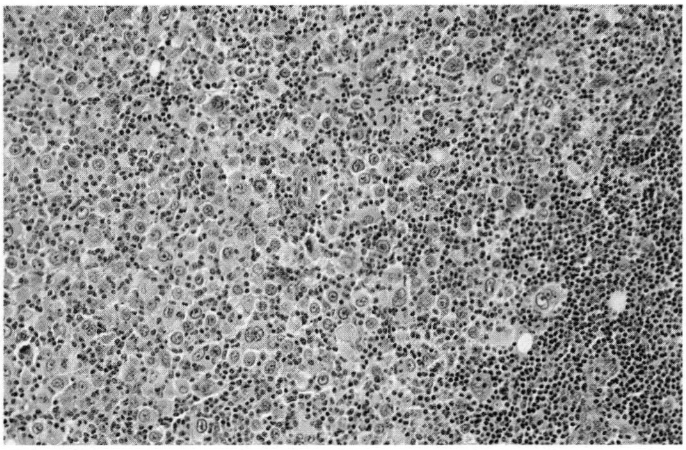

Figure 3.17 Hodgkin's disease, nodular sclerosing type, syncytial variant. Numerous Reed–Sternberg variants are disposed in cohesive clusters and sheets, simulating either metastatic carcinoma or non-Hodgkin's lymphoma

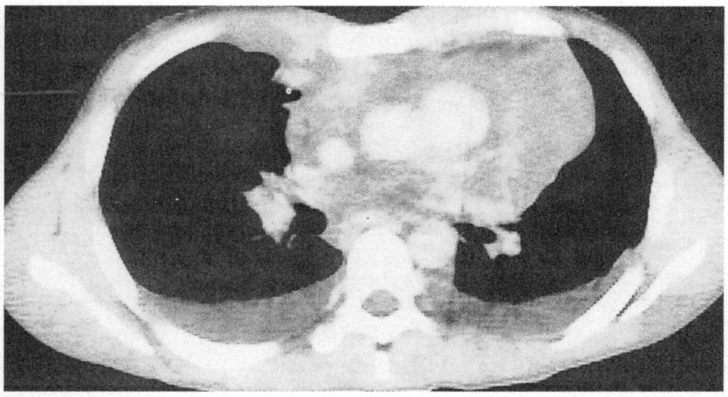

Figure 3.18 Hodgkin's disease of the thymus. The CT scan shows a very large polylobated, well-delimited mass projecting into the anterior mediastinum

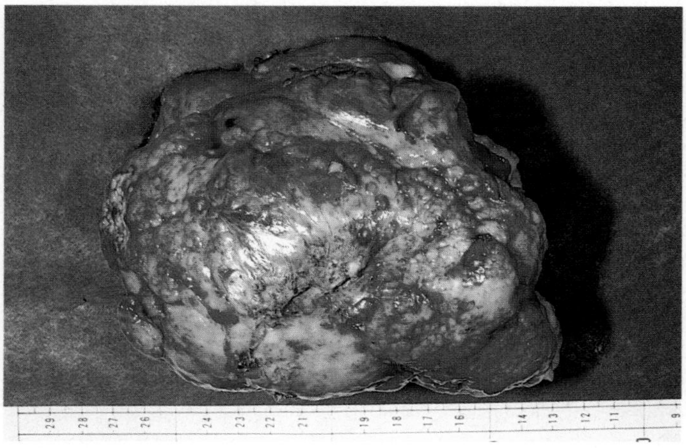

Figure 3.19 Hodgkin's disease of the thymus. Gross appearance of the same tumour

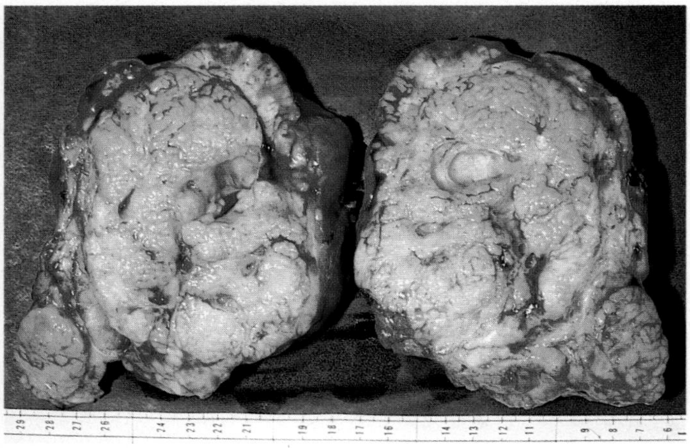

Figure 3.20 Hodgkin's disease of the thymus. Cut section of the same tumour showing fibrous bands delimiting areas of fleshy tissue. A cyst is present in the superior half of the lesion

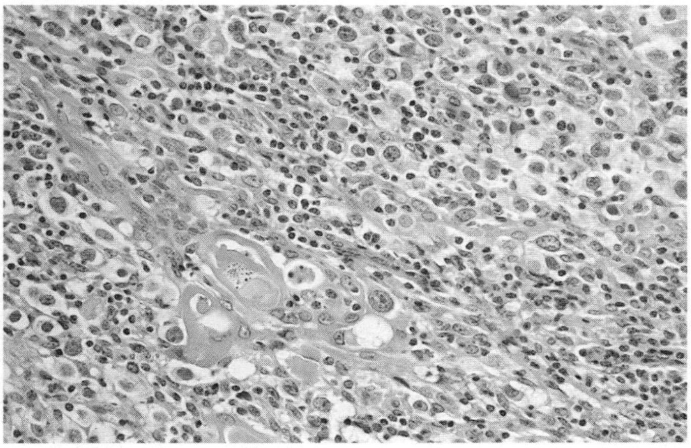

Figure 3.21 Hodgkin's disease of the thymus. The figure shows the characteristic admixture of Hodgkin's tissue and thymic epithelial remnants containing Hassall's corpuscles

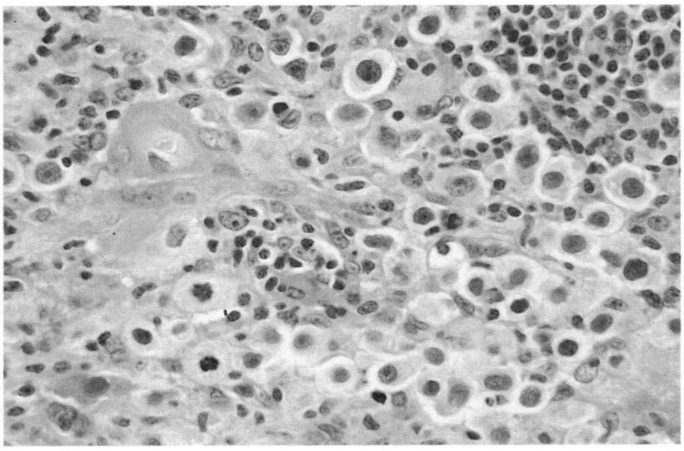

Figure 3.22 Hodgkin's disease of the thymus. Numerous large lacunar Hodgkin's cells infiltrate the proliferated thymic epithelium

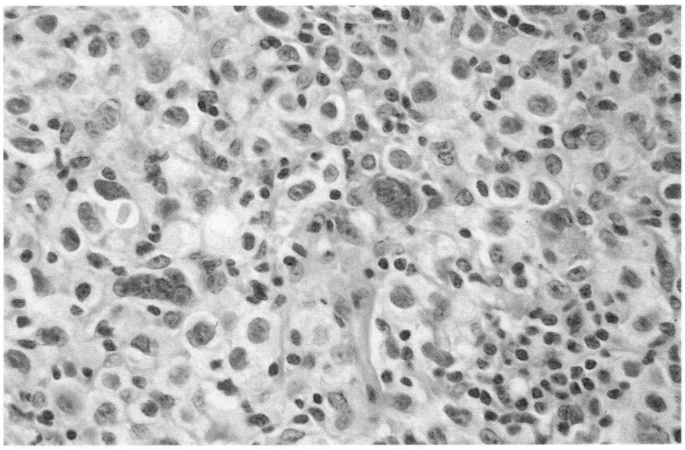

Figure 3.23 Hodgkin's disease of the thymus. Another aspect of the same tumour. The aspects shown on Figs 3.19–3.21 strongly simulate a thymoma, a carcinoma or a large-cell lymphoma

Occasionally the tumour is completely cystic, simulating a teratoma or a cystic thymoma.

Histology

Hodgkin's disease of the thymus gland is always of nodular sclerosis type. It is frequently of advanced fibrous stage, and then appears as the most sclerotic lesions observed in the mediastinum. It shows a number of morphological features that set it apart from the other localizations of the disease.

The lesions consist of an intimate combination of the features of nodular sclerosis type of Hodgkin's disease with proliferating thymic epithelium (Figs 3.21–3.24). Extensive fibrous bands tend to enclose highly cellular areas containing Reed–Sternberg cell variants, lymphocytes, histiocytes, eosinophil and plasma cells in varying proportions. The Reed–Sternberg cells are mostly of the lacunar type.

Within or adjacent to the Hodgkin's tissue, foci of thymic epithelial proliferation occur. They are characterized by well-delimited sheets of thymic epithelium composed of regular epithelial cells, with no morphological atypia, sometimes centred by a well-preserved Hassall's corpuscle (Figs 3.21–3.23). Cyst formation of different size occurs within the epithelial strands. The cysts are lined by thymic epithelium which is either flattened, assuming the appearance of stratified squamous epithelium, or of columnar, ciliated or mucus-producing type (Fig. 3.24). In rare instances cysts are very large, bordered by a mixture of thymic epithelial remnants and foci of Hodgkin's tissue giving radiologically and macroscopically the appearance of a thymic cyst. The closely intermixed Hodgkin's tissue and thymic elements produce a confusing pattern and may result in a false diagnosis of thymoma.

In some cases the Reed–Sternberg cells are very scarce and scattered throughout the tumour, whereas Hodgkin's cells are numerous and grouped together in pseudo-epithelial or seminomatous clusters (Figs 3.25 and 3.26). In these cases the differential diagnosis with a thymoma or a seminoma could be extremely difficult, and immunocytochemistry would be of interest in demonstrating the epithelial nature of the thymic remnants embracing in its network areas of Hodgkin's tissue (Fig. 3.27). Another difficulty occurs when sclerosis is extremely advanced, obliterating the typical cellular Hodgkin's granuloma.

Immunohistochemistry and histogenesis of Reed–Sternberg cell

Although the origin of the Reed–Sternberg cell is still debated, recent immunohistochemical studies have demonstrated that approximately 50% or more cases express lymphoid associated B-cell as well as T-cell antigens on Reed–Sternberg cells. Some of the remaining cases may have a similar lymphoid origin which is not detectable with current techniques (Agnarsson and Kadin, 1989).

Nodular sclerosis, mixed cellularity and lymphocyte-depleted types are more often of T-cell phenotype ($CD2^+$, $CD4^+$, less frequently $CD3^+$, $CD4^+$), whereas lymphocyte predominant type expresses mainly B-cell antigens ($CD20^+$, $CD22^+$, $LN1^+$, J $chain^+$). In addition, leukocyte common antigen (LCA) is negative on Reed–Sternberg cell in nodular sclerosing type, but positive in 50% of the cases of mixed cellularity and lymphocyte predominant type. CD19 (Leu-M1) is positive in most cases, with the exception of the lymphocyte predominant type (Fig. 3.28). Activation antigens (Ki-1, Ia, CD25, T9) are expressed in a high proportion of cases regardless of subtype (Table 3.6).

These results suggest that most cases of Hodgkin's disease are histogenetically derived from activated T cells or B cells, and confirm the distinction of the nodular lymphocyte predominant type of Hodgkin's disease from the majority of nodular sclerosing and mixed cellularity types.

The high frequency of activation antigens observed in the majority of cases of Hodgkin's disease is similar to that found in anaplastic Ki-1 lymphoma derived mostly from activated T cells and may support a common histogenesis and/or a borderline condition of these two entities (Stein *et al.*, 1985; Agnarsson and Kadin, 1989, Table 3.7).

The gene rearrangement studies performed on Hodgkin's tissues are disappointing and reveal conflicting results, since some cases show either immunoglobulin and/or T-cell receptor gene rearrangement, and different gene rearrangement patterns are demonstrated within the same histological subtypes. The heterogeneity of lineage lymphoid markers observed on Reed–Sternberg cells may explain the variable findings of the molecular genetic studies.

Prognosis and treatment

The prognosis for the different forms of localized mediastinal Hodgkin's disease is usually favourable, with an overall 5-year survival of 79%, comparable to that of patients with stage I Hodgkin's disease of the nodular-sclerosis type. Large size of the mass or direct invasion of the adjacent lung are adverse prognostic factors.

Despite the overall good prognosis, half of the patients have recurrent disease and patients with and without thymic involvement have similar rates of recurrence.

Table 3.6 Immunophenotype of RS cell

Histological type	*Lymphoid markers*	*LCA*	*Leu-M1*	*EMA*	*Activation antigens*
Lymphocyte predominant	B cell (80%)	+ 50%	−	+	+
Nodular sclerosing	T cell (40%) B cell (15%)	−	+	−	+
Mixed cellularity	T cell (70%) B and T cell (10%)	+ 50%	+	−	+
Lymphocyte depleted	mostly T cell	−	+	−	+

LCA (T200, CD45) Leukocyte common antigen. Leu M1 (CD15). EMA, Epithelial membrane antigen. Activation antigens: Ki-1 (CD30, Ber.H2); Ia (HLA-DR related antigen); Tac (CD25, interleukin-2-receptor); T9 (transferrin receptor).
According to Hsu *et al.*, 1985; Chittal *et al.*, 1988; Agnarsson and Kadin, 1989.

Table 3.7 Putative origin of neoplastic cells in Hodgkin's disease and Ki-1 lymphoma

Type of lymphoma	*Cell of origin*	*Admixture of non-malignant cells*	*Morphological features*
Hodgkin's disease	Activated T cell	Large amounts	Modular sclerosis Mixed cellularity Lymphocytic depletion
	Activated B cell	Large amounts	Lymphocyte predominant (nodular)
Ki-1 lymphoma	Activated T cell	Little	Anaplastic (bizarre) large cells
	Activated B cell	Little	

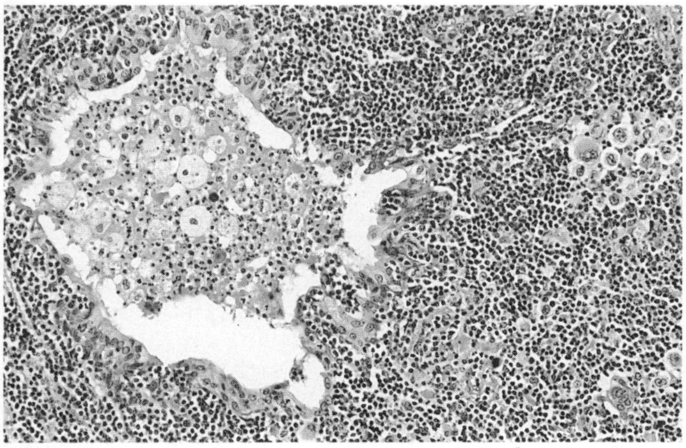

Figure 3.24 Hodgkin's disease of the thymus. A thymic cyst lined by mucus-producing epithelium is present within the tumour. A cluster of Reed–Sternberg cells may be seen on the right

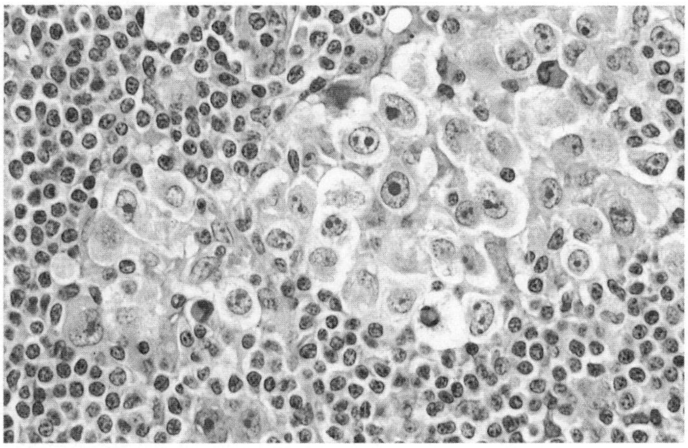

Figure 3.25 Hodgkin's disease of the thymus. Cluster of closely arranged Hodgkin's cells simulating a seminoma

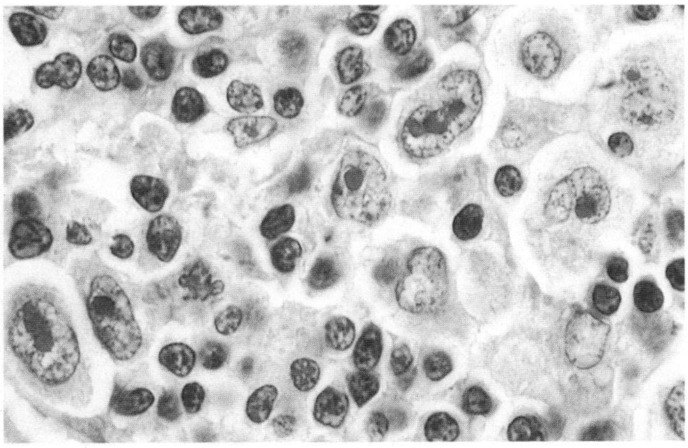

Figure 3.26 Hodgkin's disease of the thymus. Higher magnification of the same area illustrating the distinctive features of the Reed–Sternberg cells.

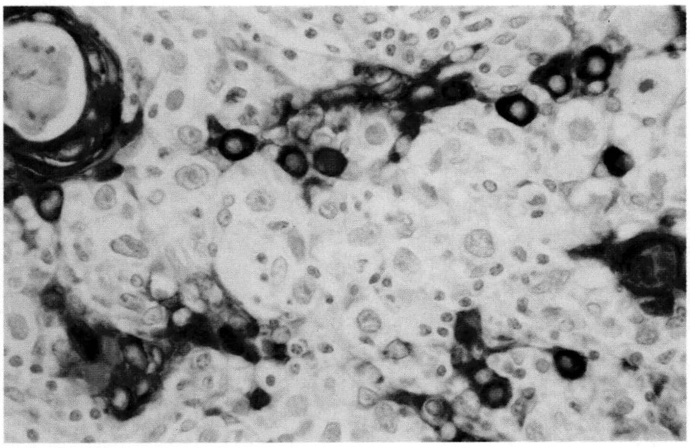

Figure 3.27 Hodgkin's disease of the thymus. The cytokeratin immunostains positively the epithelial thymic remnants surrounding the cytokeratin-negative Reed–Sternberg cells

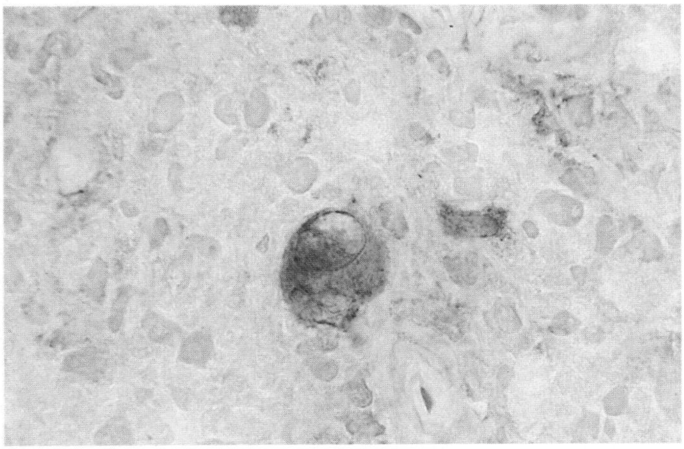

Figure 3.28 Hodgkin's disease of the thymus. Reed–Sternberg cell positively immunostained with Leu-21 (CD19)

Recurrences tend to appear in lymph node groups contiguous to the area of initial involvement, suggesting that these untreated areas may have contained foci of Hodgkin's disease initially, and supporting the radiotherapeutic practice of treating areas adjacent to the grossly involved lymph-node or thymic region. Recurrences below the diaphragm are exceptional, raising the question of the need for a staging laparotomy in patients with Hodgkin's disease limited to the mediastinum.

Although the management of patients with mediastinal involvement is still controversial, most authors recommend a combined-modality therapy (chemotherapy followed by radiotherapy) for patients with large mediastinal mass (Ferrant *et al.*, 1985).

References

Agnarsson, B. A. and Kadin, M. E. (1989). The immunophenotype of Reed–Sternberg cells. A study of 50 cases of Hodgkin's disease using fixed frozen tissues. *Cancer*, **63**, 2083–2087

Bennett, M. H., Maclennan, K. A., Easterling, M. J., Vaughan Hudson, B., Jelliffe, A. M. and Vaughan Hudson, G. (1983). The prognostic significance of cellular subtypes in nodular sclerosing Hodgkin's disease: an analysis of 271 non-laparotomized cases (BNLI report no 22). *Clin. Radiol.*, **34**, 497–501

Ben-Yehuda-Salz, D., Ben-Yehuda, A., Polliack, A., Ron, N. and Okon, E. (1990). Syncytial variant of nodular sclerosing Hodgkin's disease. A new clinicopathologic entity. *Cancer*, **65**, 1167–1172

Bergh, N. P., Gatzinsky, P., Larsson, S., Lundin, P. and Ridell, B. (1978). Tumors of the thymus and thymic region: II. Clinicopathological studies on Hodgkin's disease of the thymus. *Ann. Thorac. Surg.*, **25**, 99–106

Carbone, P. P., Kaplan, H. S., Musshoff, K., Smithers, D. W. and Tubiana, M. (1971). Report of the committee on Hodgkin's disease staging classification. *Cancer Res.*, **31**, 1860–1861

Chittal, S. M., Caveriviere, P., Schwarting, R., Gerdes, J., Al Saati, T., Rigal-Huguet, F., Stein, H. and Delsol, G. (1988). Monoclonal antibodies in the diagnosis of Hodgkin's disease. The search for a rational panel. *Am. J. Surg. Pathol.*, **12**, 9–21

Ferrant, A., Hamoir, V., Binon, J., Michaux, J.-L. and Sokal, G. (1985). Combined modality therapy for mediastinal Hodgkin's disease. Prognostic significance of constitutional symptoms and size of disease. *Cancer*, **55**, 317–322.

Hsu, S.-M., Yang, K. and Jaffe, E. S. (1985). Phenotypic expression of Hodgkin's and Reed–Sternberg cells in Hodgkin's disease. *Am. J. Pathol.*, **118**, 209–217

Katz, A. and Lattes, R. (1969). Granulomatous thymoma or Hodgkin's disease of thymus? A clinical and histologic study and a re-evaluation. *Cancer*, **23**, 1–15

Keller, A. R. and Castleman, B. (1974). Hodgkin's disease of the thymus gland. *Cancer*, **33**, 1615–1623

Lukes, R. J. and Butler, J. J. (1966). The pathology and nomenclature of Hodgkin's disease. *Cancer Res.*, **26**, 1063–1081

Lukes, R. J., Craver, L. F., Hall, T. C., Rappaport, H. and Ruben, P. (1966). Report of the nomenclature committee. *Cancer Res.*, **26**, 1311

Pinkus, G. S. and Said, J. W. (1985). Hodgkin's disease, lymphocyte predominance type, nodular – a distinct entity. *Am. J. Pathol.*, **118**, 1–6

Ree, H. J., Neiman, R. S., Martin, A. W., Dallenbach, F. and Stein, H. (1989). Paraffin section markers for Reed–Sternberg cells. A comparative study of peanut agglutinin, Leu-M1, LN-2, and Ber-H2. *Cancer*, **63**, 2030–2036

Stein, H., Mason, D. Y., Gerdes, J. *et al.* (1985). The expression of the Hodgkin's disease associated antigen Ki-1 in reactive and neoplastic lymphoid tissue: Evidence that RS cells and histiocytic malignancies are derived from activated lymphoid cells. *Blood*, **66**, 848–858

Strickler, J. G., Michie, S. A., Warnke, R. A. and Dorfman, R. F. (1986). The 'syncytial variant' of nodular sclerosing Hodgkin's disease. *Am. J. Surg. Pathol.*, **10**, 470–477

Wright, D. H. and Isaacson, P. G. (1983). *Biopsy Pathology of the Lymphoreticular System*, Chapman & Hall, London

PRIMARY NON-HODGKIN'S LYMPHOMAS OF THE MEDIASTINUM

Mediastinal involvement is noted at presentation in 15–25% of patients with both diffuse and nodular non-Hodgkin's lymphoma, in association with widespread nodal and extranodal involvement. These lymphomas have no predilection for histological subtype and will not be discussed here. Primary non-Hodgkin's lymphoma *localized to the mediastinum* is an uncommon occurrence. According to Lichtenstein *et al.* (1980) they occur in 9.2% of all lymphomas, and according to Levitt *et al.* (1982) 12% of patients with non-Hodgkin's lymphoma present with signs of intrathoracic disease and 6% have no extrathoracic disease detectable.

Until the last decade mediastinal lymphomas were predominantly related to the lymphoblastic T-cell lymphoma. During recent years there have been increasing reports of primary involvement of the mediastinum by 'non-lymphoblastic' large-cell lymphomas, which were first classified as 'histiocytic' after Rappaport's classification. With progress in immunohistochemistry the mediastinal large-cell lymphomas have been recognized as a heterogeneous group of tumours. The larger subgroup corresponds to large-cell lymphoma of B-cell type, with sclerosis, first reported by Lichtenstein *et al.* (1980). The remainder are anaplastic Ki-1 lymphoma. These mediastinal lymphomas share in common a very aggressive clinical course, a poor prognosis and a misleading histological feature.

Very recently a low-grade B-cell lymphoma of mucosa-associated lymphoid tissue arising in the thymus has also been described (Isaacson *et al.*, 1990).

Mediastinal large-cell lymphoma of B-cell type, with sclerosis

Mediastinal large-cell lymphoma of B-cell type, with sclerosis, is now a well-recognized entity, characterized by common clinical features and a deceptive histological morphology (Menestrina *et al.*, 1986). In adult patients it is the most frequent lymphoma presenting with mediastinal involvement.

Clinical aspects (Table 3.8)

The disease is characterized by the young age of the patients (15–40 years; mean 35 years) with a clear female predominance (about 2:1; Addis and Isaacson, 1986; Levitt *et al.*, 1982; Menestrina *et al.*, 1986; Trump and Mann, 1982; Perrone *et al.*, 1986).

Patients present with a predominantly extensive anterior mediastinal tumour that frequently infiltrates neighbouring structures, particularly the anterior chest wall, the sternum, and the superior vena cava (Fig. 3.29). Extrathoracic involvement at presentation is unusual. Bone marrow and peripheral lymph nodes are generally not affected. When subsequent extrathoracic spread occurs it develops to unusual sites, such as the kidneys, adrenals, liver, thyroid, gastrointestinal tract and ovaries.

Table 3.8 Mediastinal large-cell lymphoma of B-cell type: clinical features

Young age (15–40 years; mean 35)
Female predominance (ratio 2:1)
Primary anterior mediastinal involvement, presumed to originate in thymus
Locally aggressive
anterior chest wall
sternum
neighbouring mediastinal structures
superior vena cava
Involvement neither of bone marrow nor of peripheral lymph nodes
Metastases to unusual sites:
kidneys, adrenal, liver, thyroid, gastrointestinal tract, ovary
Aggressive clinical course

Morphological aspects

Large B-cell lymphomas are bulky, non-encapsulated, invasive tumours. The cut surface is grey and of fibrous consistency, with areas of necrosis. Histologically the tumours usually have a diffuse growth pattern, without evidence of nodularity (Figs 3.30 and 3.31). However, an 'alveolar' pattern is common due to the presence of thin collagen or of narrow fibrous septa dividing the tumour cell population into irregular areas of varying size, thus giving a 'compartmentalized' aspect to the whole tissue (Figs 3.32 and 3.33). Less frequently, broader bands of dense connective tissue may be present, conferring a nodular appearance similar to that seen in nodular sclerosing Hodgkin's disease.

The neoplastic cells are predominantly of large size (Figs 3.34–3.38). Their cytoplasm is abundant, most often pale and granular, with well-delimited cell membranes. Nuclei show variation in size and shape. Some are irregularly folded with dispersed chromatin and rather inconspicuous nucleoli, and have the morphology of large centrocytes. Others have more rounded nuclear outlines with two or more basophilic nucleoli applied to a conspicuous nuclear membrane and correspond to centroblasts. Mitotic activity is usually marked. Occasional cells resemble immunoblasts with large rounded nuclei and a single central nucleolus. When indentation or folding is extreme, nuclei possess two or more lobes resulting in cells that closely resemble Reed–Sternberg cells (Figs 3.35 and 3.36).

Stromal infiltrate of lymphocytes, occasional eosinophils and plasma cells may be present. Reactive histiocytes and epithelioid cells, sometimes arranged in a granulomatous pattern, are frequently seen (Fig. 3.39). Areas of necrosis are always present.

Residual thymic structures are frequently identified at the periphery of the tumours (Fig. 3.40). In some cases the thymus is heavily infiltrated, and isolated Hassall's corpuscles are the only recognizable thymic elements (Fig. 3.41). Epithelium-lined thymic cysts are found in about 25% of cases.

Differential diagnosis

The diagnosis of mediastinal large-cell lymphoma of B-cell type with sclerosis is based on a careful confrontation between clinical, histopathological and immunohistochemical data. As emphasized by Addis and Isaacson (1986), Menestrina *et al.* (1986) and Perrone *et al.* (1986), mediastinal large B-cell lymphoma often presents a diagnostic problem which is two-fold: the distinction has to be made between malignant lymphoma and other types of mediastinal tumours, and the lymphoma may be difficult to classify.

Malignant thymoma may be simulated by the presence of fibrous bands lobulating the tumour, and of occasional perivascular lymphocytic cuffs resembling the perivascular spaces characteristic of thymoma (Fig. 3.42). Residual thymic structures inside the tumour, such as entrapped Hassall's corpuscles, isolated thymic epithelial cells or thymic cysts, may be misinterpreted as evidence of neoplastic epithelial cells at the light microscopic, immunohistochemical and ultrastructural levels.

The resemblance to seminoma is due to the compartmentalization of the tumour by sclerosis, the presence of large cells with clear cytoplasm and the frequent existence of lymphoid infiltrates and histiocytic epithelioid and giant-cell reaction. But PAS stain does not reveal glycogen, and the prominent nucleoli characteristic of seminoma are lacking.

Sclerosis, tumour lobulation, presence of epithelium-lined thymic cysts, cells resembling Reed–Sternberg cells, stromal infiltrate of lymphocytes and occasional eosinophils and plasma cells, may strongly mimic Hodgkin's disease, particularly the syncytial variant of nodular sclerosis. Observance of strict criteria for Hodgkin's disease and for acceptance of Reed–Sternberg cells (large, red nucleoli and perinucleolar haloes) are indispensable, together with immunohistochemistry.

Electron microscopy may be of value in demonstrating cell junctions and cytoplasmic tonofilaments in thymoma and metastatic carcinoma. But immunohistochemical analysis appears of greater importance to define the nature of the neoplastic proliferation, and is necessary to type the lymphoma accurately. On pure morphological grounds the typing is difficult, with most tumours showing a mixture of centroblasts and large centrocytes, leading to a false impression of heterogeneity in this group of tumour. Before the advance of immunohistochemistry these lymphomas were classified as immunoblastic sarcoma of either B- or T-cell type, or follicle centre cell lymphoma of large-cleaved or non-cleaved type.

Immunohistochemistry

Even on fixed tissue and paraffin sections immunohistochemistry allows the distinction between malignant lymphoma and epithelial tumour: the neoplastic cells do not demonstrate epithelial cell markers such as cytokeratin, but are invariably reactive with the leukocyte common antibody, thus clearly defined as non-epithelial in nature.

On cryostat section, immunohistochemical studies show a phenotype characteristic of lymphocytes of B-lineage (Yousem *et al.*, 1985; Menestrina *et al.*, 1986). According to Möller *et al.* (1986, 1987), the tumours all express the B cell-restricted antigens CD19 and CD20, but CALLA and CD21 are not detectable. The neoplastic cells strongly bound PC-1, a mAB recognizing a plasma cell-associated antigen. Immunoglobulin constituents (heavy and light chains, J chain) are not detectable either in the cytoplasm or on the surface of the tumour cells, and the tumours show variable deficiencies in major histocompatibility (MHC) antigen of class I (HLA-A,B,C) and class II (HLA-D) expression. Referring to the B-cell differentiation scheme the immunophenotype LC$^+$, CD19$^+$, CD20$^+$, CD21$^-$, (Ki-1$^-$, T-cell antigens$^-$) supports a terminal B-cell differentiation. However, other studies show that numerous cases express CD20, CD45, and HLA-DR, and some cases immunoglobulin (IgG or IgA), suggesting that the tumours have not undergone terminal differentiation to the plasma cell stage, but only a post-germinal centre stage (Lamarre *et al.*, 1989).

Prognosis and treatment

Mediastinal large-cell lymphomas of B-cell type, with sclerosis, are considered as of poor prognosis by most authors (Miller *et al.*, 1981; Trump and Mann, 1982; Addis and Isaacson, 1986; Menestrina *et al.*, 1986; Perrone *et al.*, 1986). However, Jacobson *et al.* (1988), employing CHOP or CHOP-based chemotherapy (cyclophosphamide, doxorubicin, vincristine, prednisone) and consolidation radiation therapy, observe an 80% complete remission and 59% disease-free survival at 5 years.

Prognostic factors predictive of poor outcome are age under 25 years at diagnosis, extrathoracic disease at presentation and incomplete response to initial therapy. Sclerosis in the primary tumour is weakly correlated with survival. The Ann Arbor staging classification is not adequate in predicting survival (Table 3.1; Perrone *et al.*, 1986). Jacobson *et al.* (1988), however, emphasize that mediastinal mass size at diagnosis is the only significant prognostic feature, and that no other factor, including age, correlates with survival. Thus, patients with bulky

[*continued on p. 56*]

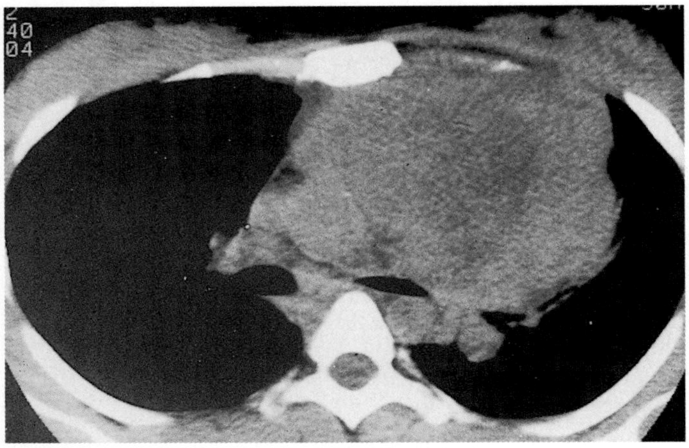

Figure 3.29 Mediastinal large B-cell lymphoma. CT scan shows a very large anteromediastinal mass, invading the surrounding structures and compressing the trachea

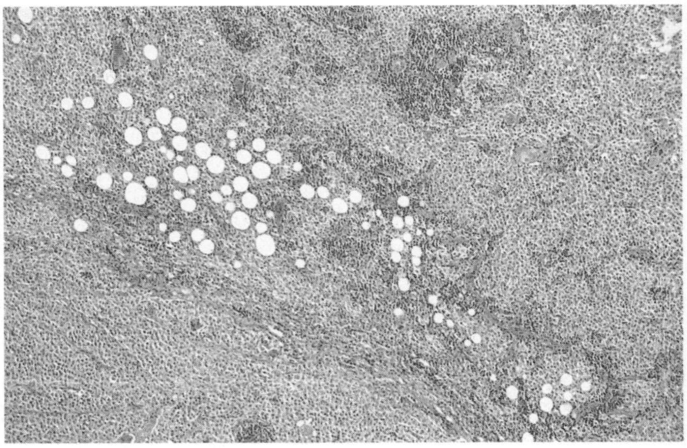

Figure 3.30 Mediastinal large B-cell lymphoma. The tumour has a diffuse growth pattern invading the thymus and the adipose tissue

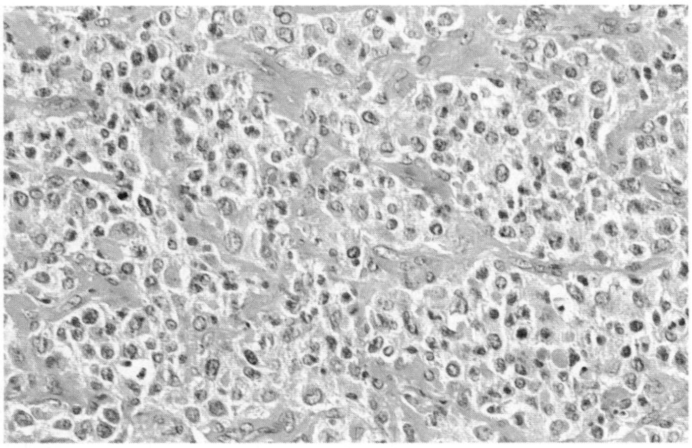

Figure 3.31 Mediastinal large B-cell lymphoma. This tumour is composed of sheets of large cells with an abundant, clear cytoplasm and well-delimited cell membranes, suggestive of a carcinoma

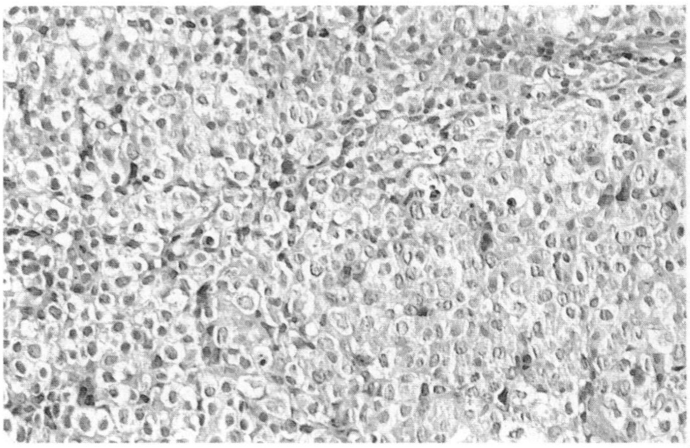

Figure 3.32 Mediastinal large B-cell lymphoma. Fibrous septa lobulate the tumour cell population and reinforce the carcinoma-like pattern of the neoplasm

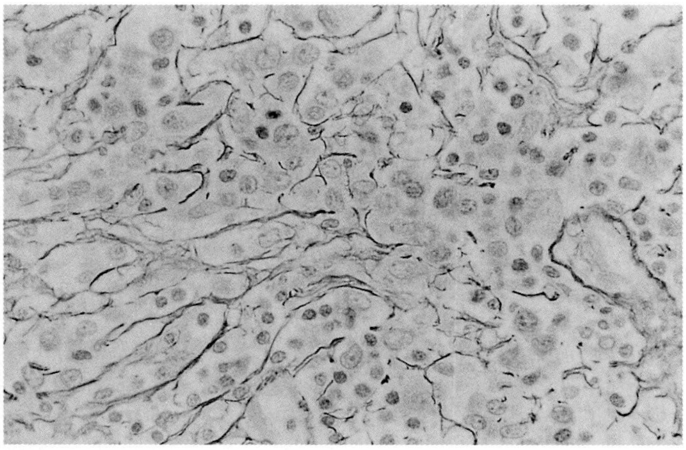

Figure 3.33 Mediastinal large B-cell lymphoma. Gordon stain underlines the 'compartmentalization' of the tumour

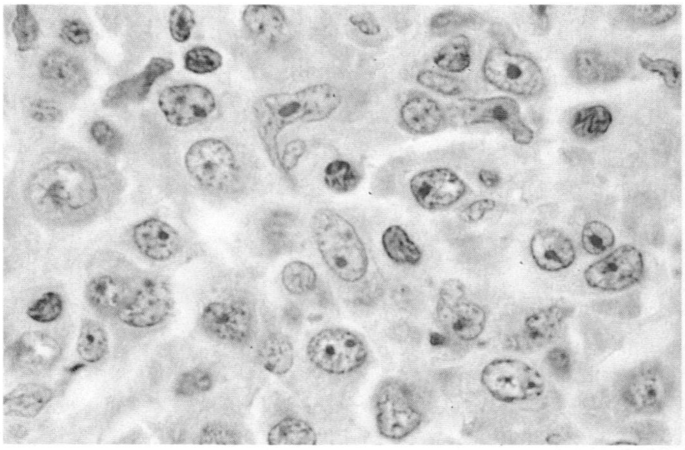

Figure 3.34 Mediastinal large B-cell lymphoma. The tumour cells are large with an abundant clear cytoplasm, round nuclei, and small nucleoli attached to the nuclear membrane

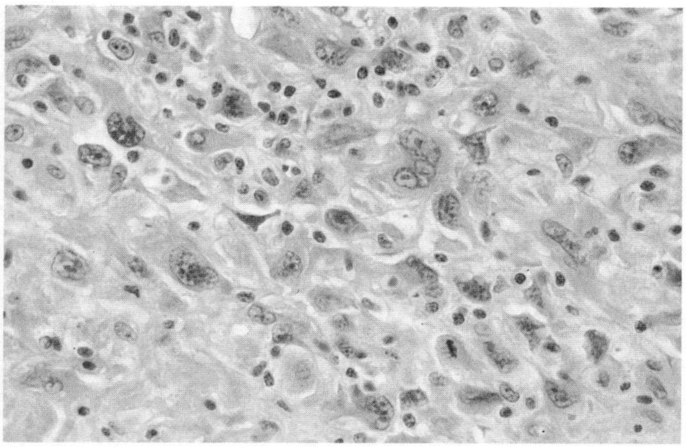

Figure 3.35 Mediastinal large B-cell lymphoma. In this tumour there are numerous atypical cells with irregular multilobed nuclei simulating Hodgkin's disease

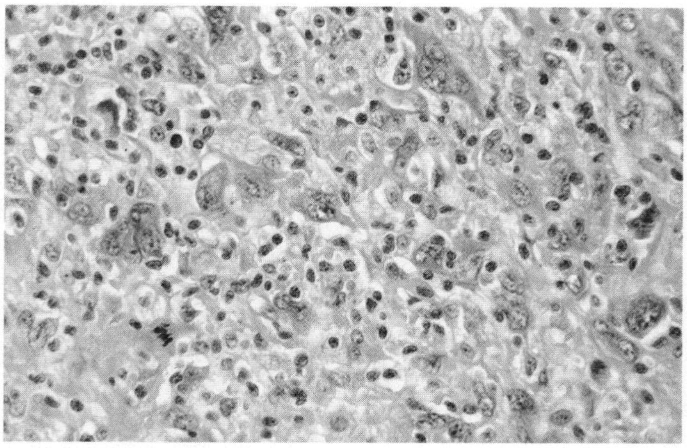

Figure 3.36 Mediastinal large B-cell lymphoma. The figure shows another aspect of the same tumour

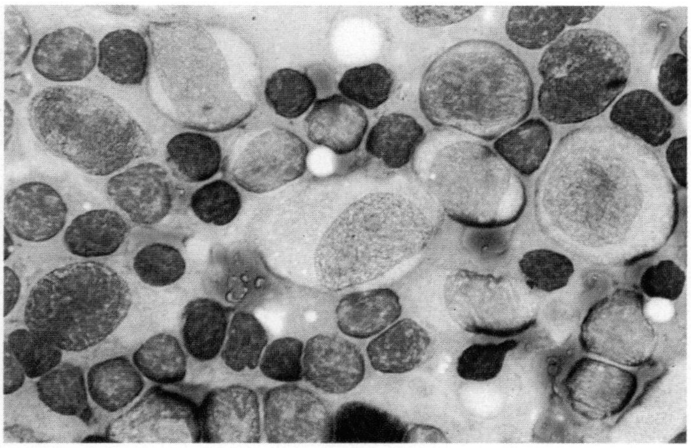

Figure 3.37 Mediastinal large B-cell lymphoma. This imprint shows the large, clear, well-delimited cytoplasm of the tumour cells, and the regularly outlined nuclei with dispersed chromatin and rather inconspicuous nucleoli

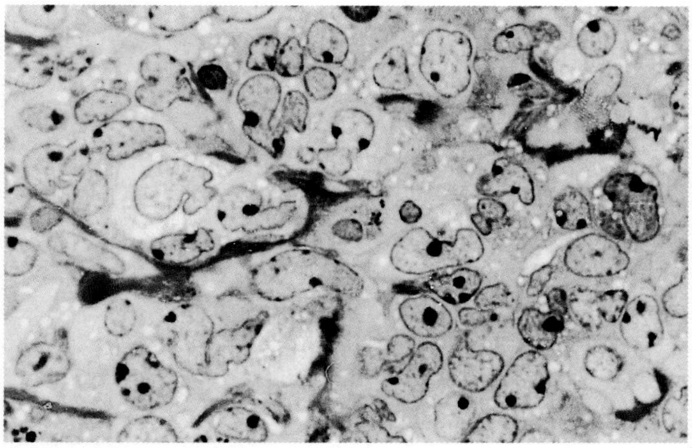

Figure 3.38 Mediastinal large B-cell lymphoma. On this half-thin section the tumour cells have irregularly folded nuclei with one or more nucleoli often on the nuclear membrane

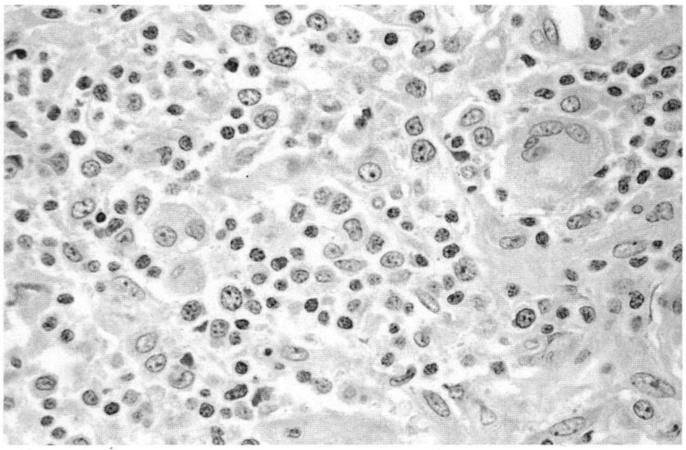

Figure 3.39 Mediastinal large B-cell lymphoma. There is an abundant stromal infiltrate of lymphocytes and reactive histiocytes with a Langhans-type giant cell on the right

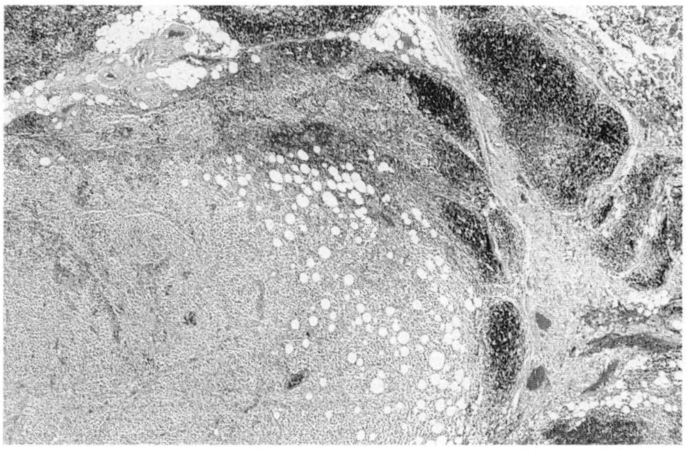

Figure 3.40 Mediastinal large B-cell lymphoma. The tumour invades the thymus, which can be recognized at the upper right of the figure

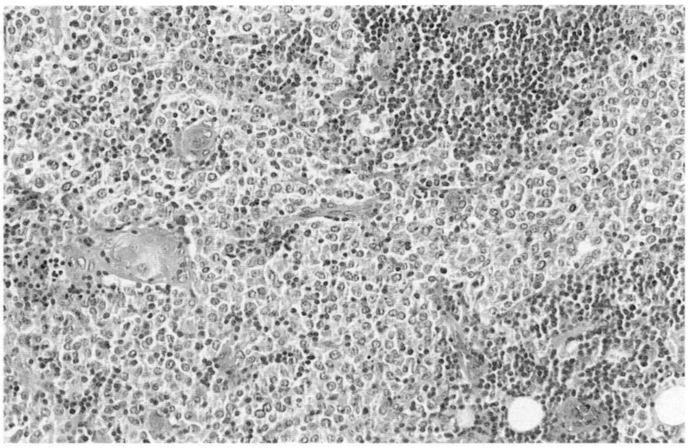

Figure 3.41 Mediastinal large B-cell lymphoma. Entrapped Hassall's corpuscles and sheets of lymphocytes within the tumour may be misinterpreted as a thymoma

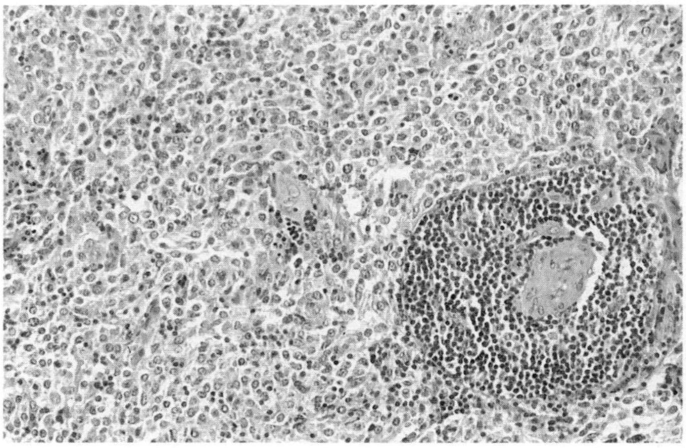

Figure 3.42 Mediastinal large B-cell lymphoma. Perivascular lymphocytic cuff resembling a perivascular space characteristic of thymoma

masses are candidates for more intense chemotherapy and/or for new treatment approaches.

References

Addis, B. J. and Isaacson, P. G. (1986). Large cell lymphoma of the mediastinum: A B-cell tumour of probable thymic origin. *Histopathology*, **10**, 379–390

Isaacson, P. G., Chan, J. K. C., Tang, C. and Addis, B. J. (1990). Low-grade B-cell lymphoma of mucosa-associated lymphoid tissue arising in the thymus. A thymic lymphoma mimicking myoepithelial sialadenitis. *Am. J. Surg. Pathol.*, **14**, 342–351

Jacobson, J. O., Aisenberg, A. C., Lamarre, L. *et al.* (1988). Mediastinal large cell lymphoma. An uncommon subset of adult lymphoma curable with combined modality therapy. *Cancer*, **62**, 1893–1898

Lamarre, L., Jacobson, J. O., Aisenberg, A. C. and Harris, N. L. (1989). Primary large cell lymphoma of the mediastinum. A histologic and immunophenotypic study of 29 cases. *Am. J. Surg. Pathol.*, **13**, 730–739.

Levitt, L. J., Aisenberg, A. C., Harris, N. L., Linggood, R. M. and Poppema, S. (1982). Primary non-Hodgkin's lymphoma of the mediastinum. *Cancer*, **50**, 2486–2492

Lichtenstein, A. K., Levine, A., Taylor, O. R., Boswell, B., Rossman, S., Feinstein, D. I. and Lukes, R. J. (1980). Primary mediastinal lymphoma in adults. *Am. J. Med.*, **68**, 509–514

Menestrina, F., Chilosi, M., Bonetti, F., Lestani, M., Scarpa, A., Novelli, P., Doglioni, C., Todeschini, G., Ambrosetti, A. and Fiore-Donati, L. (1986). Mediastinal large-cell lymphoma of B-type, with sclerosis: histopathological and immunohistochemical study of eight cases. *Histopathology*, **10**, 589–600

Miller, J. B., Variakojis, D., Bibran, J. C., Sweet, D. L., Kinzie, J. J., Golomb, H. M. and Ultmann, J. E. (1981). Diffuse histiocytic lymphoma with sclerosis. *Cancer*, **47**, 748–756

Möller, P., Lämmler, B., Herrmann, B., Otto, H. F., Moldenhauer, G. and Momburg, F. (1986). The primary mediastinal clear cell lymphoma of B-cell type has variable defect in MHC antigen expression. *Immunology*, **59**, 411–417

Möller, P., Moldenhauer, G., Momburg, F., Lämmler, B., Eberlein-Gonska, M., Kiesel, S. and Dörken, B. (1987). Mediastinal lymphoma of clear cell type is a tumor corresponding to terminal steps of B cell differentiation. *Blood*, **69**, 1087–1095

Perrone, T., Frizzera, G. and Rosai, J. (1986). Mediastinal diffuse large cell lymphoma with sclerosis: A clinicopathologic study of 60 cases. *Am. J. Surg. Pathol.*, **10**, 176–191

Trump, D. L. and Mann, R. B. (1982). Diffuse large cell and undifferentiated lymphomas with prominent mediastinal involvement. *Cancer*, **50**, 277–282

Yousem, A. S., Weiss, L. M. and Warnke, R. A. (1985). Primary mediastinal non-Hodgkin's lymphoma: A morphologic and immunologic study of nineteen cases. *Am. J. Clin. Pathol.*, **83**, 676–679

Lymphoblastic lymphoma

Lymphoblastic lymphoma is a distinct clinicopathological entity characterized by the proliferation of immature lymphoid cells that are indistinguishable from the lymphoblasts and prolymphocytes of acute lymphoblastic leukemia (Nathwani *et al.*, 1976). It is a rare form of malignant lymphoma in adults, comprising approximately 5% of all non-Hodgkin's lymphomas, but accounts for about one-third of childhood lymphomas (Streuli *et al.*, 1981). It has a mediastinal presentation in 50% of cases.

Age and sex

Although more common in children and young adults, lymphoblastic lymphoma may be seen in all age groups, with a high male-to-female ratio. This ratio is particularly high in the case of mediastinal presentation (3:1) and patients with mediastinal masses are significantly younger than patients without mediastinal involvement (age range 4–77 years; median 24; Nathwani *et al.*, 1981).

Clinical aspects (Table 3.9)

Mediastinal lymphoblastic lymphoma typically involves the thymus and supradiaphragmatic lymph nodes, and patients often have a large mediastinal mass at presentation. Although most of the patients have advanced (stage III or IV) disease at the time of diagnosis, nearly half of them are asymptomatic whereas others have symptoms of fever, weight loss or respiratory difficulties. Superior vena cava syndrome is not uncommon, and invasion of the anterior chest wall may be observed.

Table 3.9 Lymphoblastic lymphoma: clinical features

Frequent occurrence in children and young adults
High male to female ratio, 3:1
Mediastinal mass at presentation in 50% of cases
Early bone marrow and peripheral blood involvement
Frequent CNS involvement
Rapid progression of the disease with poor prognosis

With or without mediastinal localization, lymphoblastic lymphoma is recognized as the most malignant form of non-Hodgkin's lymphoma. Bone marrow is frequently involved at the time of diagnosis (22–60% of cases) as well as the peripheral blood (11–40%). Involvement of the central nervous system is frequent during the course of the disease (20–40%).

Histology (Table 3.10)

The neoplastic proliferation has a characteristic diffuse pattern, with large invasion of mediastinal tissue and a typical single-file arrangement of cells (Figs 3.43 and 3.44). Invasion of vessel walls and crush artifact distorting the nuclei of the neoplastic lymphoid cells are frequent

Table 4.6 Mediastinal embryonal carcinoma

Young adult male (15–35 years of age)
Very large circumscribed invasive anterior mediastinal tumour
Frequent haemoptysis as presenting symptom
Eventual bilateral gynaecomastia
aspermatogenic atrophy of testes
sexual precocity in infants
extensive acne
Klinefelter's syndrome
Early lymphatic and lung metastases
Serum beta-HCG occasionally elevated
Serum AFP most commonly elevated
Histologically:
glandular, tubular, papillary or solid pattern of large polygonal cells;
frequent PAS-positive hyaline globules secreting AFP;
occasional isolated syncytiotrophoblasts secreting HCG
Poor prognosis

Table 4.7 Mediastinal choriocarcinoma

Young adult male (15–35 years of age)
The rarest pure malignant GCT of the mediastinum
Unless association with other malignant germ-cell element, not very large, non-encapsulated, invasive anterior mediastinal tumour
Frequent presenting symptoms:
haemoptysis
bilateral gynaecomastia
aspermatogenic atrophy of testes
sexual precocity in infants
extensive acne
possible association with Klinefelter's syndrome
Bilateral pulmonary metastases frequent at presentation
Serum beta-HCG markedly elevated
Serum CEA occasionally elevated when immature glandular tissues are present
Histologically: association of both cytotrophoblasts and syncytiotrophoblasts secreting beta-HCG and placental lactogen
Very poor prognosis, the worst of all GCTs of the mediastinum

GCT: Germ-cell tumour

Table 4.8 Mediastinal yolk-sac tumour

Young adult male, (15–35 years of age)
Large, locally invasive anterior mediastinal tumour
Lymphatic and haematogenous metastases (liver, lungs, brain) present at diagnosis in 25% of the patients
Serum AFP markedly elevated (400–50 000 ng/ml) ($n < 20$)
Serum CEA occasionally elevated due to enteric-like differentiation ($n < 10$ ng/ml)
Histologically:
association of reticular, tubulopapillary, solid growth and polyvesicular vitelline pattern
Schiller–Duval bodies
PAS-positive hyaline globules containing alpha-fetoprotein and alpha-1-antitrypsin
hepatic- and enteric-like, and parietal yolk-sac structures
Very poor prognosis

Table 4.9 Mediastinal immature teratoma and teratocarcinoma

Young adult male, (15–35 years of age), some females
Large, multilobated mediastinal mass, sometimes well encapsulated, frequently cystic
Early haematogenous metastases
Serum alpha-fetoprotein, beta-HCG and CEA (if immature glandular tissue) occasionally elevated
Histologically: wide variety of tissues derived of all three primitive germ layers, including immature as well as mature elements, $\pm$ embryonal carcinoma component
In pure immature teratoma: uncertain prognosis, generally good, mostly depending on the age of the patient (good prognosis under the age of 15)

infection and pneumonia. In general, the size of tumour and the severity of symptoms are proportional.

Chest roentgenography is an important diagnostic aid. The typical benign teratoma appears as a well-circumscribed anterior mediastinal mass that often protrudes into one of the lung fields. The teratoma is rarely confined to the posterior mediastinum. Hilar extension may be seen in about 25% of cases. Calcification is one of the most distinctive characteristics of benign teratomas. Rim calcification along the periphery of the tumour usually indicates a benign teratoma. Diffuse pattern of calcifications is not indicative for diagnosis since it also occurs in thymomas, thyroid masses and aneurysms of the great vessels. The diagnosis of teratoma may be made with certainty in the occasional case in which bone or a tooth within the lesion is demonstrated. Rapid growth of a teratoma does not necessarily indicate malignancy because haemorrhage into a dermoid cyst can cause rapid increase in size. A benign cyst can become infected and rupture into the mediastinum, trachea, bronchi, pleural or pericardial cavity (Recondo and Libshitz, 1978).

Computed tomography (CT) and magnetic resonance imaging (MRI) demonstrate the extent of the anterior mediastinal masses and can detect calcifications or fatty or cystic areas inside the lesion, but this information will not obviate surgical resection to establish the final diagnosis (Figs 4.2–4.4).

As for benign teratomas, symptoms of malignant germ-cell tumours of the mediastinum are non-specific but, due to the rapid growth rate of the tumour, nearly all patients are symptomatic at presentation, and the time interval from clinical onset to diagnosis is short; <3 months in 88% of cases (Truong *et al.*, 1986). Besides chest pain, cough and dyspnoea, superior vena caval syndrome, anorexia, loss of weight and fever are frequently observed. Haemoptysis is a presenting symptom in embryonal carcinoma and choriocarcinoma, but not in other malignant germ-cell tumours of the mediastinum. In cases of choriocarcinomas, and less frequently in embryonal carcinomas, bilateral gynaecomastia, sexual precocity in infants, extensive acne and aspermatogenic atrophy of the testes are important clinical features. Klinefelter's syndrome, with XXY karyotype, has been reported in some instances in patients with germ-cell tumour. In these patients sexual precocity does not mean choriocarcinoma and the beta-HCG levels remain normal.

Radiological examination of the chest, CT and MRI document a large mass, usually lobulated, sometimes spherical, located in the anterior mediastinum, with protrusion to one side of the mediastinum, without any distinctive characteristics (Figs 4.5 and 4.6). The differential diagnosis for the radiologist includes a variety of neoplastic conditions, with the most important being malignant lymphoma, thymoma and metastatic carcinoma. The size of the tumours tends to be smaller in choriocarcinomas than in seminomas or embryonal carcinomas where the lesions are very large and most well circumscribed. The tumours may extend to the pleural spaces or the hilar areas or involve the surrounding structures. Seminomas have a tendency to be confined to the mediastinum without invasion of the adjacent structures, although encroachment on great vessels may occur.

Metastases are frequently present at the time of initial diagnosis. In endodermal sinus tumour they occur in more than 25% of patients, developing via the lymphatics towards the mediastinal and supraclavicular lymph nodes. Haematogenous spread, most frequently to the lung, liver, and/or brain, is common. In choriocarcinoma bilateral pulmonary metastases are frequent findings at presentation.

An atypical clinical presentation has been described by

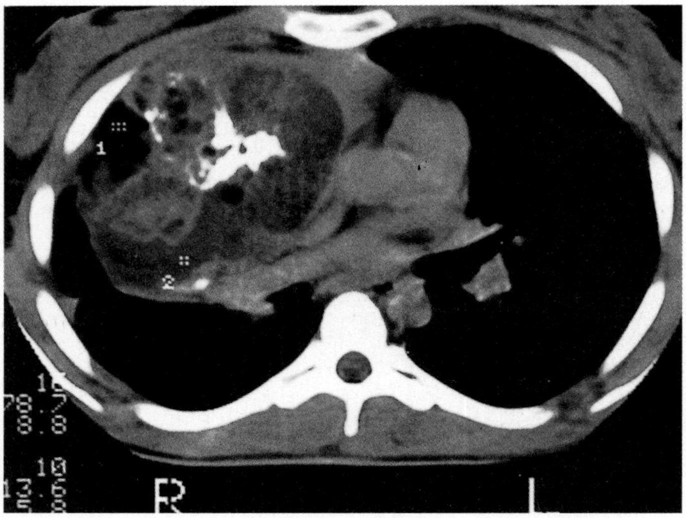

Figure 4.2 Mature teratoma. CT scan shows a large anterior mediastinal mass extending into the right hemithorax, containing fatty and cystic areas, and calcifications

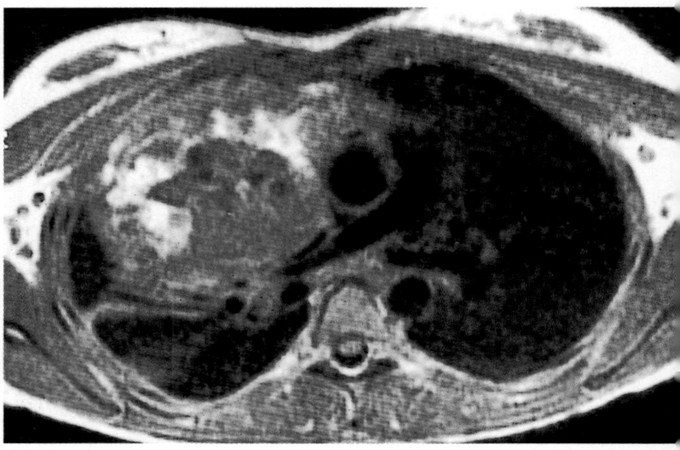

Figures 4.3 (above) **and 4.4** (below left) Magnetic resonance imaging of the same tumour in transaxial and coronal view

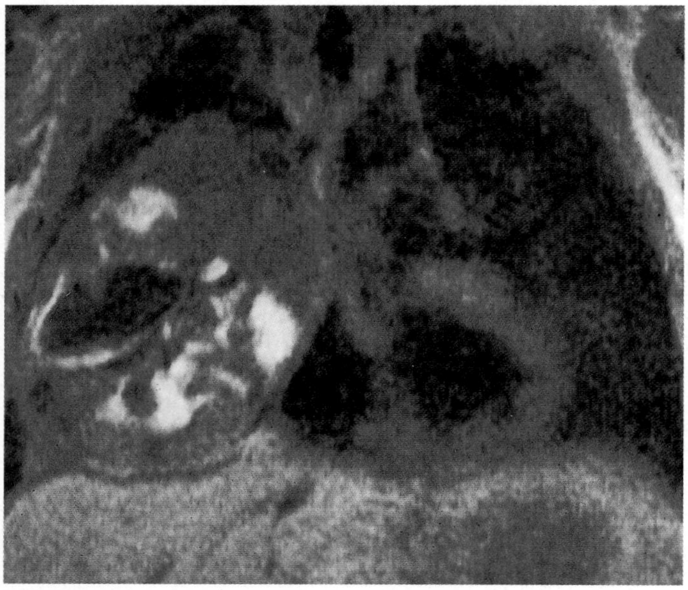

Figure 4.4

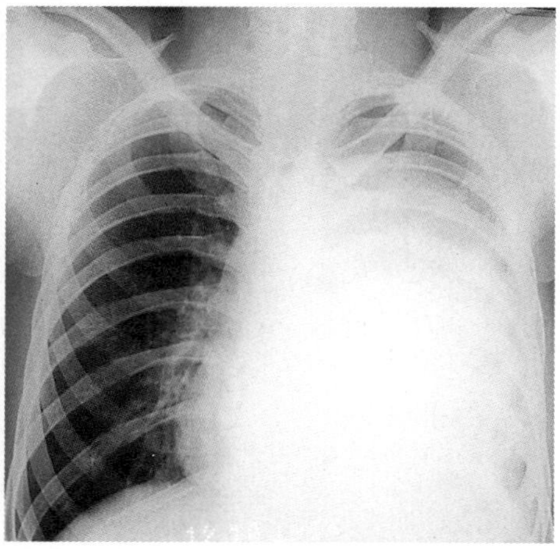

Figure 4.5
posteroanterior position

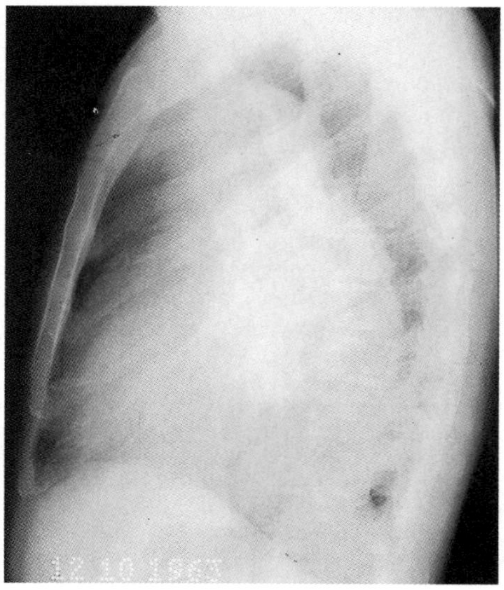

Figure 4.6
lateral position

Figures 4.5 and 4.6 Chest radiographs of a patient with yolk-sac tumour demonstrating a large lobulated mass protruding to the left hemithorax

Fox *et al.* (1979) in patients with embryonal germ-cell component. It consists of predominant symptoms and signs referring to metastatic disease in supraclavicular lymph nodes and lung with no apparent primary site. Knapp *et al.* (1985) describe two similar presentations in the case of mediastinal choriocarcinoma. In such cases the primary lesions are detected at thoracotomy or at autopsy.

All patients with germ-cell tumour containing syncytiotrophoblastic cells have elevated beta-HCG levels at presentation. Patients with yolk-sac tumour or presence of endodermal sinus tumour (EST) elements in their tumour have elevated serum alpha-fetoprotein (AFP) levels. Levels of these hormones correlate the quantity of syncytiotrophoblastic or EST elements. Embryonal carcinoma may be accompanied by slightly elevated levels of both markers. In pure seminoma AFP level is within normal limits but HCG level is sometimes elevated. In mixed tumours both markers may be elevated, proportional to the corresponding amount of each element.

Seminomas tend to produce lymph node metastases early and bony metastases later in the course of the disease. Bony metastases are rare in patients with other germ-cell tumours. In the non-seminoma group, bony metastases are more frequent with teratocarcinoma than with the other non-seminomatous tumours. Although haematogenous metastases can occur in seminomas, they are much more typical of the other germ-cell tumours. Metastases to lungs, liver, pancreas, kidney, brain, and other 'soft tissue' are the rule. Some patients have retroperitoneal nodal involvement, with normal testes at serial section, thus excluding the possibility of an occult germinal primary tumour with metastases to the retroperitoneum and suggesting retrograde spread from the mediastinum (Recondo and Libshitz, 1978).

A unique association between mediastinal germ-cell tumours and malignant haematological disorders has been occasionally reported, and was reviewed by Nichols *et al.* (1985). The syndrome involves a spectrum of haematological disorders ranging from refractory thrombocytopenia, myelodysplastic or myeloproliferative syndrome to acute megakaryocytic leukaemia. Some acute lymphocytic leukaemias have also been reported. The disorder presents simultaneously or in a brief interval from the onset of the mediastinal tumour and shares the cytogenetic abnormality of *de-novo* acute leukaemia. These chartacteristics lead the authors to conclude that the malignant haematological disorder is not a consequence of chemotherapy given for the germ-cell tumour, and that this association represents the evolution of a neoplastic disorder that initially involves a totipotent germ cell. These germ cells, when located in the mediastinum, apparently acquire haematological phenotypes and are manifested clinically as a haematological malignancy.

MORPHOLOGICAL FEATURES (Tables 4.5–4.9)

Seminoma

Gross

One-half to one-third of the mediastinal seminomas are encapsulated since the others invade the surrounding structures. On cross-section the tumours are pink–grey, firm, fleshy to rubbery, and lobulated. Areas of necrosis or cystic changes may be seen (Figs 4.7 and 4.8).

Histology

Microscopically seminomas exhibit very distinctive histological appearances (Figs 4.9–4.13). It is composed of sheets, nests or strands of large uniform cells, surrounded by varying amounts of connective tissue stroma. The tumour cells are round to polygonal and measure from 15 to 25 μm. The cytoplasm is large, eosinophilic or clear, slightly granular. The cellular borders are well defined. The nucleus is large, centrally located, round and vesicular, and has a thick nuclear membrane and a coarse clumped chromatin. It usually contains a single prominent irregularly shaped nucleolus. Mitotic activity is present, varying in amount from tumour to tumour. The cytoplasm of the tumour cells contains large amounts of glycogen, which can be demonstrated by the periodic acid-Schiff (PAS) reaction, and lipids.

The amount of connective tissue stroma present within the tumour is variable. In almost all cases it contains lymphocytes which may be sprinkled among the tumour cells or be very numerous with focal formation of lymphoid follicles (Fig. 4.9). In a considerable number of cases the stroma also contains a sarcoid-like granulomatous reaction composed of clusters of histiocytes surrounded by lymphocytes, plasma cells, and occasional giant cells both of the Langhans (Fig. 4.13) and foreign-body type. Rarely, the granulomatous reaction is so extensive that an erroneous diagnosis of tuberculosis is made. Foci of necrosis and haemorrhage are frequent, especially in large tumours.

Six to eight per cent of the tumours contain larger syncytiotrophoblastic giant cells reacting positively for human chorionic gonadotropin (HCG). These cells have a large, eosinophilic, frequently vacuolated cytoplasm and a varying number of nuclei. The presence of these cells does not justify the diagnosis of choriocarcinoma, which requires cytotrophoblasts and syncytiotrophoblasts growing in concert, and there is no evidence that seminomas containing these cells have any worse prognosis. These giant syncytial cells must be differentiated from the foreign-body and Langhans giant cells which are associated with the granulomatous reaction.

Seminoma is not infrequently associated with other neoplastic germ-cell elements. Since there is a sharp difference in prognosis and treatment between mixed and pure seminoma, the tumour must be carefully examined to exclude the presence of such components before it can be considered a pure seminoma.

Differential diagnosis

Pathological distinction of seminoma from other mediastinal tumours may be exceedingly difficult, and on small biopsy may be impossible. The tumours that are most often misdiagnosed with seminoma are the diffuse large B-cell non-Hodgkin's lymphoma, clear-cell carcinoma, undifferentiated carcinoma and certain thymomas.

Non-Hodgkin's lymphoma is the most critical diagnosis since it occurs in young adults in the same range of age, although carcinomas and thymomas are observed in older patients. Mediastinal clear B-cell lymphoma with sclerosis (see Chapter 3) may mimic seminoma by the association of large, pseudo-carcinomatous appearing cells, numerous lymphocytes and histiocytes, abundant fibrosis, and occasional mutinucleated Langhans cells. The multilobed character of the hyperchromatic nuclei of certain tumour cells and the absence of abundant well-delimited cytoplasm, rich in glycogen, together with specific lymphoid immunohistochemical characteristics, are the best criteria leading to correct diagnosis.

Epithelial thymoma and seminoma are also often confused histologically, and doubt is reflected by such previous denominations as seminomatous or pseudoseminomatous thymoma. Both tumours are composed of an admixture of large epithelial or epithelial-like cells and lymphocytes, and are subdivided into lobules by bands of collagen. Particularly helpful for the diagnosis of epithelial thymoma is the presence of perivascular spaces often containing lymphocytes, occasional formation of

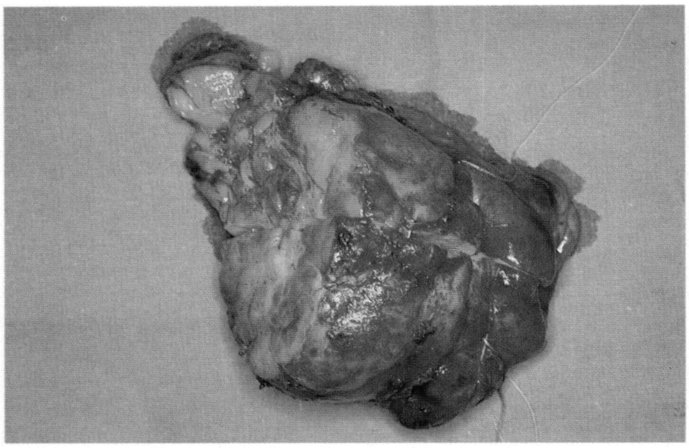

Figure 4.7 Seminoma. The tumour is lobulated and well encapsulated

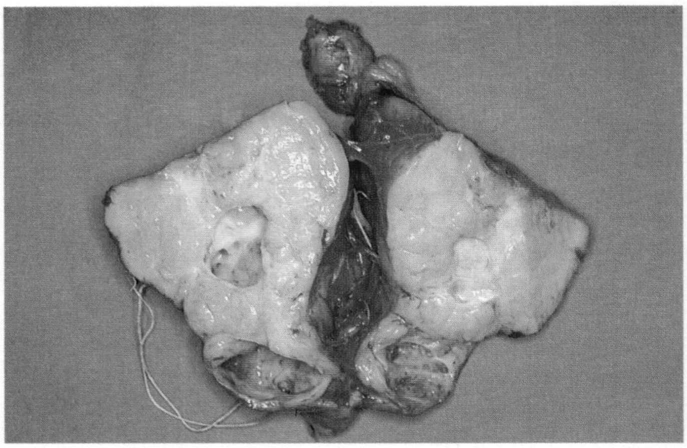

Figure 4.8 Seminoma. The cut section is pinkish. Note the presence of two well-delimited cysts

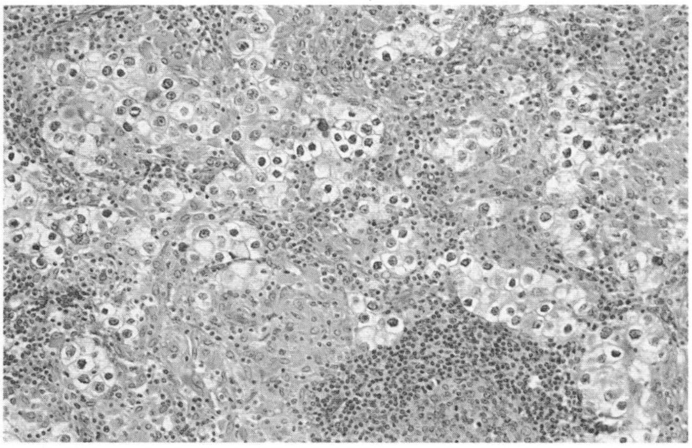

Figure 4.9 Seminoma. The tumour is composed of nests of large seminoma cells. The stroma contains a large number of histiocytes, scattered lymphocytes, and a lymph follicle

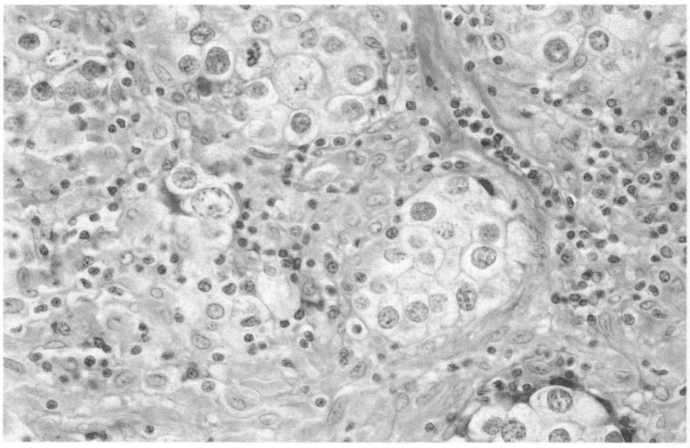

Figure 4.10 Seminoma. Higher magnification of the same area

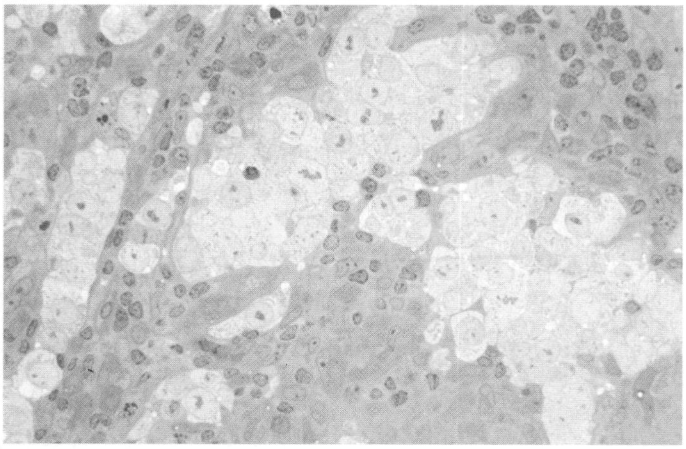

Figure 4.11 Seminoma. The half-thin section demonstrates the large pale tumour cells with a clear cytoplasm, a well-delimited nucleus, and a characteristic single prominent nucleolus

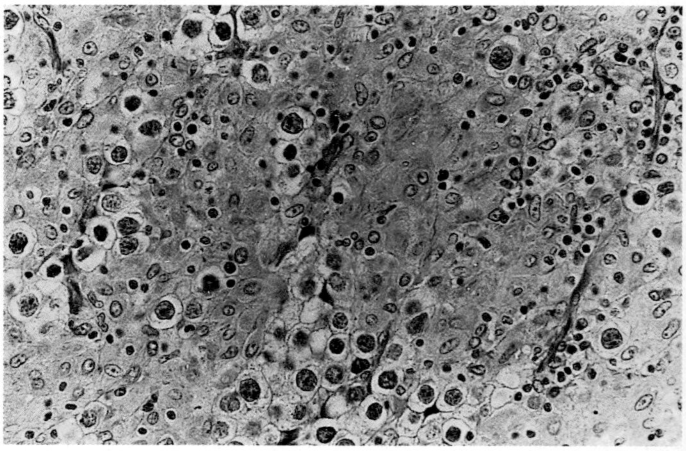

Figure 4.12 Seminoma. The tumour cells are obscured by the granulomatous reaction composed of numerous epithelioid histiocytes and some lymphocytes

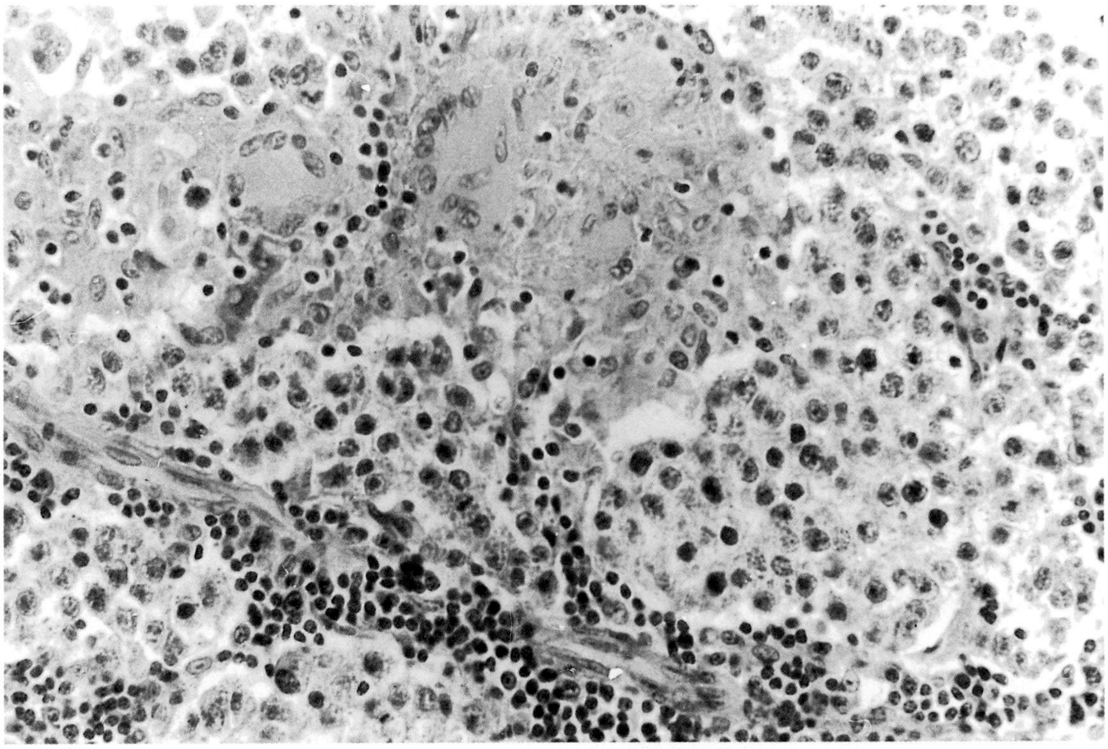

Figure 4.13 Seminoma. The figure displays a sarcoid-like reaction composed of epithelioid histiocytes and giant cells of the Langhans-type

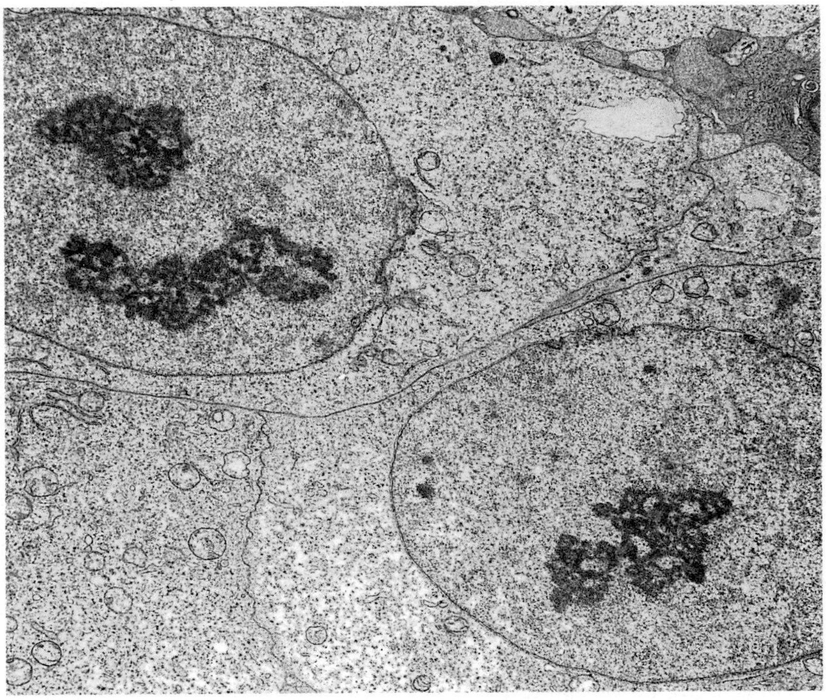

Figure 4.14 Seminoma. The electron micrograph shows the clear homogeneous cytoplasm, the round well-delimited nucleus, and the thread-like nucleolus of the tumour cells

rosettes, and broad collagen bands subdividing the lesion into large lobules. Immunohistochemically the epithelial cells are rich in cytokeratin. In doubtful cases electron microscopy shows distinct differences between the two tumours (Levine, 1973) (Fig. 4.14; Table 4.10).

Table 4.10 Ultrastructural comparison of thymoma and seminoma

	Seminoma	*Epithelial thymoma*
Nuclei	Regular, round	Irregular, oval
Nucleoli	Bizarre, complex	Relatively simple
Cell outline	Short cytoplasmic processes	Elongated cytoplasmic processes
Tonofilaments	Absent	Prominent
Desmosomes	Rare	Prominent
Basal lamina	Absent	Prominent
Organelles	Relatively scant	Well developed
Glycogen	Abundant	Absent

After Levine, 1973.

Embryonal carcinoma

Embryonal carcinoma is the least differentiated germ-cell neoplasm capable of further differentiation. This capability explains the finding that embryonal carcinoma is frequently admixed with other embryo- or extraembryo-derived elements. The combination of embryonal carcinoma and teratoma is frequently seen, and is designated teratocarcinoma.

Gross

Pure embryonal carcinoma is usually a small tumour. On cross-section it is solid, grey–white, variegated, soft, and does not appear to be encapsulated. It is frequently associated with haemorrhage and necrosis (Fig. 4.15). When embryonal carcinoma is associated with teratoma or seminoma the tumour may be larger, and in the case of teratoma may be partly cystic. Invasion of surrounding tissues is frequent.

Histology

Embryonal carcinoma is composed of large polygonal to ovoid cells with abundant pale cytoplasm and poorly distinct cytoplasmic borders. The nuclei are large, prominent, irregular, sometimes hyperchromatic and contain one or more nucleoli. Mitoses are numerous. There is marked cellular and nuclear pleomorphism.

The tumour grows in glandular, tubular, papillary or solid pattern (Fig. 4.16). Primitive mesenchymal tissue may be present in conjunction with the epithelial component. Isolated syncytiotrophoblastic cells are scattered throughout (Fig. 4.17) and are positive immunohistochemically for HCG. Hyaline bodies similar to those of the endodermal sinus tumour are present in most cases and contain alphafetoprotein. Their presence raises the question whether endodermal differentiation has occurred in the tumour. Necrosis and haemorrhage are frequently seen.

When embryonal carcinoma is combined with other neoplastic germ-cell elements, their presence should be noted and quantified.

In a number of embryonal carcinomas, organoid structures are formed, which simulate embryoid bodies (Figs 4.18–4.20). Embryoid bodies consist of a disc composed of large, epithelial-like cells, a cavity lined by flattened epithelial cells simulating an amniotic cavity, and a tubular structure resembling endoderm. This complex structure is surrounded by loose mesenchyme in which syncytiotrophoblastic (Fig. 4.20) and cytotrophoblastic cells may be seen. The tumours consisting predominantly of embryoid bodies are designated polyembryoma.

Choriocarcinoma

Pure choriocarcinoma is the least frequent and most malignant germinal tumour of the mediastinum. It accounts for about 5% of the primary malignant germ-cell tumours of the mediastinum.

All patients with choriocarcinoma have elevated beta-HCG levels. Since choriocarcinoma is not exceptionally mixed with yolk-sac tumour and/or embryonal carcinoma, serum alphafetoprotein levels should be measured at least once at presentation. These tumour markers, if elevated, should be remeasured in the follow-up in order to document a response to treatment or a recurrence.

Gross

Choriocarcinoma is grossly unresectable in most cases, and only biopsy can be obtained. In the resected cases the tumours appear frequently circumscribed but not encapsulated, and have a typical haemorrhagic and necrotic appearance. The tumorous tissue is soft and friable, greyish or brown to yellow (Fig. 4.21).

Histology

Choriocarcinoma has a unique feature composed of the association of both cytotrophoblastic and syncytiotrophoblastic cells (Figs 4.22 and 4.23). The diagnosis can be made only if the tumour is composed of both elements. The cytotrophoblastic cells are medium-sized, rounded to polygonal, with abundant clear cytoplasm and distinct cell borders. The nuclei are fairly uniform, hyperchromatic or vesicular with prominent nucleoli. Mitotic activity is abundant. These cells grow in large cellular masses bordered by syncytiotrophoblasts often forming a plexiform pattern. The syncytiotrophoblasts are very large, irregularly outlined multinucleated cells containing hyperchromatic nuclei and abundant eosinophilic somewhat vacuolated cytoplasm. The neoplastic cells characteristically lie in juxtaposition to dilated vascular sinusoids, the source of massive haemorrhage. Large areas of necrosis are present.

Immunohistochemistry studies indicate that syncytiotrophoblastic cells are positive for beta-HCG, and that they are the source of human chorionic gonadotrophin.

Differential diagnosis

The diagnosis of choriocarcinoma needs the association of both cytotrophoblastic and syncytiotrophoblastic cells. Isolated syncytiotrophoblasts does not mean choriocarcinoma and may occur in embryonal carcinoma and seminoma, explaining the occasionally elevated level of serum beta-HCG in these tumours.

In the typical cases the diagnosis of choriocarcinoma encounters no difficulty. The only problem is to exclude a mediastinal metastasis from a gonadal germ-cell tumour and to assess whether the tumour is a pure choriocarcinoma or is a mixed germ-cell tumour, requiring adequate tissue for pathological study and tumour marker determinations.

Endodermal sinus tumour (yolk-sac tumour)

Endodermal sinus tumour (EST) is a specific type of germ-cell neoplasm differentiating in the direction of extraembryonal vitelline or yolk-sac structures. In old reports it is generally referred to as embryonal carcinoma. Pure endodermal sinus tumour is a rare tumour. Nevertheless the incidence of EST elements in mediastinal tumour, as in testicular germ-cell neoplasms in adults, is certainly

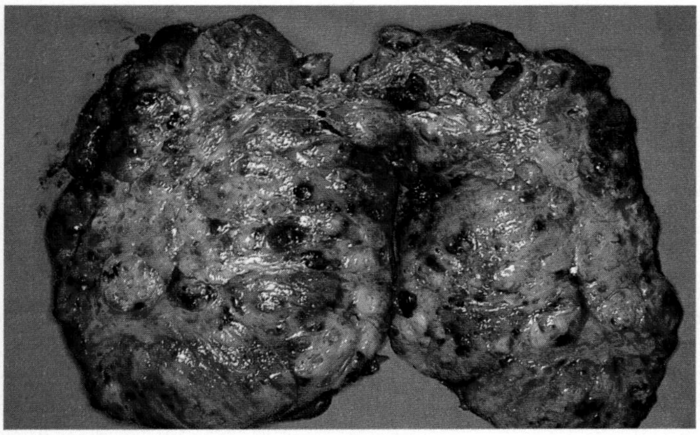

Figure 4.15 Teratocarcinoma. The cut surface is soft, variegated, with numerous haemorrhagic and necrotic areas

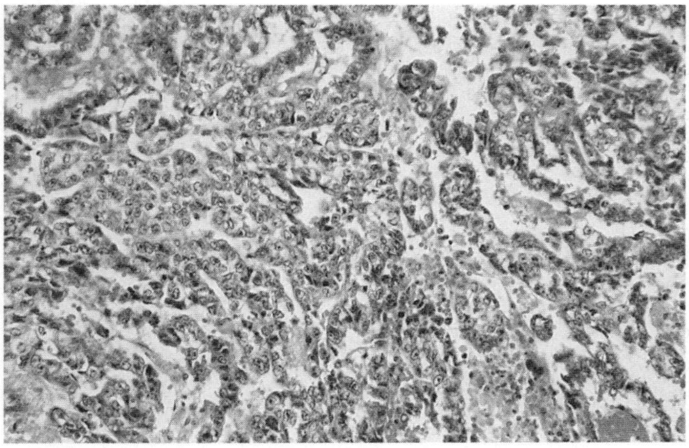

Figure 4.16 Embryonal carcinoma growing in a tubular pattern

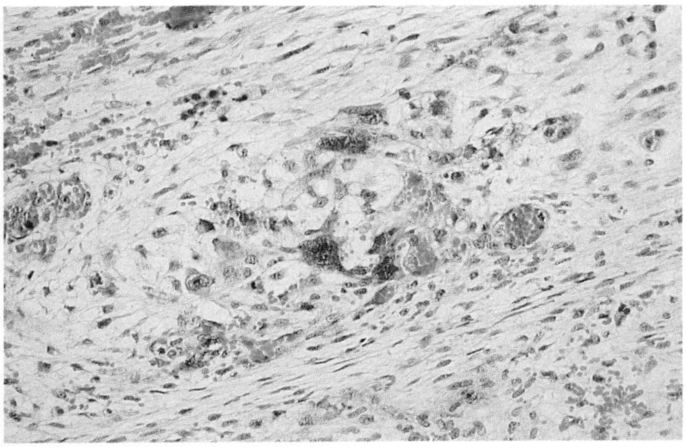

Figure 4.17 Embryonal carcinoma. Cluster of syncytiotrophoblastic cells

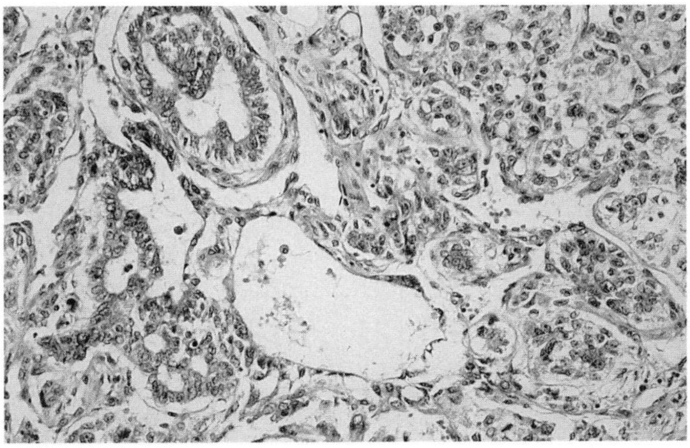

Figure 4.18 Embryonal carcinoma containing structures resembling embryoid bodies

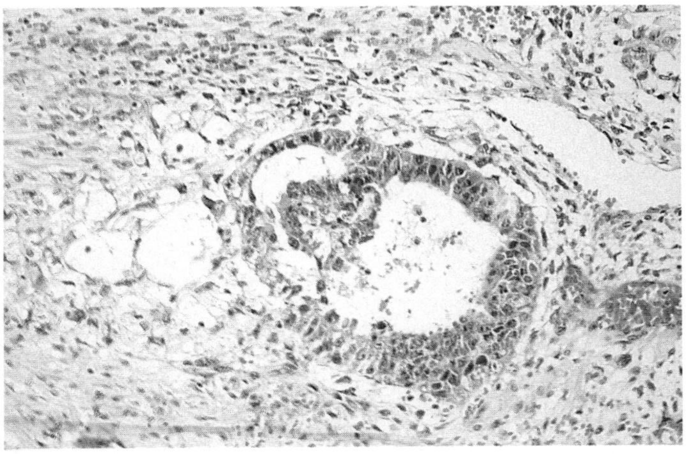

Figure 4.19 Embryonal carcinoma. Fully developed embryoid body

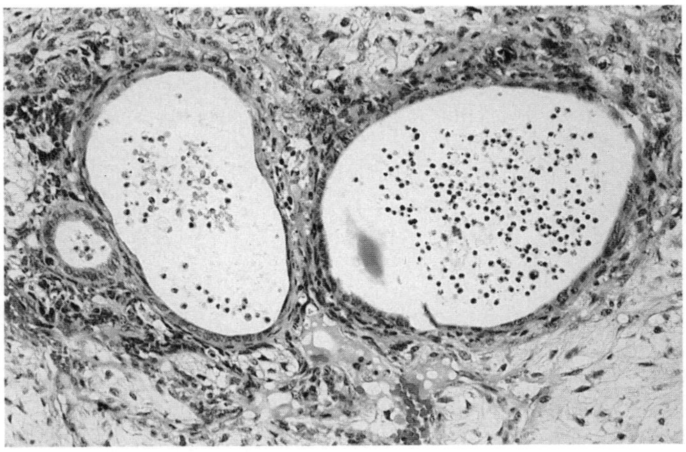

Figure 4.20 Embryonal carcinoma. Syncytiotrophoblastic cells surround the cavity on the right

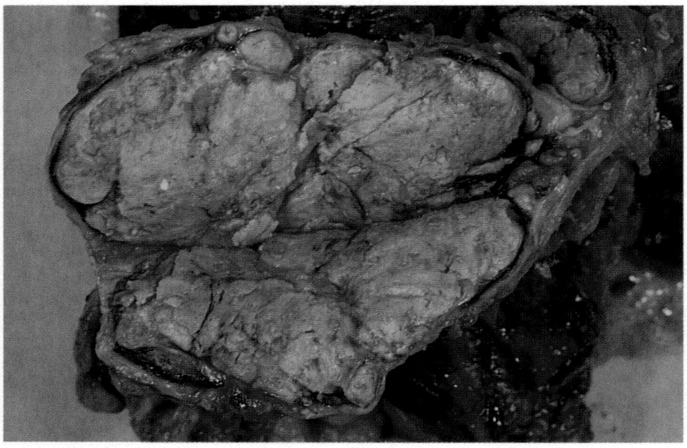

Figure 4.21 Choriocarcinoma. Large, brown, necrotic tumour invading a lung

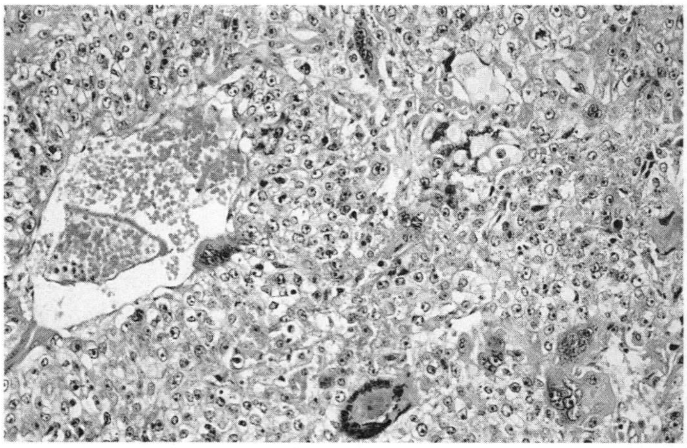

Figure 4.22 Choriocarcinoma. The tumour is composed of sheaths of medium-sized cytotrophoblasts surrounded by large, irregular syncytiotrophoblastic cells

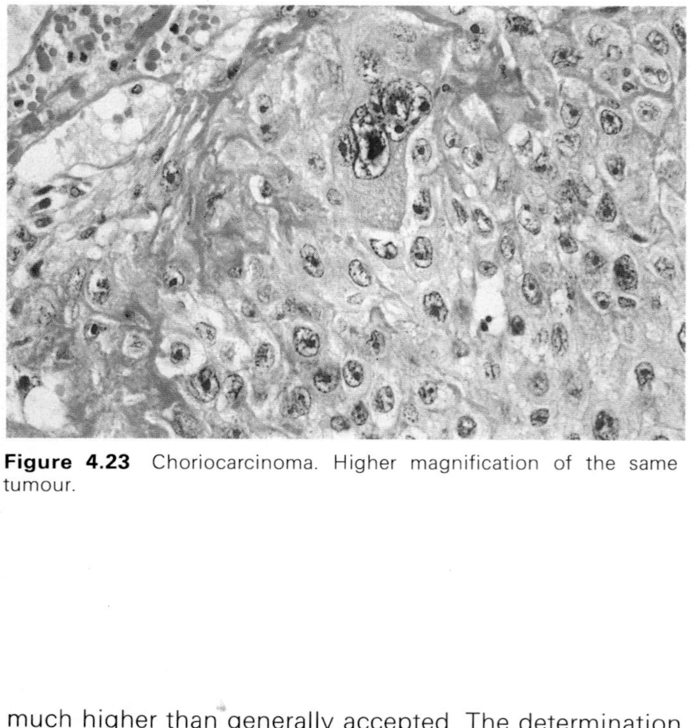

Figure 4.23 Choriocarcinoma. Higher magnification of the same tumour.

much higher than generally accepted. The determination of serum AFP levels is very useful since there is a good correlation between elevated levels of serum AFP and EST elements within the tumour (Teilum, 1976; Talerman, 1980). According to Truong *et al.*, (1986) mediastinal endodermal sinus tumours are pure in 68% of cases and are mixed in other cases with mature and/or immature teratoma components in 14% of the cases, embryonal carcinoma in 14%, seminoma in 7% and choriocarcinoma in 2%.

Gross

Currently these tumours are unresectable with local invasion and/or distant metastases. They are large tumours, round or nodular, with solid areas alternating with necrotic, haemorrhagic or cystic spaces. The neoplastic tissue is soft and friable, and grey, yellow or dark red. Areas of gelatinous degeneration are often observed. The cysts may contain gelatinous material (Fig. 4.24.).

Histology

Endodermal sinus tumour has a distinctive microscopic feature characterized by the association of two or more of four major histological patterns: reticular, tubulopapillary, solid and polyvesicular vitelline (Kurman and Norris, 1976). The first three patterns are very frequent (Fig. 4.25), the polyvesicular vitelline pattern occurs most rarely. Schiller–Duval bodies and eosinophilic PAS-positive intra- and extracellular hyaline globules are two other major features (Teilum, 1976). Other differentiations such as hepatic-like foci, enteric-like glands and parietal yolk sac structures are uncommon, but their diagnostic value has been emphasized by Ulbright *et al.* (1986).

The reticular growth pattern appears as a loose, vacuolated meshwork of communicating spaces lined by flattened, endothelial-like cells and containing mucin. The tubulopapillary pattern displays interconnecting tubular and papillary structures lined by one or several layers of columnar or cuboidal cells. The solid growth pattern shows compact sheets of cuboidal large cells. In these areas perivascular palisades of tumour cells are frequently observed. The polyvesicular vitelline growth pattern is characterized by the presence of numerous epithelial cysts with eccentric constriction. The existence of such features, not exceptional in gonadal endodermal sinus tumours, is denied in mediastinal tumours by Truong *et al.* (1986).

Schiller–Duval bodies result in the projection of simple papillae into the spaces of reticular areas. They are composed of a single central vessel lined by primitive columnar or cuboidal cells, lying within a space bordered by flattened tumour cells (Teilum, 1976; Fig. 4.26).

The PAS-positive, diastase-resistant, extra- or intracellular material is globular and more prominent in areas showing the reticular pattern (Fig. 4.27). These globules vary in size and contain alpha-fetoprotein and alpha-1-antitrypsin, as demonstrated by immunohistochemical procedures (Shirai *et al.*, 1976; Ulbright *et al.*, 1986; Truong *et al.*, 1986).

The neoplastic cells have hyperchromatic, irregular nuclei. In the reticular area they are small with elongated amphophilic cytoplasm. In the tubulopapillary and solid growth pattern the cells have large nuclei and abundant clear cytoplasm, containing glycogen. Markedly anaplastic mono- or multinucleated giant cells may be observed, particularly in the solid areas.

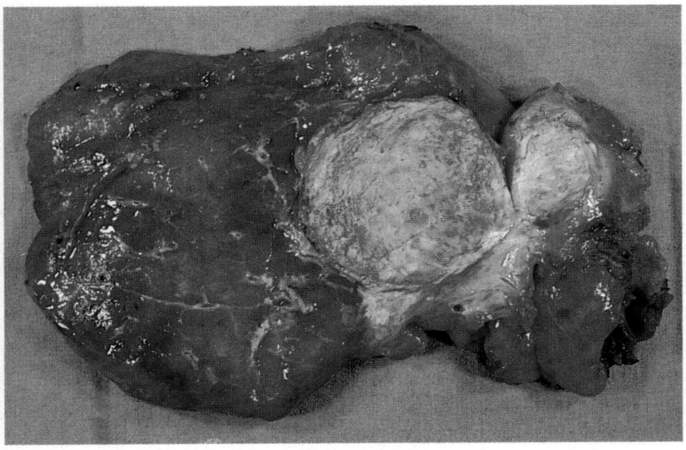

Figure 4.24 Yolk-sac tumour resected after chemotherapy. The tumour invades the left lung

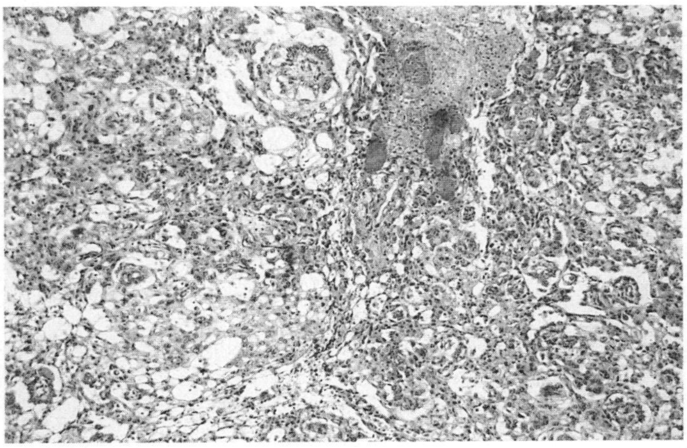

Figure 4.25 Yolk-sac tumour. Reticular and tubulopapillary growth pattern

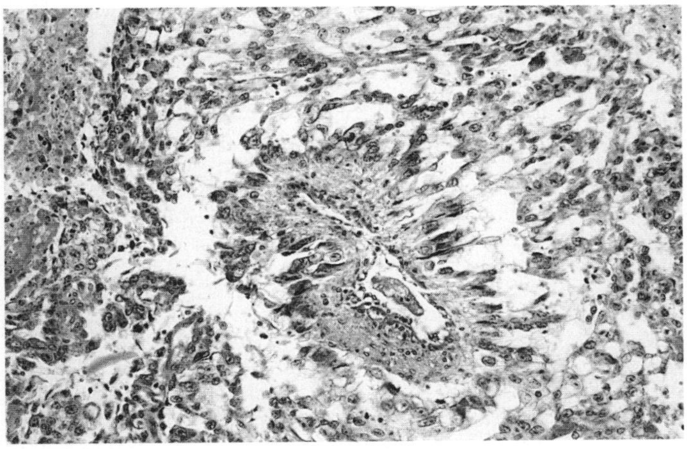

Figure 4.26 Yolk-sac tumour. Typical Schiller–Duval body

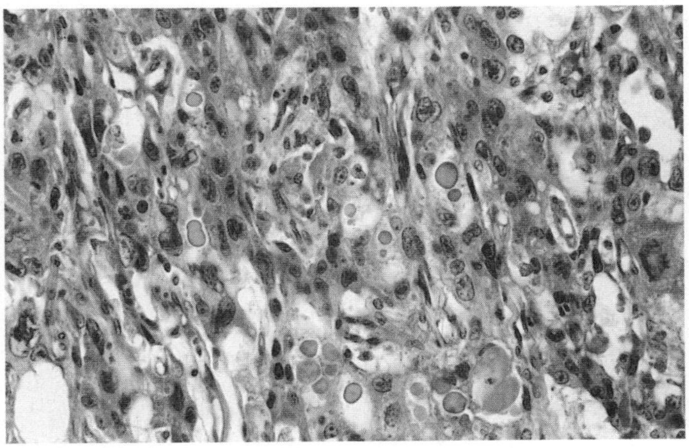

Figure 4.27 Yolk-sac tumour. The figure illustrates numerous intra- and extracellular hyaline globules

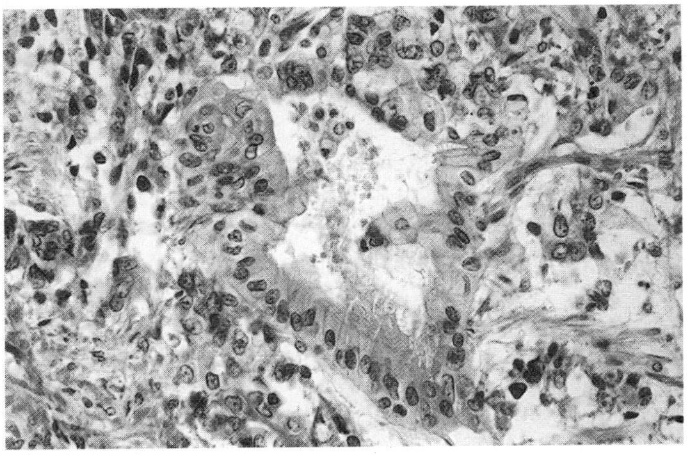

Figure 4.28 Yolk-sac tumour. Foci of enteric differentiation

Hepatic differentiation (Jacobsen and Jacobsen, 1983; Ulbright *et al.*, 1986). is characterized by small foci of cells with abundant, eosinophilic to clear cytoplasm, well-defined cell borders and round, central nuclei with prominent, single nucleoli. Hepatoid cells may contain intracytoplasmic hyaline globules and show a deep cytoplasmic immunostaining for AFP.

Enteric differentiation occurs as small glands, which are frequently in direct continuity with adjacent yolk-sac tumour tissue, particularly with the polyvesicular vitelline pattern. The glandular structures are formed by cells that have a discernible striated border (Fig. 4.28) or a mucus-containing apical cytoplasm reproducing gastric or intestinal-type cell. Foci of enteric differentiation are positively immunostained for CEA (Ulbright *et al.*, 1986). Ultrastructurally these glands have apical microvilli with associated glycocalyx or are mucus-secreting.

Parietal yolk sac differentiation (Damjanov *et al.*, 1984; Ulbright *et al.*, 1986) is characterized by the intercellular accumulation of hyaline basement membrane-like substance occurring generally as bands of eosinophilic matrix.

This matrix resembles Reichert's basement membrane described in the parietal portion of the rat yolk sac (Martinez-Hernandez *et al.*, 1982). Such material corresponds immunohistochemically to laminin and, by electron microscopy, is both intra- and extracellular, and has irregular outlines and inhomogeneous density (Gonzalez–Crussi and Roth, 1976; Nogales-Fernandez *et al.*, 1977; Ulbright *et al.*, 1986).

On electron microscopic examination the tumour cells have focal, short microvilli on the free surface, similar to those of human yolk sac epithelium at 8 weeks of development. Cell junctions occur, varying from well-formed desmosomes to interdigitation of cell membranes. The tumour cells contain large numbers of cytoplasmic glycogen granules. Electron-dense inclusions are scattered in the tumour within the cell cytoplasms and the extracellular spaces. Some are spheroidal and uniformly electron-dense, although others are irregularly shaped and not homogeneously electron-dense. Amorphous granules of lesser electron-density are present within cisternae of ergastoplasm. These inclusions correspond to hyaline bodies but their nature has not been conclusively elucidated. Some of them undoubtedly contain AFP; however, some others may be composed of material synthesized by endodermal sinus tumour, particularly basement membrane components (Gonzales-Crussi and Roth, 1976; Nogales-Fernandez *et al.*, 1977; Ulbright *et al*, 1986; Truong *et al.*, 1986).

Differential diagnosis

The distinct morphological patterns of endodermal sinus tumour make easy its differentiation from most other primary anterior mediastinal tumours occurring in the same range of age, particularly Hodgkin's and non-Hodgkin's lymphomas, but also seminoma, teratoma and choriocarcinoma. Thymoma is equally morphologically different.

The distinction from metastatic poorly differentiated adenocarcinoma is more critical, although in general metastatic adenocarcinoma occurs in older patients, displays no male predominance, and is more homogeneous in growth patterns. In these cases the presence of Schiller–Duval bodies, PAS-positive globules, immunocytochemically detectable AFP and elevated serum AFP are the best indicators for the diagnosis of endodermal sinus tumour.

In the case of endodermal sinus tumour growing mostly in a solid growth pattern the differential diagnosis with embryonal carcinoma may be difficult, since PAS-positive globules and elevated serum AFP have been occasionally described in embryonal carcinoma. Nevertheless, embryonal carcinoma is characterized by larger cells with vesicular nuclei and prominent nucleoli, and lack the recticular growth pattern and Schiller–Duval bodies. In difficult cases immunohistochemical demonstration of AFP into the tumour, and electron microscopy showing typical features, are very useful.

Teratomas

Teratomas are germ-cell tumours composed of derivatives of the three primitive germ-cell layers, endoderm, ectoderm, and mesoderm. The neoplastic component may be entirely mature, entirely immature, or both mature and immature. The maturity of the tumour may vary from area to area. Thus, teratomatous elements of different degrees of maturity are closely admixed with each other, usually without organoid arrangement. Teratoma is frequently combined with other neoplastic germ-cell elements, and its combination with embryonal carcinoma is particularly frequent (teratocarcinoma). *Stricto sensu* these cases should be excluded from the frame of teratomas. As for testicular teratomas there is a considerable difference between the histological appearances and the behaviour of tumours occurring in infants and children, and those seen in adults. Most of the teratomas occurring in children are composed of mature tissues, and in cases where immature elements are present the tumours exhibit a benign clinical course.

Immature teratoma

The immature teratoma is a malignant form of teratoma that contains immature structures resembling those of the embryo.

Gross

The tumours usually appear as large multilobated mass, sometimes well encapsulated (Fig. 4.29). On cross-section they are typically variegated in appearance with both solid and cystic areas (Fig. 4.30). The solid tissue may include recognizable cartilage or bone, greyish and soft areas corresponding to an immature neural tissue, areas of necrosis and haemorrhage. The cysts contain clear, brown–red fluid, mucus or sebaceous material and hair.

Histology

Immature teratomas contain a wide variety of tissues representing all three primordial germ layers and include immature as well mature elements (Fig. 4.31). The most predominant tissue in most tumours is neural, including neuroepithelium in the form of rosettes, glial tissue and areas resembling neuroblastoma (Figs 4.32–4.34). Immature epithelium of various types, both ectodermal and endodermal – as well as immature mesenchymal tissues, cartilage, skeletal muscle or bone – are frequently present. The immature teratoma may also contain any mature elements encountered in mature teratoma. In addition embryonal or extraembryonal tissues may be observed. Grading of immature teratoma according to the degree of differentiation and the quantity of immature tissue has been proposed by Gonzales-Crussi (1982; Table 4.3). Nevertheless, even in cases where small areas of immature tissue occur, clinical and biological surveillance is necessary since recurrence or metastases have been described in such tumours (Baldeyrou *et al.*, 1986).

Differential diagnosis

The diagnosis of immature teratoma is not difficult if careful examination of the tumour is done. The most common error is to designate an immature teratoma as mature because some of its constituents are fully differentiated, or not to recognize malignant embryonal or extraembryonal elements. As both eventualities strongly alter the prognostic and therapeutic approach, it is of the utmost importance to examine numerous sections of the tumours carefully.

Mature teratoma

Mature teratoma is composed exclusively of mature elements. Because the ectodermal component is usually predominant it is often named dermoid cyst.

Gross

Mature teratoma of the mediastinum appears as well-circumscribed, polylobated, usually well-encapsulated cystic lesion, usually of very large size (Fig. 4.35). It is composed of solid areas intermingled with more or less large cysts (Fig. 4.36). The cysts often contain yellow sebaceous material (Fig. 4.37) and hair (Fig. 4.38). Polypoid masses bordered by skin protrude into the lumen (Fig. 4.39). Teeth are frequently present, as well as

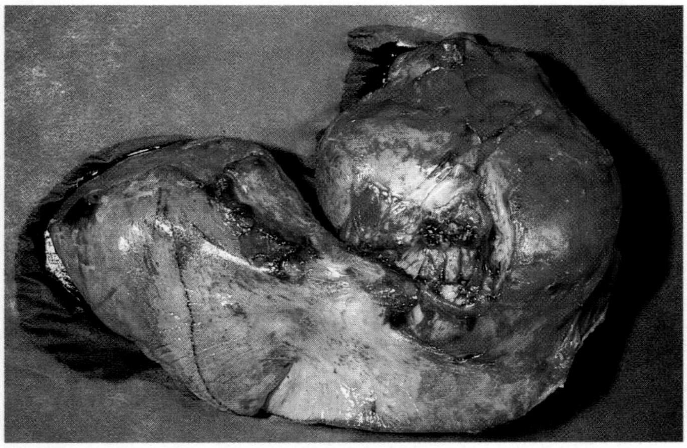

Figure 4.29 Immature teratoma. Large bosselated, irregular tumour

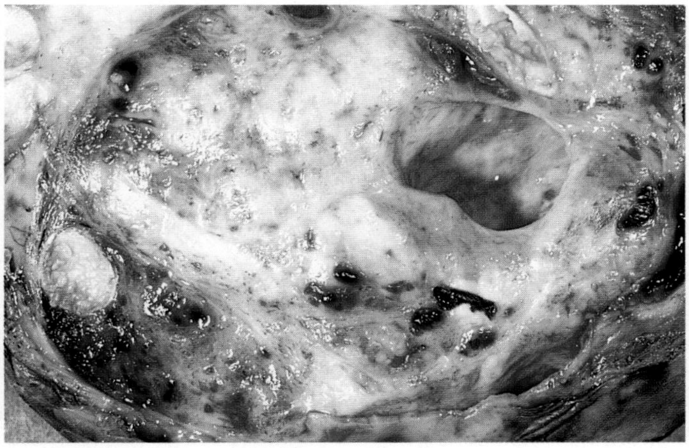

Figure 4.30 Immature teratoma. On section the tumour presents haemorrhagic foci and cystic areas

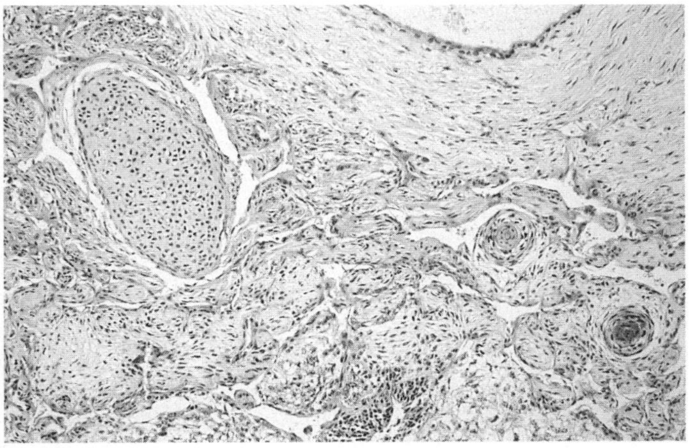

Figure 4.31 Immature teratoma. The figure shows immature connective tissue, cartilage, and hairs

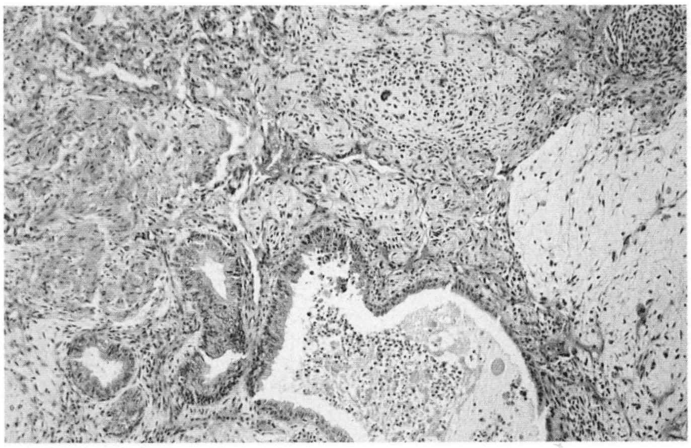

Figure 4.32 Immature teratoma. The area displays immature neural tissue, and glandular structures

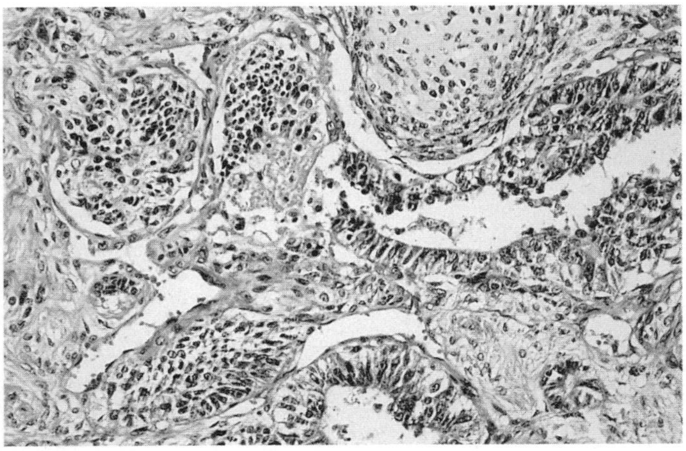

Figure 4.33 Immature teratoma. The area is composed mostly of neural tissue resembling neuroblastoma, intermingled with immature cartilage

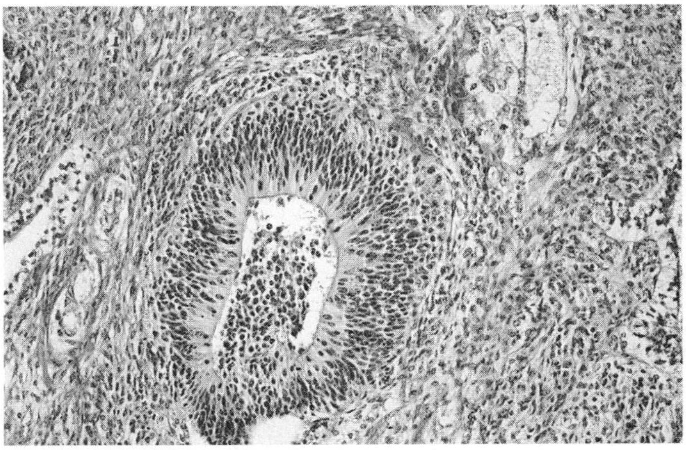

Figure 4.34 Immature teratoma. The section illustrates a primitive neural tube

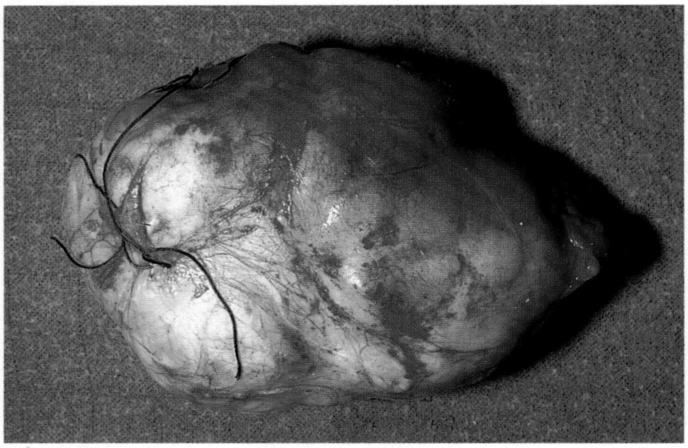

Figure 4.35 Mature teratoma. Large well-encapsulated tumour

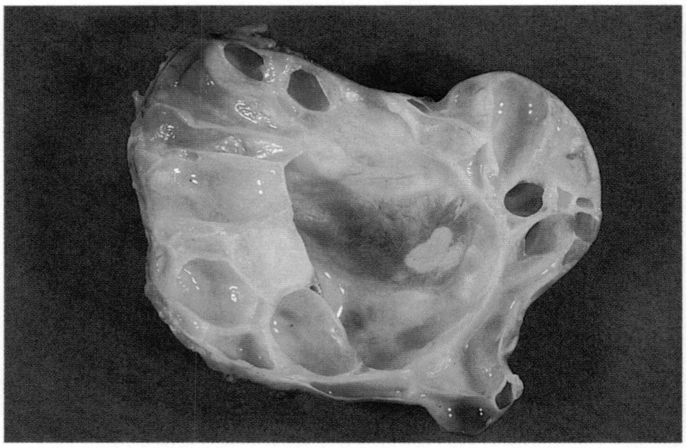

Figure 4.36 Mature teratoma. Polycystic tumour. The cysts are empty

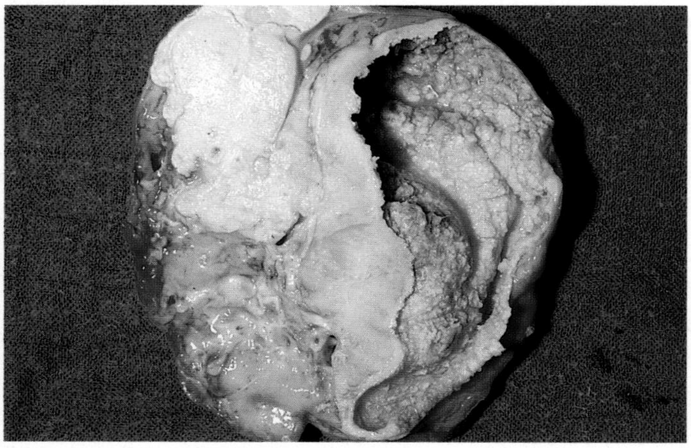

Figure 4.37 Mature teratoma. Unilocular cystic tumour. The cyst is bordered by skin and sebum (dermoid cyst)

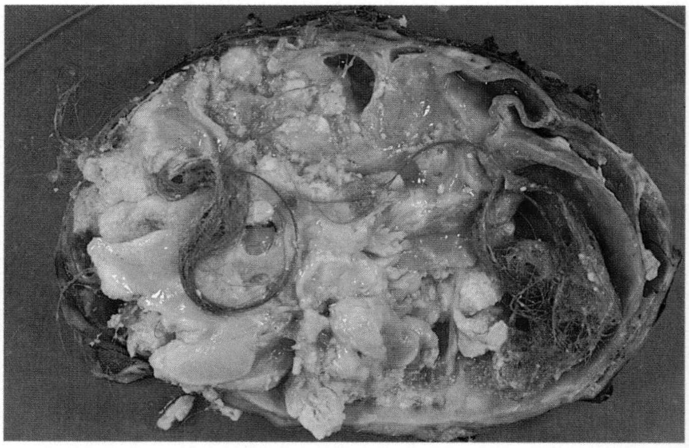

Figure 4.38 Mature teratoma. Numerous cysts contains sebum and hairs

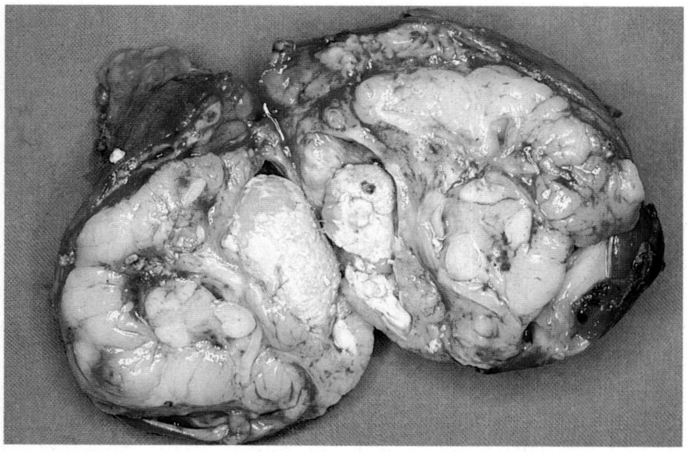

Figure 4.39 Mature teratoma. The tumour contains adipose tissue, cartilage, and polypoid mass bordered by skin and sebaceous material

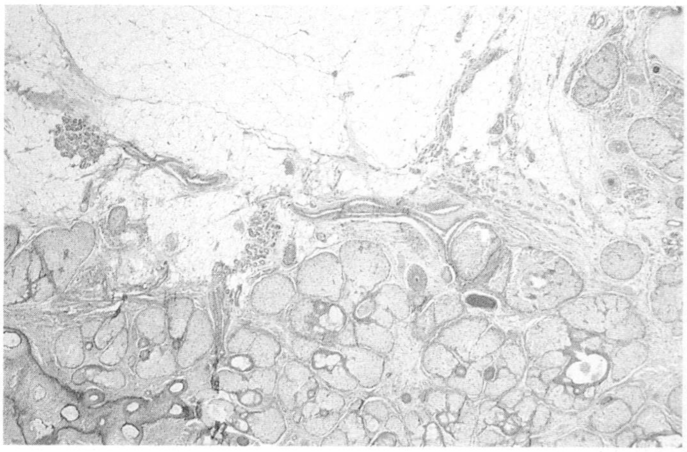

Figure 4.40 Mature teratoma. The area is composed of adipose tissue, numerous sebaceous glands, some sweat glands, and a hair follicle

bone, cartilage and adipose tissue. On occasion, partially developed organs such as limb buds or eyes can be recognized.

Histology

All normal tissues may be encountered but keratinized epidermis with sebaceous and sweat glands and hair follicles remain the main features (Figs 4.40–4.43). Very common or common are fat and smooth muscle, respiratory and gut epithelium, cartilage, bone and brain. Less frequently salivary gland, thyroid, pancreas and other tissues are encountered. All these tissues are often oriented in an organoid pattern.

Differential diagnosis

The diagnosis is obvious in many cases. The only problem is not to miss any immature teratomatous areas or any malignant germ-cell element.

Teratoma with malignant transformation

This entity corresponds to mature teratoma in which a cancer of adult rather than embryonal or extraembryonal type develops from one of the constituents. The association with malignant germ-cell tumour elements of seminoma, endodermal sinus tumour, embryonal carcinoma or choriocarcinoma type is rare, and excluded from this type of neoplasm.

Gross

The presence of cancerous areas may be suspected when solid nodular areas, patches of necrosis, red foci of haemorrhage or adhesion to surrounding organs are present in an otherwise mature teratoma.

Histology

Histologically, elements of squamous cell carcinoma, adenocarcinoma, malignant neuroepithelioma or sarcoma (Figs 4.44 and 4.45) are present in combination with mature teratomatous elements. According to Manivel *et al.* (1986), the occurrence of a sarcomatous component seems to be more common in mediastinal neoplasms.

TREATMENT

Mature teratoma

Surgical excision is the best means of treating benign teratoma. Radiation plays no role in modern management. Although these tumours are benign histologically, surgical removal is often difficult since virtually all of the tumours are densely adherent to vital adjacent intrathoracic structures. Nevertheless, even in cases of partial removal, because of adherence to vital structures, no recurrence occurs.

Malignant germ-cell tumours

A rational part of treatment planning in patients with germ-cell tumour includes the distinction between pure seminoma and germ-cell tumour with any non-seminomatous component, and a careful staging of the extent of the disease.

Determinations of HCG and AFP serum levels are crucial for their ability to detect non-seminomatous elements in a mediastinal tumour when a biopsy sample does not reflect the entire content of the tumour mass. Detection of mixed elements dictates two changes in management: (1) the use of combination chemotherapy as initial therapy if there is any elevation of AFP or marked elevation of HCG, and (2) radiation therapy for patients with seminoma presenting no or only minimal elevation of HCG (Clamon, 1983).

Prior to the advent of curative combination chemotherapy, early detection of metastatic site would have been of less importance, because an alternative therapy was not available. Even in seminoma, a patient now presenting with metastatic disease would be a candidate for chemotherapy as the initial mode of therapy. A reasonable evaluation should include a bone scan, examination of the para-aortic and retroperitoneal nodes by computed tomography and liver scanning. Shantz *et al.* (1972) advise against orchiectomy or routine testicular biopsies in patients whose testes are normal to palpation, and in their experience routine subdiaphragmatic radiation therapy does not appear necessary unless disease is apparent.

Pure seminomas are radiosensitive, and radiotherapy remains the treatment of choice for mediastinal seminomas. The current therapeutic recommendations are reduction surgery or total surgical excision if possible, followed by radiation therapy to the anterior mediastinium at dosage 3000–5000 rads (cGy) over 3–6 weeks. Adding the supraclavicular, infraclavicular and low cervical lymph nodes to the radiation fields (Economou *et al.*, 1982; Hurt *et al.*, 1982) is also advised. Due to the efficacy of radiotherapy and/or chemotherapy, extensive surgical debulking which might increase operative risk cannot be justified in invasive or very large tumours, or in patients with metastatic disease (Clamon, 1983). Metastatic spread does not preclude the possibility of cure. For these advanced cases, for patients who have relapses, or for those who have greater potential to progression of disease, combination chemotherapy with vinblastine, bleomycin, and cis-platinum (VBP) can induce a complete remission and long-term disease-free survival. The use of chemotherapy as an adjuvant to radiation therapy for mediastinal seminoma is not recommended because of the potential for severe synergistic pulmonary fibrosis induced concurrently by bleomycin and radiotherapy (Hurt *et al.*, 1982; Clamon, 1983).

Non-seminomatous germ-cell tumours are not radiosensitive. They are very aggressive tumours, most often disseminated at presentation and of very poor prognosis. Based on the results obtained in patients with testicular germ-cell tumours, aggressive combination chemotherapy is now considered as the treatment of choice also for mediastinal non-seminomatous germ-cell tumours. Different combined modality therapy has been used, generally including aggressive surgical debulking and early use of cisplatin–bleomycin-based combination chemotherapy (Economou *et al.*, 1982; Vogelzang *et al.*, 1982; Parker et al., 1983; McLeod *et al.*, 1988; Sham *et al.*, 1989; Wright *et al.*, 1990; Nichols *et al.*, 1990).

In the therapeutic approach the role of the pathologist is important. In primary resected tumour a conscientious sampling for histopathological examination, and a meticulous identification of all kinds of tissues composing the tumour and their amount and disposition within the tumour, is needed. A practical classification is suggested by Gonzalez-Crussi (1982) (Table 4.3). The morphological data must be correlated with the patient's age and sex, and with the presence of biochemical markers such as HCG and AFP corresponding to the presence of EST or choriocarcinomatous elements.

The histopathological study of post-chemotherapy resected specimens is also useful and of prognostic significance, since 40% will be found to have necrotic, non-viable tumour, an additional 40% will have a benign teratoma (Figs 4.46–4.50), and only 20% will have viable, active disease. When sarcomatous transformation is present, chemotherapy protocols have to be altered to include sarcoma-oriented drug for this particular group of patients (Manivel *et al.*, 1986).

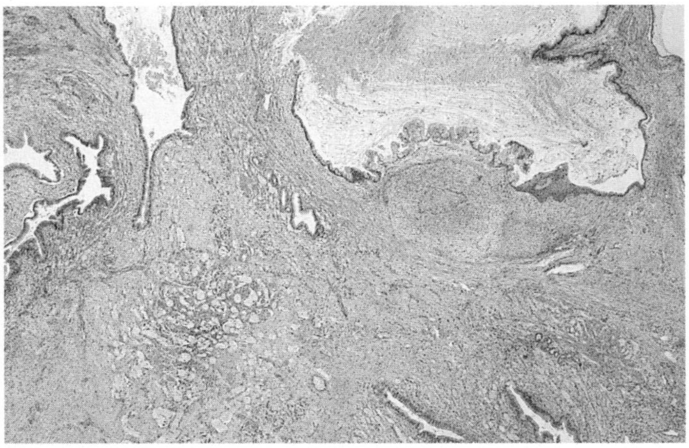

Figure 4.41 Mature teratoma. Dense connective tissue, enteric and respiratory cavities, and differentiating cartilage are illustrated

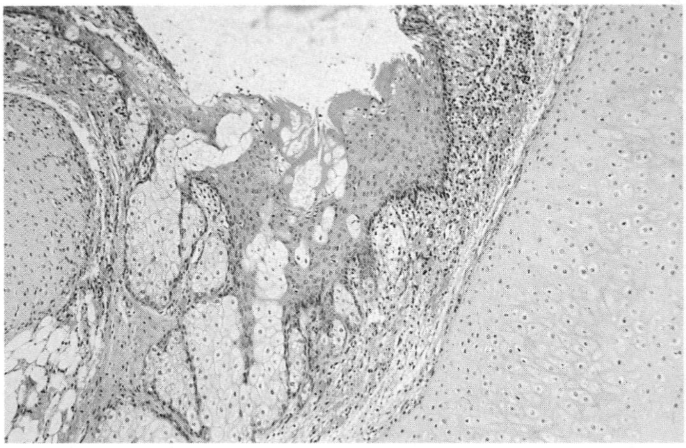

Figure 4.42 Mature teratoma. Skin and cartilage are present

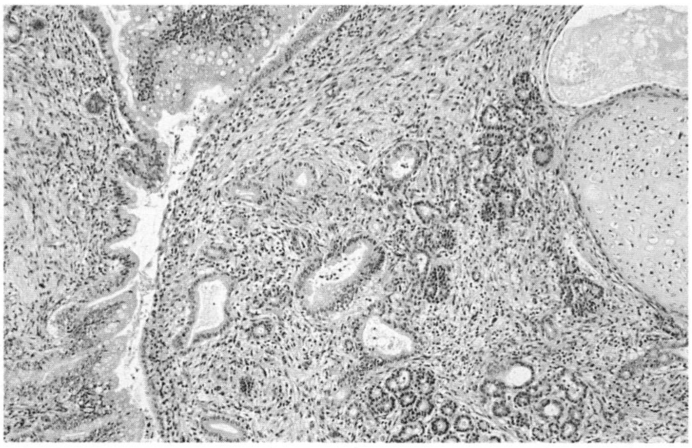

Figure 4.43 Mature teratoma. The section shows enteric cavities, glands, and cartilage

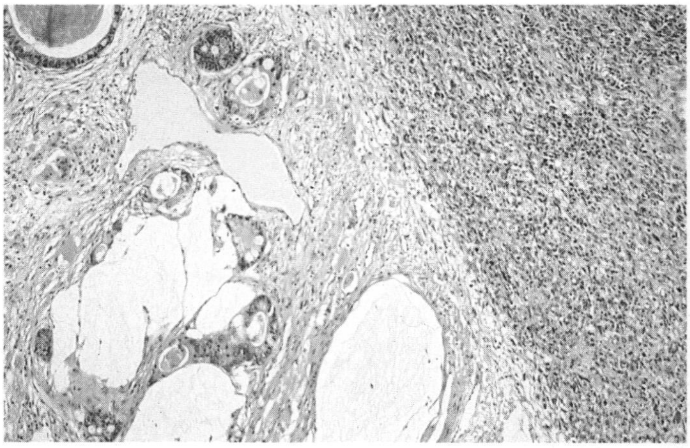

Figure 4.44 Teratoma with sarcomatous transformation. The figure shows the teratomatous elements (left) and the malignant area (right)

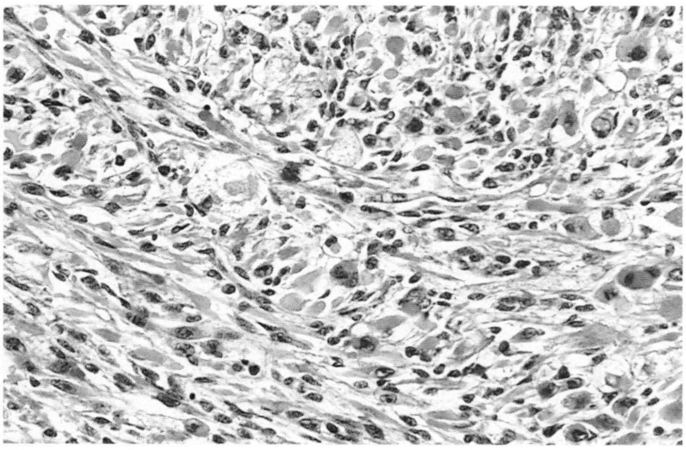

Figure 4.45 Teratoma with sarcomatous transformation. At higher magnification the tumour is a rhabdomyosarcoma

PROGNOSIS

The prognosis of a germ-cell tumour depends largely on the presence and quantity of primitive, undifferentiated cells and tissues within the tumour, but the relative prognostic significance of the different type of immature or undifferentiated tissues is not the same. The histological types, in order of increasing malignant behaviour, are: (1) seminoma (germinoma, dysgerminoma), (2) immature teratoma, (3) embryonal carcinoma, (4) yolk-sac tumour (endodermal sinus tumour), and (5) choriocarcinoma. Mixed tumours are defined as those containing at least 10% of two or more distinct histological types (Brodeur *et al.*, 1981). In a mixed-cell tumour the behaviour and prognosis depend on the most aggressive component regardless of its proportion in the tumour. Mixed-cell tumours containing choriocarcinoma plus teratocarcinoma, embryonal carcinoma, or seminoma almost always have metastases containing choriocarcinoma alone (Recondo and Libshitz, 1978).

Although *mediastinal seminomas* carry a worse prognosis than testicular lesions, because they present at a more advanced stage, prognosis is generaly good, with a

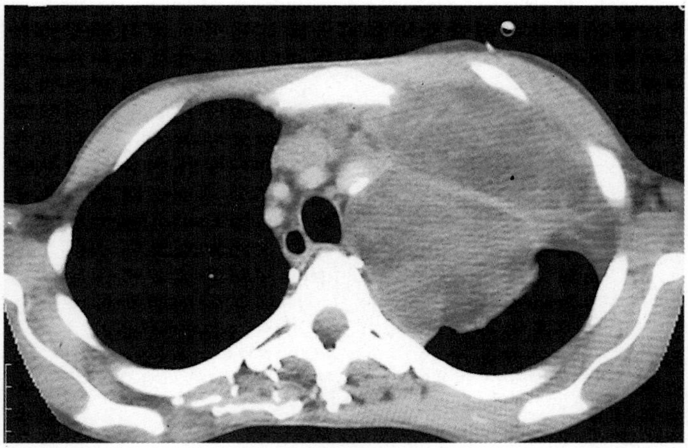

Figure 4.46 CT scan of a patient with a mixed germ-cell tumour. At presentation the serum AFP and HCG levels were elevated (46 000 ng/ml and 1200 ng/ml). The patient was treated by cisplatin-based chemotherapy with a complete serological remission

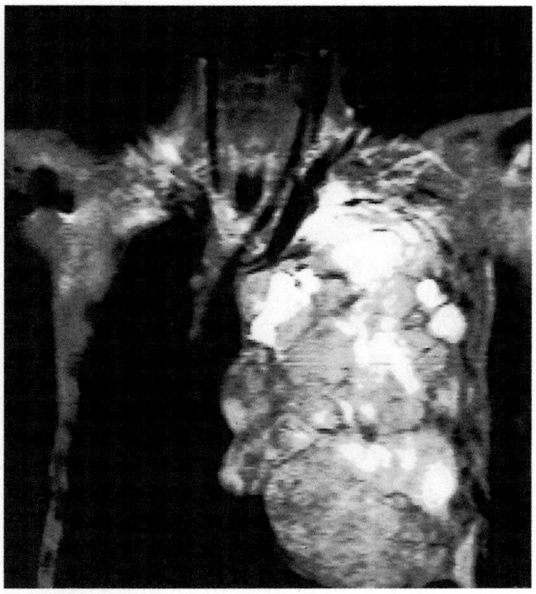

Figure 4.47

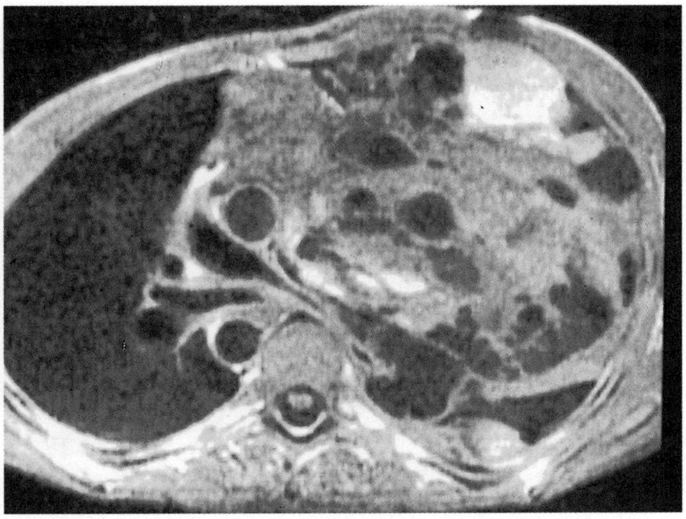

Figures 4.47 and 4.48 Magnetic resonance image from the same patient, 6 months later, showing a bulky, multicystic recurrent tumour

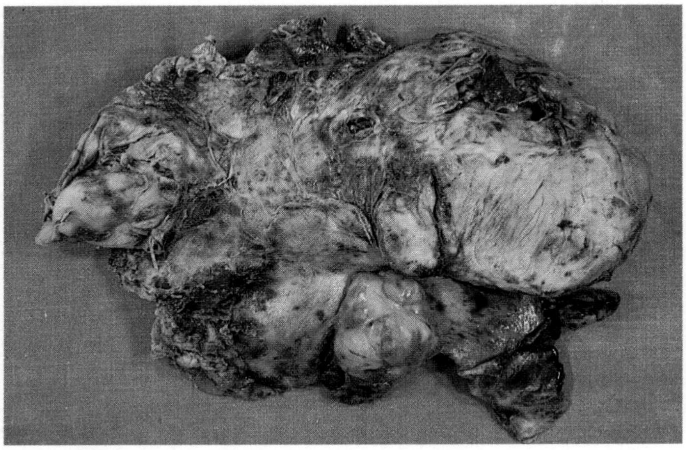

Figures 4.49 and 4.50 Teratoma was found only on post-chemotherapy surgical resection

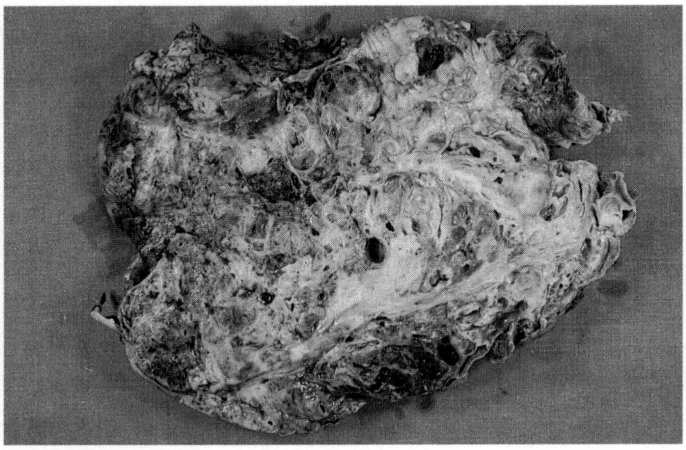

Figure 4.50

5-year survival rate of more than 75%. According to Hurt *et al.* (1982) patients with poorer prognosis are those who at time of diagnosis are 35 years old or older, those who present with fever or superior vena caval obstruction, and those who have supraclavicular, cervical or hilar adenopathy. Further metastases develop to the skeletal system, lungs, liver and other organs. Although in most cases the metastases are composed of seminoma, in some cases the metastases do not reflect the appearance of the primary tumour but contain other neoplastic germ-cell elements. The presence of other neoplastic germ-cell elements in the metastases is associated with a poorer prognosis.

Immature teratomas are always potentially malignant, although a majority of the tumours are fundamentally benign in behaviour (Gonzalez-Crussi, 1982). Among the histological findings the degree of immaturity and the extent of immature elements are considered to be the most important prognostic parameters. Moreover, immature somatic tissues have variable prognostic values. Neuroectodermal immature tissues are frequently encountered in teratomas. They reproduce the morphology of neuroblastoma in various stages of differentiation and, as in neuroblastoma, have the capacity to differentiate to mature nervous tissue. The prognostic significance of other immature tissues, such as nephrogenic tissue, embryonic lung derivatives and undifferentiated mesenchyme, is more debated. All immature tissues are potentially malignant but even well-differentiated teratoma may later metastasize.

It is difficult to predict the benign or malignant nature of immature teratomas since the biological behaviour of these tumours depends not only on the histological appearance but also on the anatomical site of the tumour and the age of the patient at diagnosis. Thus, in infants, immature teratomas originating in the mediastinum appear to behave in a manner different from both their gonadal and sacrococcygeal counterparts. Age seems to be the best-defined prognostic factor for these tumours. The immature teratomas that occur in infants under 15 years of age behave as mass lesions, as do the mature teratomas, and the patients have a benign clinical course. As a result adequate sampling of the tumour is important to exclude the presence of frankly malignant elements. In patients age 15 years or older, the immature teratomas behave as aggressive tumours similar to embryonal carcinoma (Carter *et al.*, 1982).

Other primary mediastinal non-seminomatous germ-cell tumours are highly malignant neoplasms, and before the development of cisplatin-based chemotherapy the prognosis was exceedingly poor. Modern multimodality therapy has improved the outcome considerably. Results from recent series suggest that approximately 50% of patients will be cured with intense cisplatin-based chemotherapy coupled with adjunctive surgery if needed (Wright *et al.*, 1990; Nichols *et al.*, 1990). Normalizing serum tumour marker levels with chemotherapy before resection is a significant favourable prognostic factor, whereas adverse factors are the usually advanced disease of the mediastinal non-seminomatous germ-cell tumours at presentation, and their propensity to develop non-germ-cell solid tumour or haematological malignancies (Nichols *et al.*, 1985).

References

Baldeyrou P., André-Bougaran, J. and Lemoine, G. (1986) Les tumeurs germinales primitives du médiastin chez l'enfant (séminome exclu). A propos de 7 cas. *Ann. Chir.: Chir. Thorac. Cardiovasc.*, **40**, 578–582

Brodeur, G. M., Howarth, C. B., Pratt, C. B., Caces, J. and Hustu, H. O. (1981) Malignant germ cell tumors in 57 children and adolescents. *Cancer*, **48**, 1890–1898

Carter, D., Bibro, M. C. and Touloukian, R. J. (1982). Benign clinical behavior of immature mediastinal teratoma in infancy and childhood: Report of two cases and review of the literature. *Cancer*, **49**, 398–402

Clamon, G. H. (1983) Management of primary mediastinal seminoma. *Chest*, **83**, 263–267

Damjanov, I., Amenta, P. S. and Zarghami, F. (1984) Transformation of an AFP-positive yolk sac carcinoma into an AFP-negative neoplasm. Evidence for in vivo cloning of the human parietal yolk sac carcinoma. *Cancer*, **53**, 1902–1907

Economou, J. S., Trump, D. C., Holmes, E. C. and Eggleston, J. E. (1982). Management of primary germ cell tumors of the mediastinum. *J. Thorac. Cardiovasc. Surg.*, **83**, 643–649

Fox, R. M., Woods, R. L., Tattersall, M. H. N. and McGovern, V. J. (1979) Undifferentiated carcinoma in young men: the atypical teratoma syndrome. *Lancet*, **1**, 1316–1318

Friedman, N. B. (1951) The comparative morphogenesis of extragenital and gonadal teratoid tumors. *Cancer*, **4**, 265–276

Gonzalez-Crussi, F. (1982) Extragonadal teratomas. Atlas of Tumor Pathology, 2nd series, Fasc. 18. Armed Forces Institute of Pathology, Washington, DC

Gonzalez-Crussi, F. and Roth, L. M. (1976) The human yolk sac and yolk sac carcinoma: An ultrastructural study. *Hum. Pathol.*, **7**, 675–691

Hurt, R. D., Bruckman, J. E., Farrow, G. M., Bernatz, P. E., Hahn, R. G. and Earle, J. D. (1982) Primary anterior mediastinal seminoma. *Cancer*, **49**, 1658–1663

Jacobsen, G. K. and Jacobsen, M. (1983) Possible liver cell differentiation in testicular germ cell tumours. *Histopathology*, **7**, 537–548

Knapp, R. H., Hurt, R. D., Payne, W. S., Farrow, G. M., Lewis, B. D., Hahn, R. G., Muhm, J. R. and Earle, J. D. (1985) Malignant germ cell tumors of the mediastinum. *J. Thorac., Cardiovasc. Surg.*, **89**, 82–89

Kurman, R. J. and Norris, H. J. (1976) Endodermal sinus tumor of the ovary. A clinical and pathologic analysis of 71 cases. *Cancer*, **38**, 2404–2419

Kurman, R. J., Scardino, P. T., McIntire, K. R., Waldmann, T. A. and Javadpour, N. (1977) Cellular localization of alphafetoprotein and human chorionic gonadotropin in germ cell tumors of the testis using an indirect immunoperoxidase technique. *Cancer*, **40**, 2136–2151

Lack, E. E., Weinstein, H. J. and Welch, K. J. (1985) Mediastinal germ cell tumors in childhood. A clinical and pathological study of 21 cases. *J. Thorac. Cardiovasc. Surg.*, **89**, 826–835

Levine, G. D. (1973) Primary thymic seminoma – a neoplasm ultrastructurally similar to testicular seminoma and distinct from epithelial thymoma. *Cancer*, **31**, 729–741

Lewis, B. D., Hurt, R. D., Payne, W. S., Farrow, G. M., Knapp, R. H. and Muhm, J. R. (1983) Benign teratomas of the mediastinum. *J. Thorac. Cardiovasc. Surg.*, **86**, 727–731

Manivel, C., Wich, M. R., Abenoza, P. and Rosai, J. (1986) The occurrence of sarcomatous components in primary mediastinal germ cell tumors. *Am. J. Surg. Pathol.*, **10**, 711–717

Martinez-Hernandez, A., Miller, E. J., Damjanof, I. and Gay, S. (1982) Laminine-secreting yolk sac carcinoma of the rat. Biochemical and electron immunohistochemical studies. *Lab. Invest.*, **47**, 247–257

McLeod, D. G., Taylor, H. G., Skoog, S. J., Knight, R. D., Dawson, N. A. and Waxman, J. A. (1988) Extragonadal germ cell tumors. Clinicopathologic findings and treatment experience in 12 patients. *Cancer*, **61**, 1187–1191

Mostofi, F. K. and Sobin, L. H. (1977) Histological typing of testicular tumours, In: International histological classification of tumours, No. 16. World Health Organization, Geneva, pp. 27–31

Nichols, C. R., Hoffman, R., Einhorn, L. H., Williams, S. D., Wheeler, L. A. and Garnick, M. B. (1985) Hematologic malignancies associated with primary mediastinal germ-cell tumors. *Ann. Intern. Med.*, **102**, 603–609

Nichols, C. R., Saxman, S., Williams, S. D., Loehrer, P. J., Miller, M. E., Wright, C. and Einhorn, L. H. (1990) Primary mediastinal nonseminomatous germ cell tumors. A modern single Institution experience. *Cancer*, **65**, 1641–1646

Nogales-Fernandez, F., Silverberg, S. G., Bloustein, P. A., Martinez-Hernandez, A. and Pierce, G. B. (1977) Yolk sac carcinoma (endodermal sinus tumor). Ultrastructure and histogenesis of gonadal and extragonadal tumors in comparison with normal yolk sac. *Cancer*, **39**, 1462–1474

Parker, D., Holford, C. P., Begent, R. H. J., Newlands E. S., Rustin, G. J. S., Makey, A. R. and Bagshawe, K. D. (1983) Effective treatment for malignant mediastinal teratoma. *Thorax*, **38**, 897–902

Patcher, M. R. and Lattes, R. (1964) 'Germinal' tumors of the mediastinum: A clinicopathologic study of adult teratomas, teratocarcinomas, choriocarcinomas and seminomas. *Dis. Chest*, **45**, 301–310
Recondo, J. and Libshitz, H. I. (1978) Mediastinal extragonadal germ cell tumors. *Urology*, **11**, 369–375
Sham, J. T., Fu, K. H., Chiu, C. S. W. *et al.* (1989) Experience with the management of primary endodermal sinus tumor of the mediastinum. *Cancer*, **64**, 756–761
Shantz, A., Sewall, W. and Castleman, B. (1972) Mediastinal germinoma. A study of 21 cases with an excellent prognosis. *Cancer*, **30**, 1189–1194
Shirai, T., Itoh, T., Yoshiki, T., Noro, T., Tomino, Y. and Hayasaka, T. (1976). Immunofluorescent demonstration of alpha-fetoprotein and other plasma proteins in yolk sac tumor. *Cancer*, **38**, 1661–1667
Sickles, E. A., Belliveau, R. E. and Wiernik, P. H. (1974) Primary mediastinal choriocarcinoma in the male. *Cancer*, **33**, 1196–1203
Talerman, A. (1980) Germ cell tumors of the testis. In *Progress in Surgical Pathology*, vol. 1, Fenoglio, C.M. and Wolff, M. (eds) Masson, New York, pp. 175–204
Teilum, G. (1965) Classification of endodermal sinus tumor (mesoblastoma vitellinum) and so called 'embryonal carcinoma' of the ovary. *Acta Pathol. Microbiol. Scand.*, **64**, 407–429
Teilum, G. (1976) *Special Tumours of the Ovary and Testis – Comparative pathology and histological identification*, 2nd edn. Munskgaard, Copenhagen, pp. 31–93
Teilum, G., Albrechtsen, R. and Norgaard-Pedersen, B. (1974) Immunofluorescent localization of alpha-fetoprotein synthesis in endodermal sinus tumor (yolk sac tumor). *Acta Pathol. Microbiol. Scand. (A)*, **82**, 586–588
Truong, L. D., Harris, L., Mattioli, C., Hawkins, E., Lee, A., Wheeler, T. and Lane, M. (1986) Endodermal sinus tumor of the mediastinum. A report of seven cases and review of the literature. *Cancer*, **58**, 730–739
Ulbright, T. M., Roth, L. M. and Brodhecker, C. A. (1986) Yolk sac differentiation in germ cell tumors. A morphologic study of 50 cases with emphasis on hepatic, enteric, and parietal yolk sac features. *Am. J. Surg. Pathol.*, **10**, 151–164
Vogelzang, N. J., Raghavan, D., Anderson, R. W., Rosai, J., Levitt, S. H. and Kennedy, B. J. (1982) Mediastinal nonseminomatous germ cell tumors: The role of combined modality therapy. *Ann. Thorac. Surg.*, **33**, 333–339
Wright, C. D. Kesler, K. A., Nichols, C. R. *et al.* (1990) Primary mediastinal nonseminomatous germ cell tumors. Results of a multimodality approach. *J. Thorac. Cardiovasc. Surg.*, **99**, 210–217
Wychulis, A. R., Payne, W. S., Clagett, O. T. and Woolner, L. B. (1971) Surgical treatment of mediastinal tumors. A 40 year experience. *J. Thorac. Cardiovasc. Surg.*, **62**, 379–392

DEFINITIONS

Germ-cell tumours: all tumours derived from primitive multipotent germ cell.

Seminoma: according to the authors, tumours derived from primitive unipotent gonadal cell without competence to differentiate into teratomatous elements **or:** initial stage in differentiation of primitive multipotent germ cell.

Embryonal carcinoma: poorly differentiated germ-cell neoplasm derived from embryonic multipotential cell.

Yolk-sac tumour (endodermal sinus tumour, mesoblastoma): extra-embryonal derivative of embryonal carcinoma, differentiating in the vitelline or yolk-sac direction.

Choriocarcinoma: extra-embryonal derivative of embryonal carcinoma, differentiating in the cyto- and syncytiotrophoblast direction.

Teratoma: germ cell composed of derivatives of the three primitive germ-cell layers: endoderm, ectoderm and mesoderm. They may be of varying degrees of maturity and thus may exhibit only slight somatic differentiation (immature teratoma), or may be composed of perfectly mature tissues (mature teratoma). Malignant transformation in an otherwise mature teratoma characterizes the entity 'teratoma with malignant transformation'

Mature teratoma: tumour composed of mature embryo-derived tissues.

Immature teratoma: tumor composed of immature embryo-derived tissues.

Teratoma with malignant transformation: malignant transformation of somatic tissues within a mature teratoma.

Neural Tumours 5

Intrathoracic neurogenic tumours arise from the peripheral nervous system or from the diffuse neuroendrocrine system. The peripheral nervous system is composed of sensory neurons, motor neurons, and autonomic neurons that are found outside of the central nervous system. The Schwann cell is a pluripotential supporting cell of the cell processes, or 'axons', of the peripheral nerves. Undifferentiated neural crest cells contribute most of the cells of the nerve sheaths and most of the neuroblasts and chromaffin or paraganglionic cells of the autonomic nervous system (Hajdu, 1979). The diffuse neuroendocrine system also derives from the neural crest. All tumours are embryologically related, accounting for the possible overlapping between the different types of tumours (Table 5.1).

Nervous tumours are among the most common mediastinal neoplasms accounting for 15–35% of all mediastinal tumours, including cysts. They are mainly situated in the posterior mediastinum where they represent about 75% of the tumours of this compartment. The descending order of frequency is schwannoma and neurofibroma, ganglioneuroma, neurosarcoma, and neuroblastoma. Other tumours are very uncommon (Parish, 1971; Davidson *et al.*, 1978). The majority are benign. Their classification is still debated. The classification used in this book is indicated in Table 5.2.

Table 5.1 Histogenesis of neuroectodermal tumours

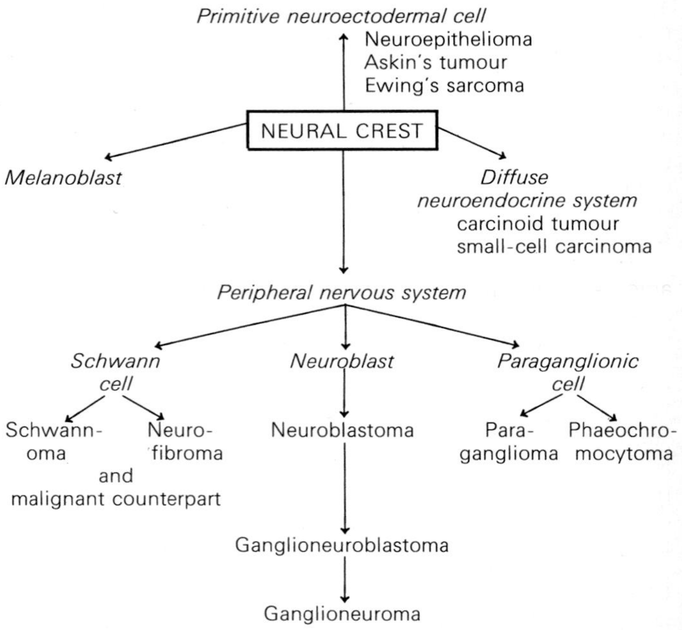

Modified from Hajdu (1979)

Table 5.2 Intrathoracic neural tumours classification

1. Tumours of nerve sheath origin
   - Benign
     - Schwannoma
     - Neurofibroma
     - Neurofibromatosis
   - Malignant
     - Malignant tumour of nerve sheath origin (malignant schwannoma)
2. Tumours of the nerve cells
   - Neuroblastic
     - Neuroblastoma
     - Ganglioneuroblastoma
     - Ganglioneuroma
   - Paraganglionic (paraganglioma)
     - Chemodectoma
     - Phaeochromocytoma
3. Primitive neuroectodermal tumours and related neoplasms
   - Peripheral neuroectodermal tumour (neuroepithelioma)
   - Malignant small-cell tumour (Askin's tumour)
   - Ewing's sarcoma
4. Tumours of the diffuse neuroendocrine system
   - Carcinoid tumour
   - Differentiated neuroendocrine tumour (atypical carcinoid)
   - Poorly differentiated neuroendocrine tumour (small-cell carcinoma)
5. Tumours of uncertain classification
   - Melanotic neuroectodermal tumour
   - Granular cell tumour (myoblastoma)

TUMOURS OF NERVE SHEATH ORIGIN

The normal peripheral nerve sheath

The nerve sheath of peripheral nerves is composed of Schwann cells, endoneurium, and perineurium. Schwann cells surround the axons, both myelinated and unmyelinated. They possess basement membrane, microfibrils and microtubules. They are pluripotential primitive cells, which are capable of transforming into fibroblasts and histiocytes. They can also assume forms of various mesenchymal cells, e.g. myoblasts, chondroblasts, and osteoblasts. The endoneurium is a fibromucinous matrix that occupies the space between nerve fibres and perineurial cells. It contains collagen fibres, scattered fibroblasts (endoneurial cells), and occasional histiocytes and mast cells. The perineurium is a tubular structure composed of concentric alternating layers of perineurial cells and collagen bundles. Perineurial cells are considered as a close relative to Schwann cells. They have a discontinuous basement membrane and contain numerous micropinocytic vacuoles. They may function as facultative fibroblasts and produce collagen.

The epineurium is the outermost sheath encompassing several nerve fascicles. It is made up of longitudinally arranged fibroblasts with abundant interspersed collagen fibrils.

Tumours of nerve sheath origin are the most frequent neurogenic neoplasms of the mediastinum, representing about 80% of these tumours. The great majority are benign and correspond to schwannoma and neurofibroma. Sometimes the two tumour types occur as a composite tumour, and this mixed pattern is best accepted as a benign nerve sheath tumour without attempting a supplementary classification. The malignant counterpart of these tumours is termed 'malignant tumour of nerve sheath origin' or 'malignant schwannoma'. 'Malignant tumour of nerve sheath origin' is a generic term indicating a common histogenesis of a number of malignant neoplasms with a wide spectrum of microscopic appearances. Both benign and malignant tumours of nerve sheath origin are generally believed to arise from Schwann cells, but differ by the diverse contribution of other components of the nerve sheath.

Clinical features

Intrathoracic benign nerve sheath tumours occur at all ages with a predilection of adults from 20 to 50 years of age and a roughly equal sex ratio. They affect left and right sides of the chest with equal frequency and are distributed from the apex of the thorax to the diaphragm with a predilection of the upper portion of the mediastinum (Luosto *et al.*, 1978; Davidson *et al.*, 1978). Most of them are located in the posterior mediastinum, developing from the spinal roots and the sympathetic chain. Less frequently the tumours arise from intercostal nerves of the lateral chest wall and only occasionally from the phrenic and vagus nerves (Strickland and Wolverson, 1974; Dabir *et al.*, 1990; Heitmiller *et al.*, 1990). Intrathoracic neurofibromas, but also schwannomas, may be either solitary or multiple as manifestations of von Recklinghausen's disease (Parish, 1971).

In benign tumours most of the patients are asymptomatic at presentation and the tumours are generally discovered on routine chest radiography. Respiratory symptoms, such as cough or dyspnoea, are mainly associated with large tumours. Pneumonia, stridor, haemoptysis, hoarseness, and dysphagia have occasionally been described, but are not specific. Signs of spinal cord compression may be observed in tumours developed both in the posterior mediastinum and the vertebral canal. Horner's syndrome has been observed in tumours situated in the right superior mediastinum and recurrent nerve paralysis in tumours arising from the vagus nerve. These neurological manifestations are rare and do not necessarily indicate malignancy.

On chest X-ray the tumour appears as a well-delimited lesion of uniform density located either along the lateral chest wall or more frequently in the left or right paravertebral region. Rib deformity or erosion adjacent to the lesion and vertebral anomalies are sometimes found. Widening of intravertebral foramina, together with signs of spinal cord compression, characterize a dumb-bell extension. Myelography, computed tomography (CT) and magnetic resonance imaging (MRI) delimit better the degree of intravertebral extension (Ricci *et al.*, 1990; Figs 5.1–5.3).

Intrathoracic malignant tumours of nerve sheath origin are infrequent and arise either *de novo* or from a preexisting benign tumour, usually a neurofibroma. They develop independently or, more frequently, in association with neurofibromatosis. Half of the cases occur in patients with von Recklinghausen's disease. Occasional reports of malignant schwannoma occurring in an area of prior radiation therapy have also been reported. The development of malignancy occurs from 6 to 25 years following radiation therapy, with a median time of 14 years (Sordillo *et al.*, 1981).

Pain, increasing symptomatology due to compression, rapid growth of the tumour or sudden enlargement of a pre-existing mass are indicative of the onset of sarcomatous changes. Radiologically, the tumours appear as large, round or oval masses that invade the mediastinum, the adjacent structures, the bones, and that may extend through the intervertebral foramina.

Intrathoracic neural tumours and neurofibromatosis of von Recklinghausen's disease

Von Recklinghausen's disease is a phakomatosis of dominant inheritance that is related to migration and differentiation abnormalities of cells of the neural crest (Hajdu, 1979; Enzinger and Weiss, 1988). The inherited dysgenesis involves the neuroectoderm and probably the mesoderm. Von Recklinghausen's disease is characterized by lesions of the skin (café-au-lait pigmented cutaneous patches due to melanin deposits in the basal epidermal layer), bones and joints (scoliosis, pseudoarthrosis), central nervous system (glial and meningeal neoplasms), and the peripheral nervous system with formation of multiple nerve sheath tumours (usually neurofibromas, but also schwannomas, and neurogenic sarcomas). In the majority of cases the manifestations of the disease remain mild with lesions limited in number ('formes frustes') and there are no universally accepted diagnostic criteria for these mild forms. The diagnosis usually depends on clinical manifestations supported by the family history: presence of two or more neurofibromas or six or more café-au-lait spots 1.5 cm or larger (Crowe *et al.*, 1956).

Whereas neurofibromatosis is a relatively common disorder, the intrathoracic neural manifestations of the disease are rare. Nerve sheath tumours occurring in patients with neurofibromatosis differ clinically and biologically from those occurring in patients without the disease. They are mostly neurofibromas, frequently multiple, and central rather than peripherally located. There is a higher predisposition to the development of sarcomas that occur in younger patients and that are clinically aggressive (Manoli *et al.*, 1969; Sordillo *et al.*, 1981; Enzinger and Weiss, 1988; Table 5.3).

Table 5.3 Comparison of mediastinal schwannoma and neurofibroma

	Schwannoma	*Neurofibroma*
Age	20–50 years	20–40 years; younger age in RD
Location	Posterior mediastinum, less often intercostal nerves	Posterior mediastinum, phrenic and vagus nerves
Histology	Encapsulated tumour, Antoni A and B patterns	Often plexiform, not encapsulated
Degenerative changes	Common	Occasional
S-100 protein	Intense and uniform staining	Weak and variable staining
Occurrence in RD	Uncommon	Plexiform or multiple neurofibromas characteristic of RD
Malignant transformation	Extremely rare	Rare in solitary form, more common in RD

RD: von Recklinghausen's disease.
Modified from Enzinger and Weiss, 1988

Schwannoma

Schwannoma is a benign, slowly growing encapsulated neoplasm that originates from a nerve and is composed of Schwann cells proliferating in a collagenous matrix. The lesion is confined by the perineurium and eccentrically compresses the nerve.

Macroscopy

Schwannomas are well encapsulated, round or fusiform tumours, attached to a nerve that can be recognized at either end of the tumour (Fig. 5.4). The tumours are firm. On section they are tan—yellow, grey or pink, with a myxoid or gelatinous surface (Fig. 5.5). Occasionally,

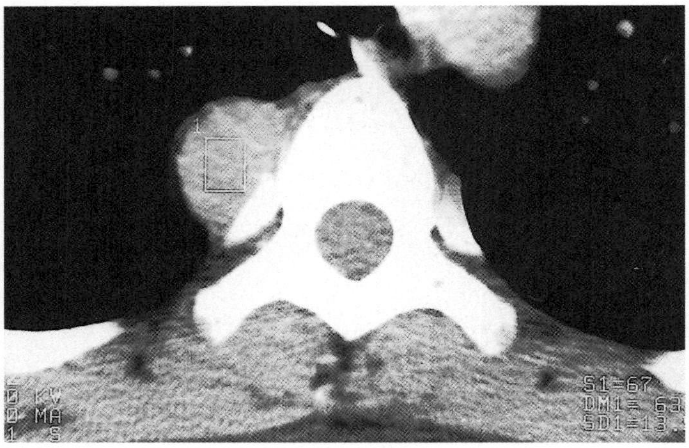

Figure 5.1 Schwannoma: CT scan shows a well-limited mass located in the right paravertebral region

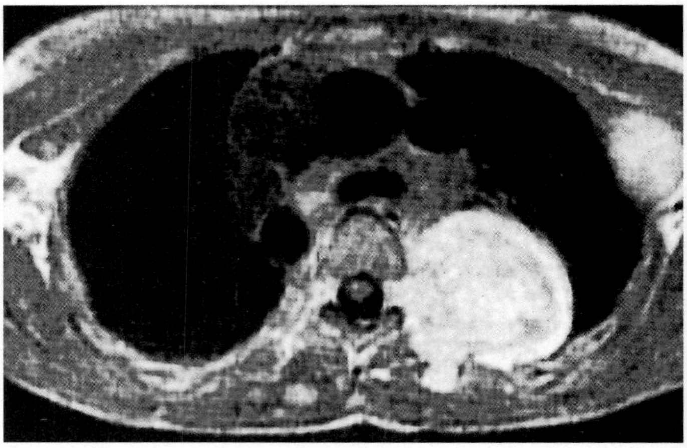

Figure 5.2 Neurofibroma: MRI from a patient with von Recklinghausen's disease showing the dumbbell extension through the fifth intervertebral foramina. Transaxial view

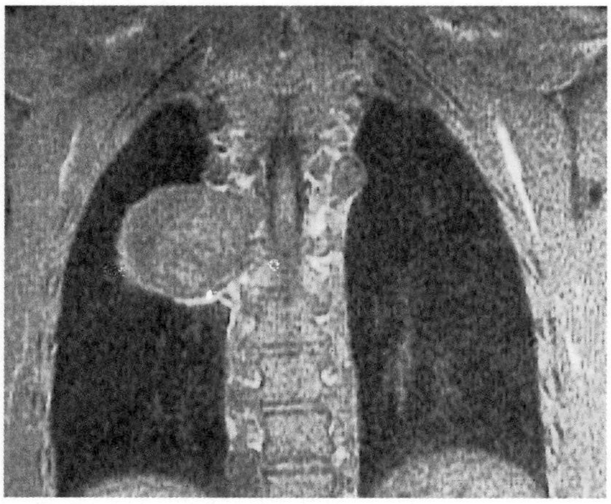

Figure 5.3 Neurofibroma: MRI, coronal view from the same patient

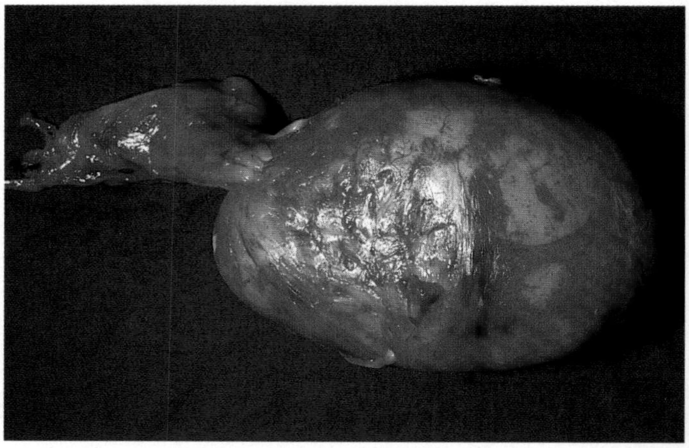

Figure 5.4 Schwannoma. Well-encapsulated ovoid tumour attached to a nerve that can be seen on the left of the figure

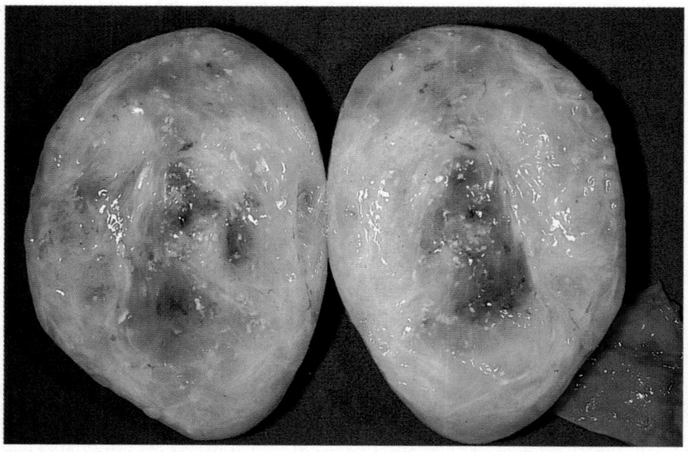

Figure 5.5 Schwannoma. The cut section is pink and gelatinous

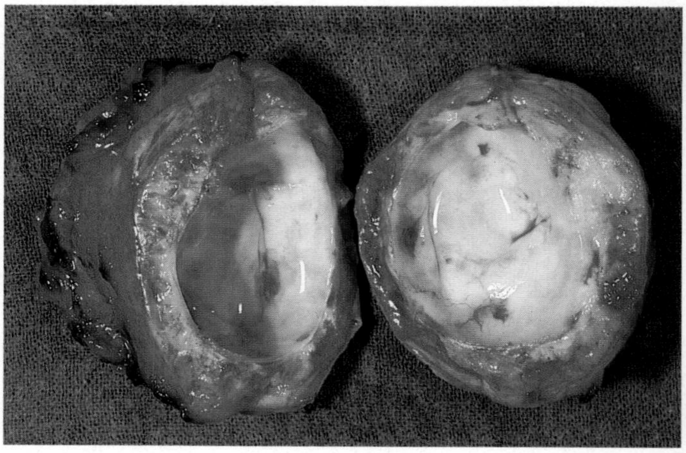

Figure 5.6 Schwannoma. Large cystic degeneration

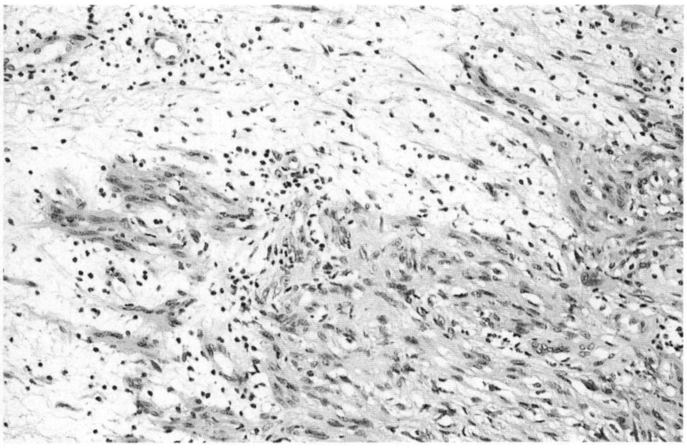

Figure 5.7 Schwannoma. The figure shows the sharply separated Antoni A (right) and Antoni B (left) areas

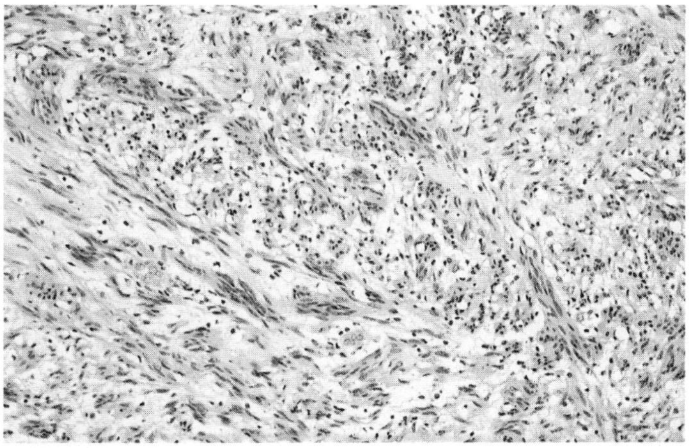

Figure 5.8 Schwannoma. The tumour cells are arranged in short palisades

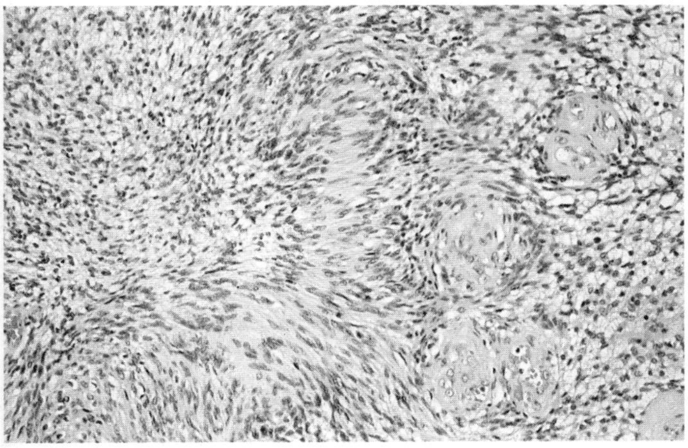

Figure 5.9 Schwannoma. Verocay bodies

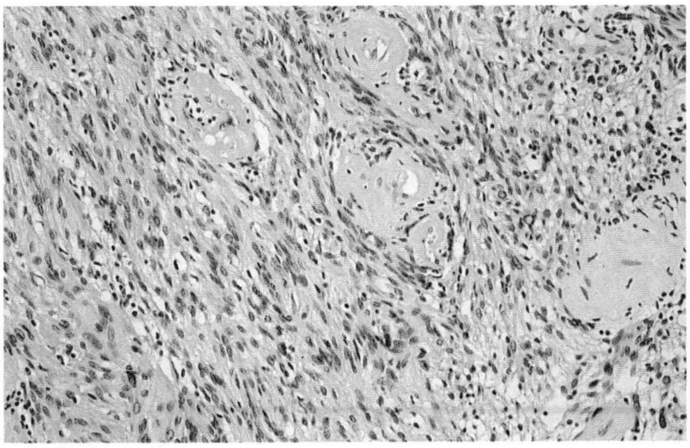

Figure 5.10 Schwannoma. The vessels have thick hyalinized walls

areas of calcifications or cystic degeneration occur (Fig. 5.6).

Histology

Schwannomas are composed of spindle cells with long oval, cigar-shaped nuclei, and moderately abundant amphophilic cytoplasm with indistinct borders. The cells are arranged in various patterns, classified as Antoni A and Antoni B types. The relative amounts of these two types vary, and they either merge progressively or are sharply separated (Fig. 5.7). Neurites are generally not demonstrable within the tumour substance.

Antoni A areas are composed of cells with indistinct cytoplasmic borders, compactly arranged in interlacing fascicles. The cells are frequently oriented with their long axes parallel to one another, and the nuclei may be disposed in palisades that are separated by fibrillar cytoplasmic processes (Fig. 5.8). *Verocay bodies* are oval formations composed of two rows of parallel well-aligned tumour cell nuclei (Fig. 5.9). Hyalinized nodules surrounded by palisades of Schwann cells are also frequently observed.

Antoni B areas have a less cellular pattern which is characterized by widely separated polymorphic tumour cells embedded in a myxomatous pale-staining matrix. The Schwann cells are disposed either in tortuous cords or in coarse fascicles resembling those seen in neurofibromas. They are elongated and twisted, and show distinct cytoplasmic borders. The matrix is loose, myxoid and does not stain with Alcian blue.

Numerous small or prominent ectatic vessels with thick hyalinized walls are a characteristic feature of schwannoma (Fig. 5.10). They often show thrombosis and subintimal deposits of fibrinoid. Cystic degeneration, foci of lipid-laden histiocytes and areas of haemorrhagic infarction are also observed.

Cellular schwannoma is a rare form composed almost exclusively of Antoni A areas and show hypercellularity and nuclear atypies. The tumours are characterized by a compact growth of spindle-shaped cells. They suggest some nuclear palisading but do not demonstrate well-formed Verocay bodies or loose Antoni B pattern. The atypical Schwann cells are frequently intermingled with numerous small, round, lymphocytoid cells. These tumours are likely to be confused with sarcomas. However, despite their marked cellularity, they have practically no mitotic activity and the prognosis is similar to that of other schwannomas. In *ancient schwannoma* there are also large atypical hyperchromatic nuclei, irregularly scattered throughout the tumour. Although these histological aspects may cause concern, the tumours are benign.

Plexiform schwannoma, a variant described by Reed and Harkin (1983), is composed of compactly aggregated foci of Schwann cells arranged in short palisades corresponding to a diffuse endoneurial proliferation with an exaggerated potential for invasive growth. The lesion may be the expression of a minimally deviant malignant schwannoma.

Neurofibroma

Neurofibroma is a well-limited benign neoplasia originating from a nerve and principally composed of Schwann cells intermingled with fibroblastic endoneurial cells, perineurial cells, fascicles of collagen, and neurites, interspersed in a mucinous matrix. The neurofibroma usually extends through the epineurium of the nerve into the adjacent soft tissues and does not remain encapsulated. The variable contribution of the different cells and the admixture with various amounts of the matrix are responsible for the diverse patterns of neurofibromas, including circumscribed fibrous or mucinous neurofibromas, plexiform neurofibromas, diffuse neurofibromas or 'paraneurofibromas' with tactoid bodies and plexiform epithelioid neurofibromas.

Solitary intrathoracic neurofibromas are rare, whereas multiple intrathoracic neurofibromas as manifestations of von Recklinghausen's disease are more frequent. Plexiform neurofibromas are particularly frequent in neurofibromatosis and virtually pathognomonic of the disease (Enzinger and Weiss, 1988).

Macroscopy

Circumscribed neurofibromas are well-limited, globoid or fusiform rubbery firm masses. The cut surface is homogeneous, pale grey and translucent. In many instances a nerve can be seen entering the tumour.

Plexiform neurofibromas are well-defined, non-encapsulated tumours that tend to involve an entire nerve trunk or a nerve plexus. The nerves appear to be thickened, swollen, giving the appearance of a 'bag of worms', and disappear in the tumour. The cut surface is shiny, translucent, and fibrous (Figs 5.11–5.13).

Histology

The circumscribed neurofibroma is composed of elongated spindle cells that are arranged in wavy thin fascicles and of bundles of collagen, separated by a loose myxomatous matrix. The neurofibroma also contains mast cells, lymphocytes and fibrocytes. Some tumours have loose hypocellular zones with numerous 'myxoma' cells, abundant mucoid matrix, and a few Schwann cells, thus simulating a myxoma (Fig. 5.14).

The plexiform neurofibroma is characterized by the proliferation of all the elements of a normal nerve, arranged in a distorted fashion. There are coarse bundles of collagen and tightly packed Schwann cells grouped in fascicles and dispersed in a mucinous matrix, associated with a diffuse proliferation of spindle and stellate cells apparently of perineurial or epineural origin (Fig. 5.15). In the early stage the nerves may simply have an increased endoneurial matrix, resulting in a wide separation of the nerve fascicles. In advanced lesions the matrix is densely fibrous and neurofibromas can be partially or completely hyalinized (Fig. 5.16). Schwannomas arising in neurofibromas are not rare. In some plexiform neurofibromas, multifocal nodules of compactly aggregated Schwann cells are irregularly distributed. The lesions are qualified as neurofibromas with multifocal schwannomatosis (Reed and Harkin, 1983). In plexiform neurofibromas hypercellularity and nuclear pleomorphism may be encountered, particularly in recurrent lesions. It is the presence of mitotic figures, however, that is indicative of malignant changes (Enzinger and Weiss, 1988).

Neurofibromas generally have neither markedly thickened vessels nor cysts, in contrast to the pattern of schwannomas. Axons, trapped by the growing tumour, are often found traversing a twisted course within the tumour. They are best demonstrated after Bodian stain. The matrix is rich in acid mucopolysaccharides and stains positively with Alcian blue.

The Schwann and perineurial cells, the melanocytes and the mesenchymal cells being embryologic relatives of neural crest origin, some unusual features such as rosettes, mucin-producing glands, and epithelioid melanin-containing cells may occur.

Malignant tumour of nerve sheath origin

The terminology for malignant tumours of nerve sheath origin remains confusing, as a result of the controversy concerning the cell of origin of the tumours, and there are a number of synonyms including malignant schwannoma, neurogenic sarcoma and neurofibrosarcoma. Although the term 'malignant schwannoma' is probably a misnomer in many instances, it is today extensively used by most authors.

Macroscopy

Malignant schwannoma usually arises within a plexiform neurofibroma or a major nerve. The tumour develops in the posterior mediastinum, or sometimes from the phrenic and vagus nerves in patients with neurofibromatosis. Thickening of the nerve of origin at one or both extremities indicates spread of the neoplasm along the epineurium and perineurium and results in a large fusiform, tortuous, well-circumscribed, occasionally lobulated mass. In von Recklinghausen's disease several malignant tumours may develop simultaneously or successively. Regardless of the clinical setting, the gross appearance of malignant schwannoma is not distinctive and resembles many sarcomas. The tumour is usually large, measuring more than 5 cm in diameter. The cut surface may be soft, fleshy, or firm, grey–white to tan–yellow, and frequently shows haemorrhagic and necrotic areas (Figs 5.17 and 5.18).

Histology

Malignant tumours of nerve sheath origin are spindle-cell tumours with a spectrum of histological patterns ranging from lesions that retain distinctive features of Schwann cell differentiation to poorly differentiated lesions that simulate fibrosarcomas, which can be hardly identified as neurogenic sarcoma (Figs 5.19–5.23).

Most malignant schwannomas are composed of plump fusiform cells arranged in whorls, interlacing fasicles or in herring-bone pattern. The nuclei are plump or elongated often twisted with a characteristic wavy or comma shape. They have a coarse chromatin distribution and a moderate pleomorphism. Mitoses are numerous. The cytoplasm is lightly stained and usually indistinct.

A characteristic feature of these tumours is *the wide variation in organization* that is greater than in fibrosarcomas. Thus, densely cellular fascicles alternate with hypocellular and myxoid zones where cells lose their parallel orientation, with a whorled arrangement simula-

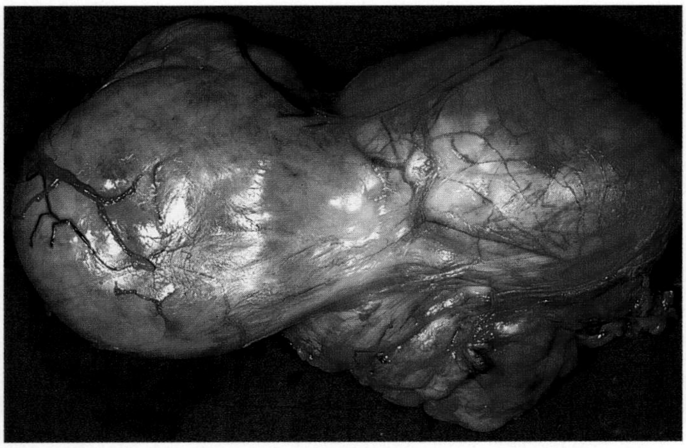

Figure 5.11 Plexiform neurofibroma. Large lobulated, well-circumscribed, non-encapsulated mass

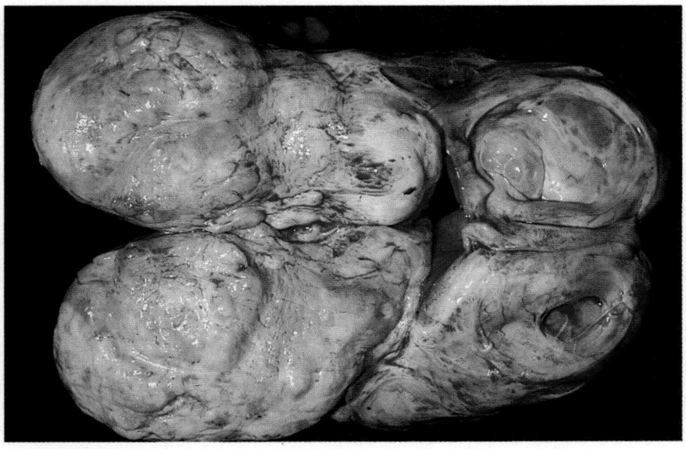

Figure 5.12 Plexiform neurofibroma. On section the tumour has a variable appearance with fibrous and cystic areas

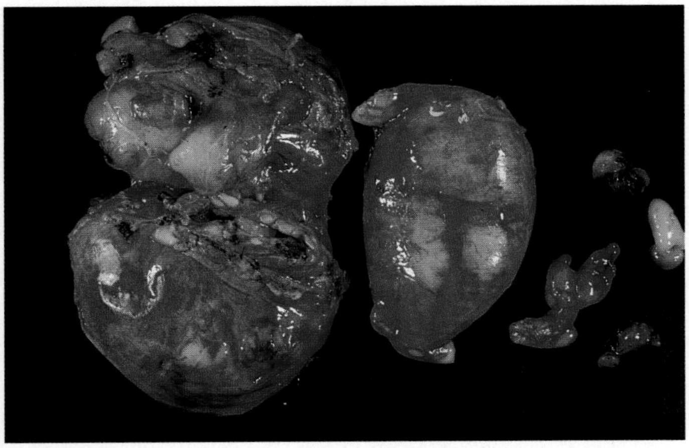

Figure 5.13 Plexiform neurofibroma. Multiple nodules of varying size, involving a nerve

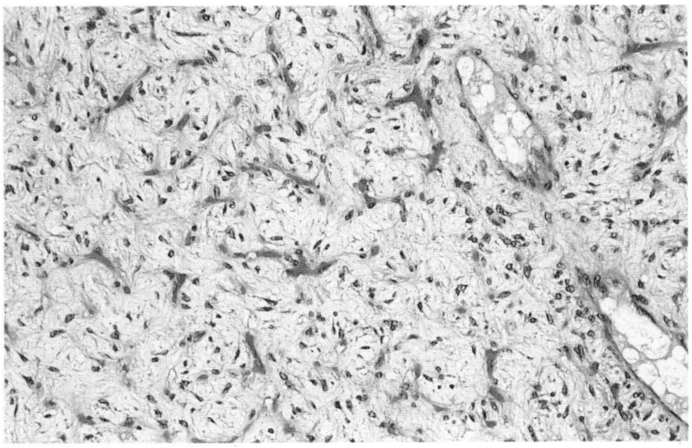

Figure 5.14 Myxoid neurofibroma containing only sparse collagen fibrils

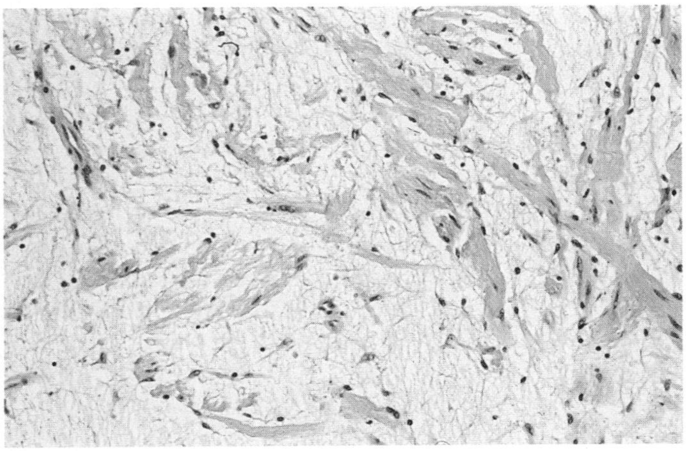

Figure 5.15 Plexiform neurofibroma consisting of Schwann cells, and wire-like collagen fibrils in a myxoid background

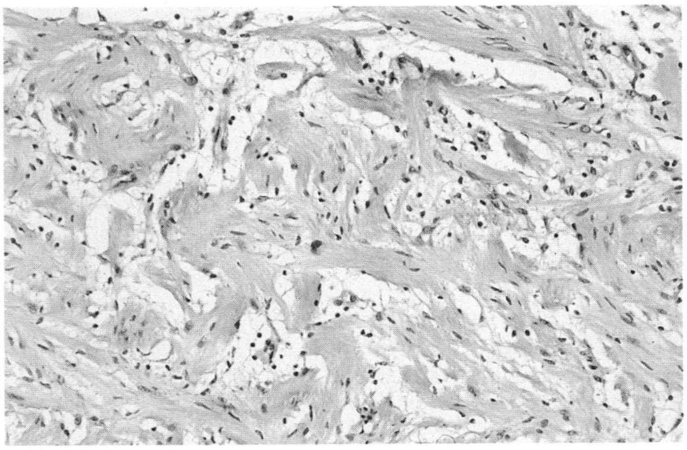

Figure 5.16 Hyalinized neurofibroma showing many thick collagen bundles.

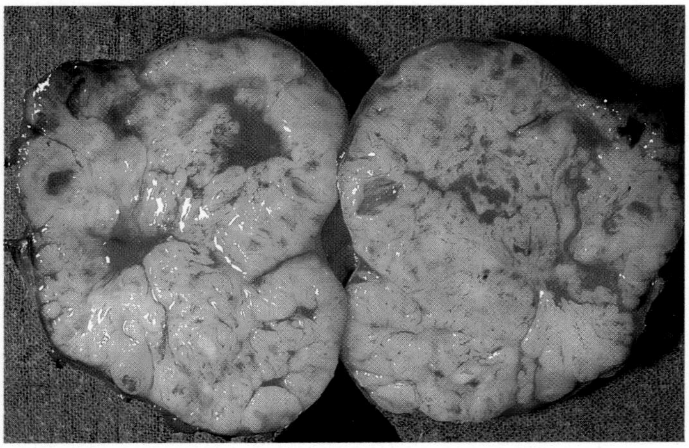

Figure 5.17 Malignant schwannoma in a patient with von Recklinghausen's disease. Large well-circumscribed tumour of fleshy appearance with haemorrhagic areas

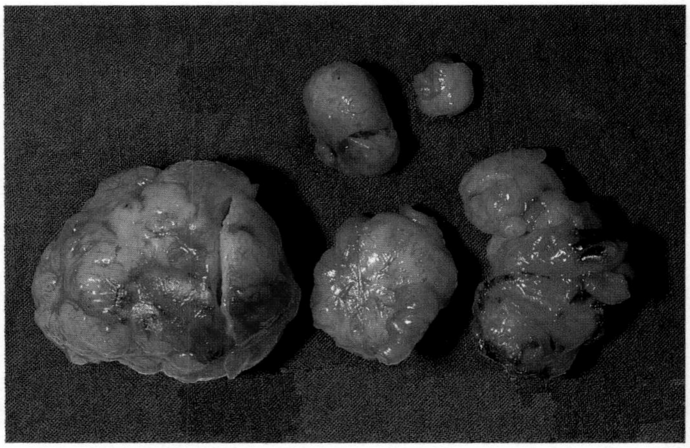

Figure 5.18 Recurrence 21 months later in the same patient. Five tumours developed simultaneously

ting tactoid differentiation, or with nuclear palisading reminiscent of the Antoni A pattern of benign schwannoma. Other typical features of malignant schwannomas are areas of necrosis bordered by cells arranged in palisades, and perithelial growth of the tumour. The blood vessels are often numerous and may show cellular proliferation and thickening of their walls. Occasional areas of prominent branching vascular channels reminiscent of a haemangiopericytoma may also be seen.

More uncommon but distinctive features of malignant schwannomas, particularly occurring in patients with neurofibromatosis, are hyaline bands and nodules, extensive spread of the tumour within epithelioid areas, clumps of melanocytic cells, and heterologous elements such as islands of cartilage and bone, skeletal muscle (Triton tumours), mucin-secreting glands and squamous differentiation (Enziner and Weiss, 1988).

Immunohistochemistry

S-100 protein is an acidic protein common to supporting cells of the central and peripheral nervous system (Steffansson *et al.*, 1982; Nakajima *et al.*, 1982; Enzinger and Weiss, 1988) and is constantly demonstrated in schwannomas, particularly in the Antoni A areas. It is strongly expressed by most cells of the tumours, in contrast to the cells of neurofibromas, which variably express the antigen. Although S-100 protein is not specific for neuroectodermal-derived cells, and has also been identified in other tissues, it is an important diagnostic tool for the recognition of severely degenerated fibrous schwannomas and the distinction from leiomyosarcomas.

In malignant schwannomas S-100 protein is identified in 50–90% of tumours. Typically the staining is rather focal and the number of immunoreactive cells is small compared with benign schwannomas and neurofibromas.

Electron microscopy

Schwannomas are composed principally of cells showing ultrastructural features of normal Schwann cells (Waggener, 1966; Razzuk *et al.*, 1973; Erlandson and Woodruff, 1982; Enzinger and Weiss, 1988). Cellular type A schwannomas consist of tightly packed, thin, elongated cells with complex entangled processes that are enveloped by a continuous external lamina and separated by dispersed collagen fibrils. Basal lamina is not present between apposed cytoplasmic processes. The cytoplasm contains scattered cytoplasmic organelles intermingled with microfilaments, microtubules, and small vesicles. Cell junctions are rare. Antoni type B areas are composed of widely spread cells similar to those described in type A schwannoma. A large extracellular compartment contains a loosely textured substance and scattered clusters of collagen fibrils. Small vessels are enveloped by thickened or reduplicated basement membranes.

Neurofibromas have an ultrastructural appearance distinct from that of schwannomas because of the participation of several cell types (Waggener, 1966; Enzinger and Weiss, 1988). The predominant cell is the perineurial cell surrounded by a discontinuous or fragmented basal lamina (Erlandson and Woodruff, 1982). They are intermingled with Schwann cells and a significant number of fibroblasts. The fibroblasts are distinguished from the perineurial and Schwann cells by their prominent endoplasmic reticulum and their lack of basal lamina. The cells are widely distributed in a loose fibrillar stroma containing random bundles of collagen fibrils and myelinated or nonmyelinated nerves entrapped within the tumour. The vessels are surrounded by one to three layers of spindle-shaped pericytes coated with a thin, continuous basal lamina in contrast to the thickened or reduplicated basal laminae enveloping vessels from Antoni type B schwannomas.

Malignant tumours of nerve sheath origin show varying degrees of ultrastructural differentiation (Taxy *et al.*, 1981; Erlandson and Woodruff, 1982; Chitale and Dickersin, 1983). The cells of well-differentiated tumours share some features with Schwann and perineurial cells. But most of the malignant peripheral nerve sheath tumours are poorly differentiated and resemble fibrosarcomas. The features suggesting a neuroectodermal derivation are the presence of broad cell processes covered by a discontinuous external lamina, of microtubules, microfilaments and primitive cell junctions, and of occasional myoid, squamous or epithelioid differentiations. In the highly anaplastic tumours the diagnosis is based only on the origin from nerves.

Differential diagnosis

The encapsulation, the presence of the two components Antoni A and Antoni B, the uniformly intense immunostaining for S-100 protein and the ultrastructural features, along with the clinical setting, distinguish schwannoma from neurofibroma (Enzinger and Weiss, 1988; Table

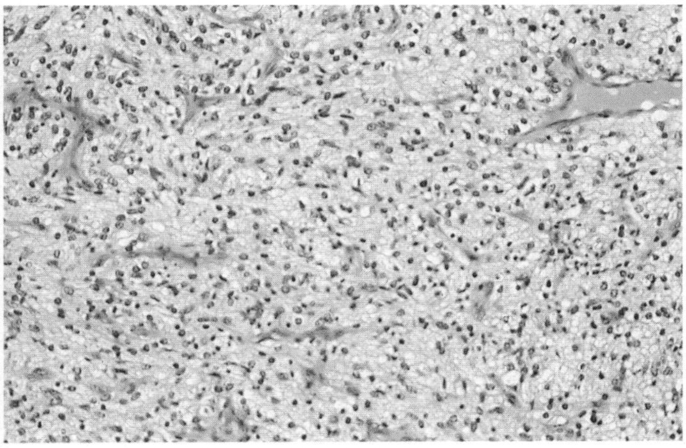

Figure 5.19–5.23 Recurrent malignant schwannoma from a patient with von Recklinghausen's disease

Figures 5.19 and 5.20 Primary sarcoma. Figure 5.19 shows minimal malignant features whereas Fig. 5.20 shows necrosis and nuclear atypia

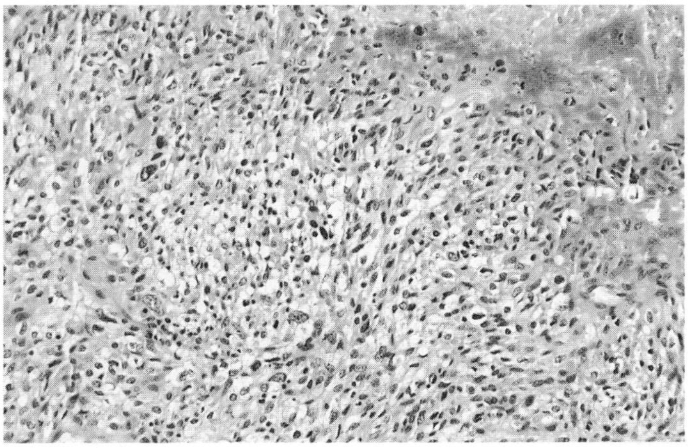

Figure 5.20

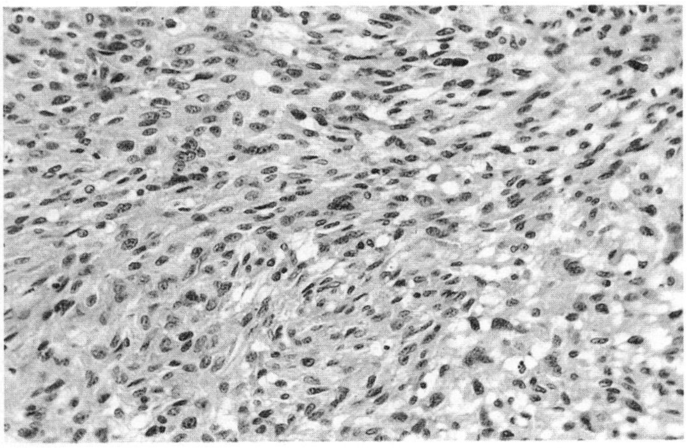

Figure 5.21 3 months later the tumour increases in cellularity

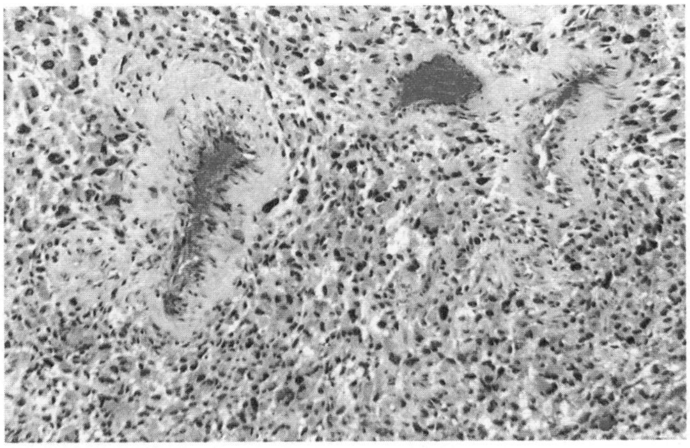

Figure 5.22 second recurrence, 3 months later. The nuclear atypia are obvious. Note the thick hyalinized walls of the vessels

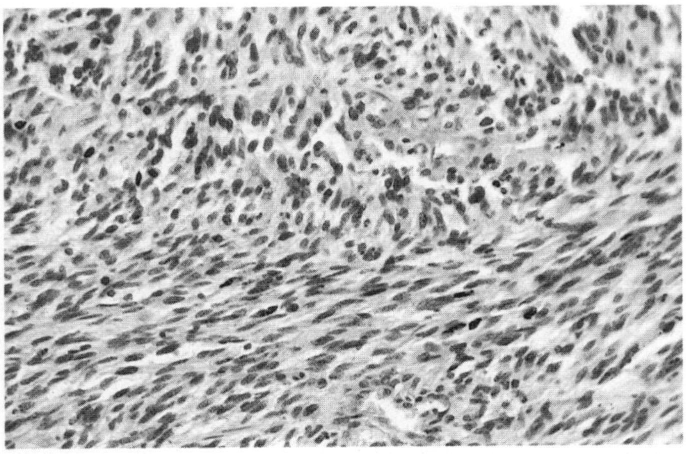

Figure 5.23 after 4 months the tumour recurred again in the form of a poorly differentiated lesion simulating a fibrosarcoma. The patient died shortly after

5.3). S-100 protein expression is also a valuable tool in diagnosing ancient schwannoma with pronounced degenerative changes, and in distinguishing schwannoma from leiomyoma in which immunostaining for S-100 protein is negative.

The diagnosis of malignant tumours of nerve sheath origin depends on the application of criteria both for nerve sheath origin and for malignancy (Trojanowski *et al.*, 1980; Horàk *et al.*, 1983). The presence of von Recklinghausen's disease or the origin of the tumour from a nerve, a neurofibroma or a schwannoma are strong indicators of a neurogenic sarcoma. In such cases the greatest difficulty is in predicting the biological behaviour of the lesion and in making the distinction between a benign and a malignant tumour (Nash, 1989). Plexiform neurofibromas, and occasionally schwannomas, may show increased cellularity and nuclear pleomorphism. Moreover, neurofibromas sometimes recur after surgical resection, and may grow along the nerve. However, these tumours rarely attain the large size of malignant schwannoma, do not invade the surrounding tissues and histologically, lack the presence of significant mitotic activity.

Malignant schwannomas occurring sporadically without the clinical setting of von Recklinghausen's disease are difficult to distinguish from other spindle-cell sarcomas. In such cases the existence of some areas with the typical histological features of malignant schwannoma, the presence of electron microscopic properties of Schwann cells, and the positivity of S-100 protein are the best diagnostic criteria.

Prognosis and treatment

Intrathoracic solitary schwannoma is a benign tumour that is cured by surgical excision. Dumb-bell extension into intervertebral foramina may lead to a simultaneous neurosurgical approach. Following complete excision the schwannoma in patients with neurofibromatosis is more likely to recur than is the solitary schwannoma. However, transformation of an intrathoracic benign schwannoma into a sarcoma rarely, if ever, occurs.

Solitary neurofibroma also follows a benign clinical course and simple excision of the tumour is considered to be an adequate therapy. In patients with intrathoracic tumours and von Recklinghausen's disease the multiplicity of lesions or the diffuse ill-defined feature of plexiform neurofibroma often make complete surgical therapy impossible. The prognosis is more severe than in other localization. Recurrences are not uncommon and the risk of malignant transformation is high. In the intrathoracic neurofibroma the quoted incidence is about 10% of cases (Manoli *et al.*, 1969).

Malignant tumours of nerve sheath origin are aggressive tumours, especially those which arise in the setting of neurofibromatosis. In patients with von Recklinghausen's disease the 5-year survival is shorter than in patients with solitary malignant schwannoma (23% versus 47%). There are often multifocal primary malignancies originating within pre-existing neurofibromas and the course tends to be that of multiple local recurrences. Distant metastases are usually haematogenous and the lung is the most frequent site of metastasis (Manoli *et al.*, 1969; Sordillo *et al.*, 1981). Malignant schwannomas developed in an area of prior radiation therapy appear even more aggressive, with a very poor median survival after diagnosis (14.5 months; Sordillo *et al.*, 1981). Malignant tumours of nerve sheath origin should be treated by radical surgery. However, the central intrathoracic location of the tumours, the occasional multiple sarcomas, or the diffuse changes of the nerve frequently restrict the local control of the lesions (Storm *et al.*, 1980).

References

Chitale, A. R. and Dickersin, G. R. (1983) Electron microscopy in the diagnosis of malignant schwannomas. *Cancer*, **51**, 1448–1461.

Crowe, F. W., Schull, W. J. and Neel, J. V. (1956) *A Clinical, Pathological and Genetic Study of Multiple Neurofibromatosis*, Charles C. Thomas, Springfield, IL.

Dabir, R. R., Piccione, W. and Kittle, C. F. (1990) Intrathoracic tumors of the vagus nerve. *Ann. Thorac. Surg.*, **50**, 494–497.

Davidson, K. G., Walbaum, P. R. and McCormack, R. J. M. (1978) Intrathoracic neural tumours. *Thorax*, **33**, 359–367.

Enzinger, F. M. and Weiss, S. W. (1988) *Soft Tissue Tumors*, 2nd edn., C. V. Mosby, St Louis, MI.

Erlandson, R. A. and Woodruff, J. M. (1982) Peripheral nerve sheath tumours: An electron microscopic study of 43 cases. *Cancer*, **49**, 273–287.

Hajdu, S. I. (1979) *Pathology of Soft Tissue Tumors*. Lea & Febiger, Philadelphia, PA.

Heitmiller, R. F., Labs, J. D. and Lipsett, P. A. (1990) Vagal schwannoma. *Ann. Thorac. Surg.*, **50**, 811–813.

Horàk, E., Szentirmay, Z. and Sugàr, J. (1983) Pathologic features of nerve sheath tumors with respect to prognostic signs. *Cancer*, **51**, 1159–1167.

Luosto, R., Koikkalainen, K., Jyrälä, A. and Franssila, K. (1978) Mediastinal Tumours. A follow-up study of 208 patients. *Scand. J. Thor. Cardiovasc. Surg.*, **12**, 253–259.

Manoli, A., Potter, R. T., Perfetto, J. and Coleman, A. (1969) Thoracic manifestations of Recklinghausen's disease. *New York State J. Med.*, **69**, 3014–3018.

Nakajima, T., Watanabe, S., Sato, Y. *et al.* (1982) An immunoperoxidase study of S-100 protein distribution in normal and neoplastic tissues. *Am. J. Surg. Pathol.*, **6**, 715–727.

Nash, A. D. (1989) *Soft Tissue Sarcomas: histological diagnosis*. Raven Press, New York.

Parish, C. (1971) Complications of mediastinal neural tumours. *Thorax*, **26**, 392–395.

Razzuk, M. A., Urschel, H. C., Martin, J. A., Kingsley, W. B. and Paulson, D. L. (1973) Electron microscopical observations on mediastinal neurolemoma, neurofibroma, and ganglioneuroma. *Ann. Thorac. Surg.*, **15**, 73–83.

Reed, R. J. and Harkin, J. C. (1983) Tumors of the peripheral nervous system. Supplement. In *Atlas of Tumor Pathology*, 2nd series, fasc. 3. Armed Forces Institute of Pathology, Washington, DC.

Ricci, C., Rendina, E. A., Venuta, F., Pescarmona, E. O. and Gagliardi, F. (1990) Diagnostic imaging and surgical treatment of dumbbell tumors of the mediastinum. *Ann. Thorac. Surg.*, **50**, 586–589.

Sordillo, P. P., Helson, L., Hajdu, S. I., Magill, G. B., Kosloff, C., Golbey, R. B. and Beattie, E. J. (1981) Malignant schwannoma – clinical characteristics, survival, and response to therapy. *Cancer*, **47**, 2503–2509.

Steffansson, K., Wollmann, R. and Jerkovic, M. (1982) S-100 protein in soft tissue tumors derived from Schwann cells and melanocytes. *Am. J. Pathol.*, **106**, 261–268.

Storm, F. K., Eilber, F. R., Mirra, J. and Morton, D. L. (1980) Neurofibrosarcoma. *Cancer*, **45**, 126–129.

Strickland, B. and Wolverson, M. K. (1974) Intrathoracic vagus nerve tumours. *Thorax*, **29**, 215–222.

Taxy, J. B., Battifora, H., Trujillo, Y. and Dorfman, H. D. (1981) Electron microscopy in the diagnosis of malignant schwannoma. *Cancer*, **48**, 1381–1391.

Trojanowski, J. Q., Kleinman, G. M. and Proppe, K. H. (1980) Malignant tumors of nerve sheath origin. *Cancer*, **46**, 1202–1212.

Waggener, J. D. (1966) Ultrastructure of benign peripheral nerve sheath tumors. *Cancer*, **19**, 699–709.

TUMOURS OF THE NERVE CELLS

These tumours are designated by Harkin and Reed (1969) as neuroectodermal tumours of primitive type (blastomas) which have the potential to develop into nerve cells. Although the division is artificial, and pathways between the different tumours are possible, they may be subdivided into two groups according to their main expression, namely neuroblastic or chromaffin (paraganglionic) lineage (Table 5.1).

Tumours of neural crest origin can secrete a variety of catecholamines and their metabolites, mostly epinephrine and norepinephrine, or related substances, as do normal cells found in the adrenal medulla and sympathetic nervous system ganglions. These products are liberated into the blood stream; their metabolites are excreted in the urine, and may be present in quantities that are of diagnostic significance.

Tumours of neuroblastic (sympathetic) origin

According to the increasing degree of differentiation these tumours comprise neuroblastoma, differentiated neuroblastoma (ganglioneuroblastoma), and ganglioneuroma. Neuroblastomas, like many other blastomas, are more in the nature of poorly organized malformations rather than neoplasms. Although most behave in a malignant fashion, they have the capacity to differentiate or mature in a manner similar to the transformation of embryonal tissue to adult tissue. Ganglioneuroblastomas exhibit an intermediate degree of maturation of tumour cells into neurons (ganglion cells), and ganglioneuroma is a mature and benign tumour composed of nerve fibres and mature ganglion cells. Carachi *et al.* (1983) subdivide neuroblastomas into differentiated and undifferentiated neuroblastomas (Table 5.4). The capacity to differentiate is latent, but may occur spontaneously or be induced by treatment.

Table 5.4 Histological grading of neuroblastic tumours

Grade I	Ganglioneuroma: fibroblasts, collagen, and Schwann cells with clumps of ganglion cells. No neuroblasts
Grade II	Ganglioneuroblastoma: neuroblastoma cells usually well differentiated, mixed with recognizable ganglion cells. Cases included in this group show a range of appearances from those in which ganglioneuromatous areas predominate to those in which the tumour is mostly composed of neuroblasts
Grade III	Differentiated neuroblastoma: neuroblastoma cells showing recognizable differentiation, predominantly the formation of neurofibrillary (axonal) material between tumour cells and with no differentiated ganglion cells visible
Grade IV	Undifferentiated neuroblastoma: characterized by diffuse sheets of neuroblasts without significant neurofibrillary differentiation at light microscopy level, but with neurosecretory granules of characteristic appearance on electron microscopy

According to Carachi *et al.*, 1983

Neuroblastoma and ganglioneuroblastoma

These tumours develop mainly in young children, generally less than 8 years of age, and represent 8–10% of all cancer observed in patients up to 15 years of age. They are thus one of the most common malignancies of childhood. Occasionally they may occur in adults (Kaye *et al.*, 1986).

They usually originate in the adrenal medulla but may arise in the sympathetic nervous system ganglions. In 20% of cases they occur in the thorax, representing about 10% of all intrathoracic neural tumours.

Most of the thoracic neuroblastomas (60%) present before the age of 2 years, without sex predilection. A family history of malignancy or a premalignant condition is not uncommon. Thus, neurofibromatosis is not infrequently found in a parent, or is associated in the patient with the neuroblastoma.

Clinical features

The children are symptomatic in two-thirds of cases. The symptoms are neurological signs: spinal cord compression, weakness or paralysis of one upper limb, clonus, Horner's syndrome, or respiratory symptoms such as wheezing, cough, respiratory distress or respiratory infection. In 30% of cases the disease is discovered incidentally at X-ray examination for an unrelated affection.

On chest X-ray the tumours are situated in the posterior mediastinum, in the left or right paravertebral region. Intravertebral extension causing widening of one or more intravertebral foraminae is not infrequent. Spinal cord compression is demonstrated by a block on myelogram. Calcifications, rib erosion, or rib notching are frequent findings. CT scanning is very useful for assessing tumour masses, and radionuclide bone scans and skeletal X-rays allow definite clinical staging (Table 5.5).

Biochemistry

Primitive tumours of sympathetic origin are biochemically active and secrete high levels of catecholamine (3,4-dihydroxyphenylalanine (DOPA) and dopamine, and their derivates, norepinephrine and epinephrine). Their metabolites (homovanillic acid and vanilmandelic acid) are excreted in the urine. The highest concentrations of dopamine metabolites in the urine correlate with the most malignant tumours (Table 5.6).

From the standpoint of catecholamine metabolism, neuroblastomas can be either biochemically differentiated or undifferentiated (Romansky *et al.*, 1978; Abramowsky *et al.*, 1989). Biochemically differentiated neuroblastomas are those in which the metabolic pathway proceeds efficiently to the end from DOPA through vanilmandelic acid. Biochemically undifferentiated neuroblastomas show a dopamine—norepinephrine pathway block, and have higher levels of early metabolites such as DOPA and dopamine along with homovanillic acid, suggesting a block at the step catalysed by dopamine β-hydroxylase (Laug *et al.*, 1978; Abramowsky *et al.*, 1989). These results are of prognostic significance and correlate with nuclear content of the tumours (Abramowsky *et al.* 1989) and with the numbers of neurosecretory granules

Table 5.5 Neuroblastoma and ganglioneuroblastoma: clinical staging

Stage I	Tumours limited to organ of origin
Stage II	Tumours with regional spread that does not cross the midline
Stage III	Tumours extending over the midline
Stage IV	Patients with metastases to distant lymph nodes, bone, brain, or lung
Stage IV-s	Patients with a small primary tumour (stage I or II) and distant metastases limited to the liver, skin, and/or bone marrow without evidence of bony metastases

According to Evans *et al.*, 1971

Table 5.6 Pathways of catecholamine metabolism

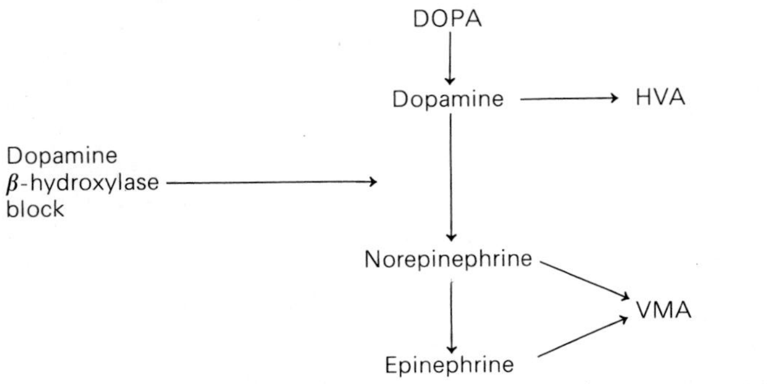

HVA: Homovanillic acid; VMA: vanilmandelic acid.
Patterns predictive of a poor prognosis are high levels of HVA relative to VMA.
According to Abramowsky *et al.*, 1989

observed under the electron microscope (Romansky *et al.*, 1978).

Morphologic features

Grossly, neuroblastomas — undifferentiated and differentiated — are friable, non-encapsulated tumours, sometimes well limited in some regions, but not demarcated in others. The cut surface is dark red with large areas of necrosis, haemorrhage, and cystic degeneration (Figs 5.24 and 5.25).

Histology

Neuroblastoma is a malignant, densely cellular, poorly differentiated neoplasm composed of diffuse sheets of small round cells or slightly elongated cells with large hyperchromatic nuclei, ill-defined borders, and prominent mitotic activity (Figs 5.26 and 5.27). The nuclei are often pyknotic and the specimens frequently seem to be poorly preserved. The immature neuroblasts appear grouped in diffuse sheets, or arranged in single file disposed into a fibrillar matrix that resembles glial tissue. They tend to form rosettes (Homer-Wright rosettes) or pseudorosettes centred by a mesh of cell processes or by an acellular fibrillar material (Fig. 5.28).

Ganglioneuroblastoma (differentiated neuroblastoma) shows an admixture of primitive neuroblasts and immature ganglion cells. The immature ganglion cells are large cells with an abundant, pink cytoplasm, and a round vesicular eccentric nucleus with prominent nucleoli. The fibrillar, glial-like background is characteristic and prevails in the more mature areas.

Ganglioneuroblastoma shows a wide spectrum of appearances from those in which the tumour is composed mainly of poorly differentiated neuroblasts with a scarce fibrillar matrix, to those in which immature differentiating ganglion cells predominate with abundant neurofibrillary material (Figs 5.29 and 5.30). In more mature tumours the lesion is made of large neuroblast and mature and immature ganglion cells disposed in a vacuolated matrix. Areas of necrosis, and calcifications, are frequent (Fig. 5.31).

The histopathological grading of neuroblastoma and ganglioneuroblastoma is indicated in Table 5.7.

Immunohistochemistry may be an adjunct in establishing the tumour diagnosis, but is not specific since the antigens expressed by neuroblastoma are also found in other tumours of neuronal origin (Table 5.8).

Tumour cells are partially positive for neuron-specific enolase (NSE), but the number of positive cells and the intensity of staining vary. The staining for S-100 protein is more distinct and clearly localized in elongated cells situated in the thin stromal septa. Undifferentiated neuroblasts are negative. The number of S-100 protein-positive tumours is usually low and correlates with the differentiation of the tumour and the prognosis. Leu-7 is usually positive. Neurofilament (NF) positivity is infrequently seen in small areas as thin thread-like neural structures in the fine fibrillary background between tumour cells.

Leukocyte common antigen (LCA) positivity correlates with lymphoid-cell infiltration and varies considerably. It is seen mainly in the more differentiated neoplastic tissue. In poorly differentiated tumours only a few LCA-positive cells are seen within the neuroblastic tissue.

Electron microscopy

Electron microscopic aspects of neuroblastoma are well documented (Gonzalez-Angelo *et al.*, 1965; Yokoyama *et al.*, 1971; Tomisawa *et al.*, 1975; Romansky *et al.*, 1978) and the main distinctive feature is the presence of cytoplasmic neuritic processes containing neurotubules and dense-core neurosecretory granules. Intermediate neurofilaments within the cytoplasm and synaptic junctions may also be evident.

In the undifferentiated neuroblastoma, tumorous cells display irregularly lobulated or indented nuclei and a very high nuclear to cytoplasmic ratio. The cytoplasm is scanty and contains very few cytoplasmic organelles and intermediate filaments. Neurosecretory granules, measuring about 100 nm in diameter, are scarce and most commonly found within neurotic processes. The cytoplasmic processes are few in number, and neurotubules averaging 20–24 nm, in diameter are rare and poorly organized.

With advancing maturation from neuroblastoma to ganglioneuroblastoma nuclei tend to be larger, occasionally multilobulated or multinucleated, and the amount of cytoplasm increases. Also the cytoplasmic organelles increase in number, the dense-core neurosecretory granules and cytoplasmic neuritic processes become more numerous, and the microtubules are better organized.

DNA ploidy

Studies of nuclear DNA content in neuroblastoma have shown that tumours with an aneuploid DNA content are clinically less aggressive in contrast to tumours with a

Table 5.7 Neuroblastoma and ganglioneuroblastoma: histopathological grading

Grade 1	>50% differentiating elements
Grade 2	5% to 50% differentiating elements
Grade 3	<5% differentiating elements
Grade 4	no recognizable neurogenesis

Differentiation defined as nuclear enlargement, cytoplasmic enlargement with eosinophilia and distinct borders, and cell processes evident in routinely stained sections.
According to Beckwith and Martin, 1968

Table 5.8 Histo- and immunohistochemistry in neuroblastoma, neuroepithelioma, Askin's tumour and Ewing's sarcoma

	Glycogen	*NSE*	*S-100 protein*	*NF*	*Leu-7*	*Vimentin*	*Cyto-keratin*
Neuroblastoma	(+)	++	+	(+)	++	(+)	–
Neuroepithelioma	+	+	+	+	+	+	(+)
Askin's tumour	(+)	+	+				
Ewing's sarcoma	++	(+)	(+)	(+)	(+)	+	+

(+): Positive in some cases; +: positive in most cases: ++: positive in every case (according to Fujii *et al.*, 1989; Pinto *et al.*, 1989; Ushigome *et al.*, 1989).

NSE (neuron-specific enolase) was interpreted initially as highly specific for neurons and neuroendocrine cells, but it has been recently found in normal and neoplastic tissues other than of neuronal origin. It is now regarded as non-specific.
S-100 protein is constantly found in tumour derived from Schwann's cells and melanocytes, including neurofibromas, schwannomas, naevi and melanomas, as well as granular cell myoblastomas. However, S-100 protein is not specific for neuroectodermal-derived cells and has also been identified in a number of different tissues.
NF (neurofilament) is an intermediate filament present in the nerve cells and in neurogenic tumours. NF consists of three subcomponents: 68, 150, and 200 kD. The 68 kD subcomponent shows best positivity in neuroectodermal-derived tumours.
Leu-7 (HNK-1) reacts positively with the neuroectodermal cells and is consistently positive in central and peripheral nervous system tissues and tumours.
Vimentin is an intermediate filament protein found in all forms of mesenchymal and some epithelial tissues. It is also present in developing glial cells, as well as meningiomas, schwannomas, haemangioblastomas, melanomas, lymphomas, and medulloblastomas.
Cytokeratin is an intermediate filament in epithelial tissues.

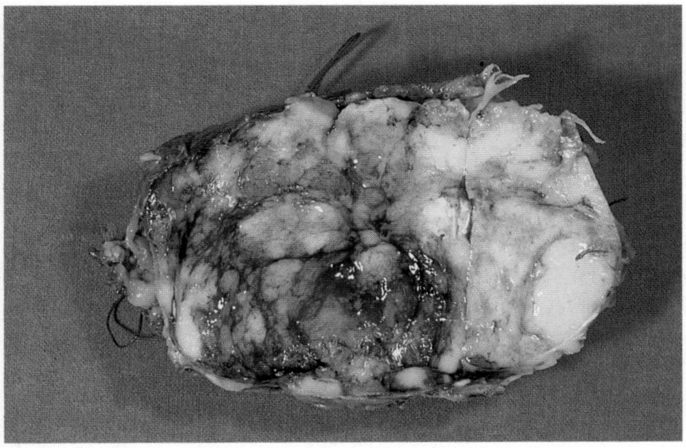

Figure 5.24 Neuroblastoma. Friable, well-delimited, non-encapsulated tumour showing large haemorrhagic and necrotic areas

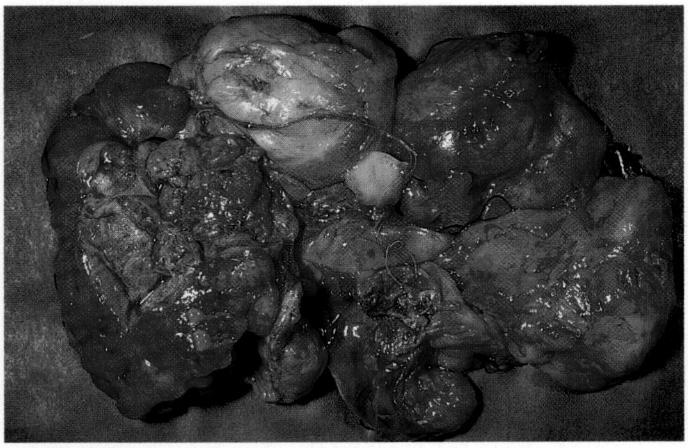

Figure 5.25 Ganglioneuroblastoma. Large lobulated, irregular and non-encapsulated tumour

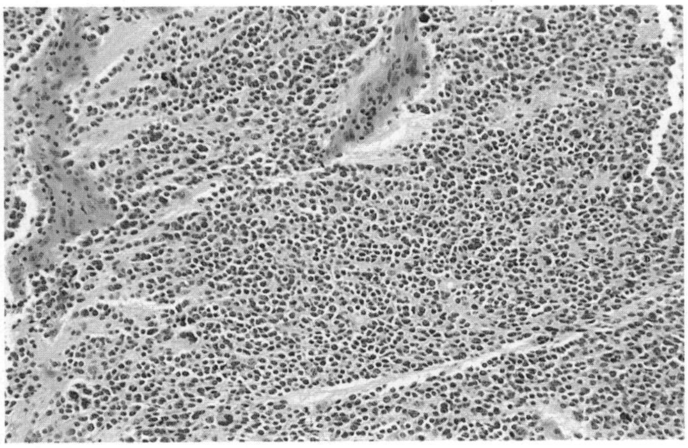

Figure 5.26 Neuroblastoma. The tumour is composed of sheets of immature neuroblasts disposed into a sparse fibrillar matrix

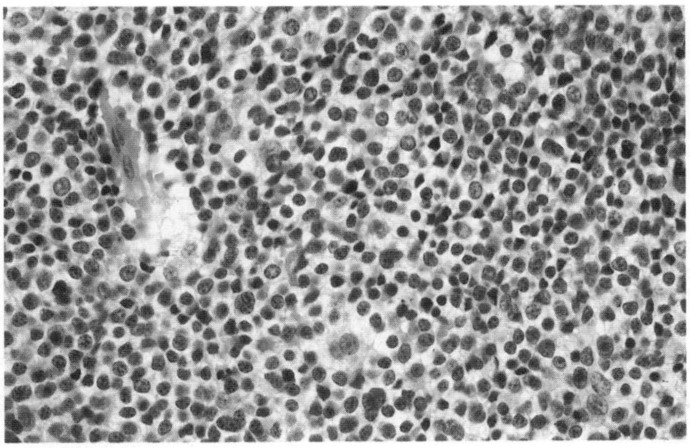

Figure 5.27 Neuroblastoma. The neuroblasts are small round cells with large hyperchromatic nuclei and ill-defined cytoplasmic borders. Mitoses are present

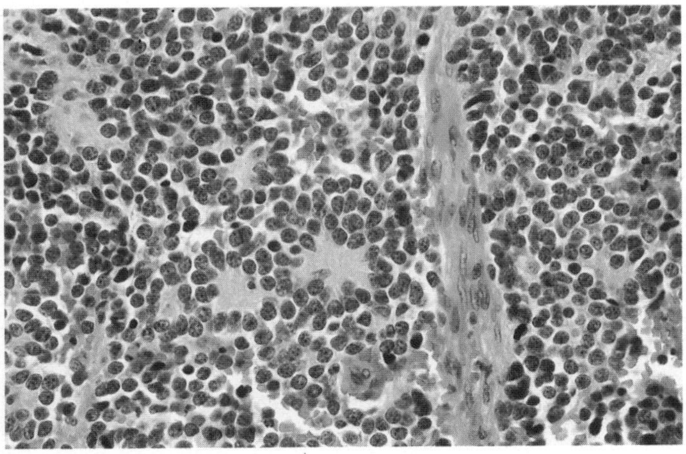

Figure 5.28 Neuroblastoma. Homer–Wright rosettes centred by a mesh of cell processes

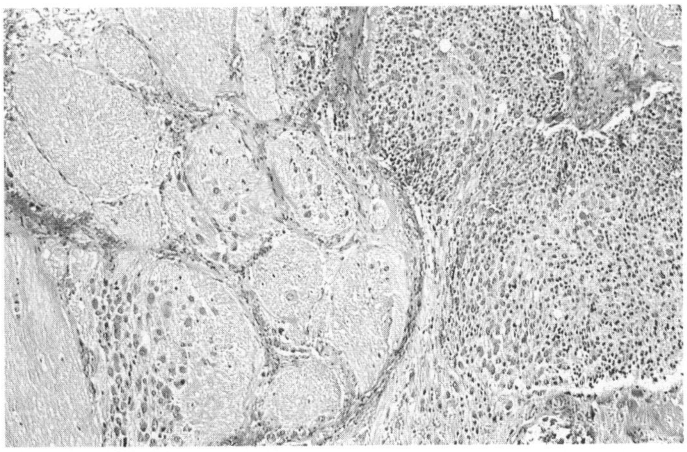

Figure 5.29 Ganglioneuroblastoma. The figure shows a sheet of poorly differentiated neuroblasts (right) and a cluster of differentiating ganglion cells disposed in an abundant fibrillar material (left)

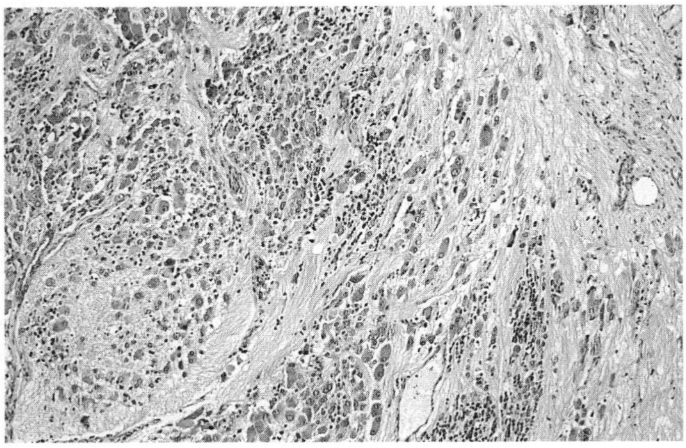

Figure 5.30 Ganglioneuroblastoma. Another aspect of the same tumour

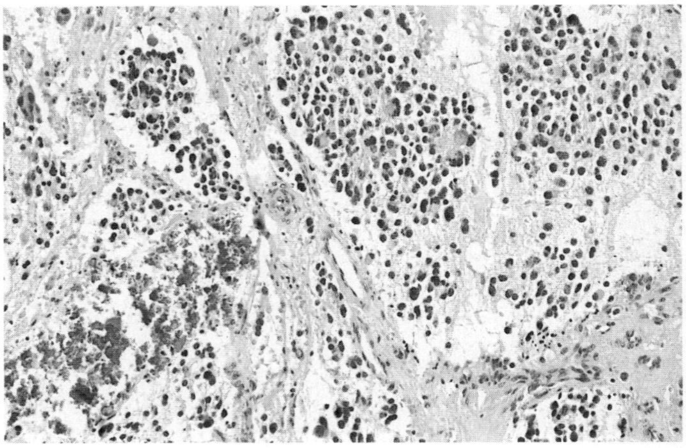

Figure 5.31 Ganglioneuroblastoma. Cluster of calcifications in a poorly differentiated tumour

non-aneuploid (diploid) content (Abramowsky *et al.*, 1989). Aneuploid tumours are significantly associated with the more favourable stages I, II or IV-s, whereas the tumours with non-aneuploid DNA content are mostly in stages III or IV.

N-myc oncogene

N-myc oncogene was initially isolated from human neuroblastoma cell lines. Although N-myc oncogene is present as a single copy localized on chromosome 2p23 to 24 in normal cells, it is mainly amplified in tumours of neural origin, neuroblastoma and retinoblastoma, and also in small-cell cancer. Amplification of N-myc oncogene is not observed in all neuroblastomas and occurs more frequently in advanced stages II and IV and in undifferentiated types of tumours than in less malignant types. No amplification is detected in ganglioneuroma and ganglioneuroblastoma. Thus, amplification of the oncogene and the number of N-myc copies in neuroblastic tumours is now regarded as a reliable prognostic factor, independent of the other prognostic indicators (Tsuda *et al.*, 1987; Garvin *et al.*, 1990; Nakagawara *et al.*, 1990).

Differential diagnosis

The diagnosis of ganglioneuroblastoma is generally easy in the presence of admixture of neuroblastic cells, ganglion cells at different stage of differentiation and abundant neurofibrillary material.

The differential diagnosis of neuroblastoma includes the group of the so-called malignant small round-cell tumours. In children with thoracic neuroblastoma, the differential diagnosis with Ewing's sarcoma, lymphoma and rhabdomyosarcoma (although less frequent in the mediastinum) should be considered. In adults the most frequent diagnosis to discuss is lymphoma and small-cell carcinoma. In children and young adults peripheral neuroepithelioma and Askin's tumour are also to be considered.

In this diagnostic approach the determination of catecholamine levels in the urine and the electron microscopic study are most useful. Except for rare cases of small-cell carcinoma, elevation of catecholamine occurs only in neuroblastic tumours. Measurements of catecholamine metabolites should be made in timed urine collections since catecholamine secretion by the tumour may fluctuate, rendering spot urine tests unreliable. The value of electron microscopy in the differential diagnosis of neuroblastoma has been strongly emphasized by several authors, and the comparative ultrastructure of malignant round-cell tumours has been carefully described by Henderson and Papadimitriou (1982). Electron microscopy further allows a distinction between highly undifferentiated neuroblastomas and more differentiated ganglioneuroblastomas.

The presence of N-myc amplification and lack of 11:22 chromosomal translocation are other features that can help to distinguish neuroblastomas from primitive neuroectodermal and related tumours, such as neuroepithelioma, Askin's tumour, and Ewing sarcoma (Table 5.9). Immunohistochemistry provides strong arguments against lymphoma and rhabdomyosarcoma.

Table 5.9 Biochemistry and cytogenetics in neuroblastoma, neuroepithelioma, Askin's tumour and Ewing's sarcoma

	Catecholamine secretion	*N-myc expression*	*11:22 Chromosomal translocation*
Neuroblastoma	Yes	Yes	No
Neuroepithelioma	No	No	Yes
Askin's tumour	No		
Ewing's sarcoma	No	No	Yes

Prognosis

Neuroblastoma has a highly varying degree of malignancy and the behaviour of the tumour remains unpredictable. It has a high tendency to be aggressive and yet to mature into the benign form of ganglioneuroma.

The best-recognized prognostic factors are the patient's age at diagnosis, tumour stage and histological grade, and the primary site of the tumour (Adam and Hochholzer, 1981). The patient's age is the best prognostic indicator. In the series of Oppedal *et al.* (1988), 72% of infants under 1.5 years of age at diagnosis survive, in contrast to only 11% in the age group 1.5–5 years, and none at age over 5 years, regardless of stage at presentation. Primary tumour site in the mediastinum (77% survival rate versus 23% for tumour below the diaphragm) and tumour differentiation are also related to a better prognosis (Carachi *et al.*, 1983). Tumours of stage IV-s stand apart in that the disease tends to undergo spontaneous maturation and involution, and therefore has a much more favourable prognosis than would be predicted from its widespread distribution. Most patients with stage IV-s disease are younger than 1 year of age at diagnosis and generally have an excellent 2-year survival of 70–90% regardless of treatment.

Biological indicators include urinary catecholamine excretion, DNA-ploidy and N-myc amplification. Unfavourable prognostic factors are non-aneuploid nuclear content versus aneuploid DNA content, high levels in urine and tumour homogenates of DOPA, dopamine and homovanillic acid with apparently a dopamine – norepinephrine pathway block suggesting a deficiency of dopamine β-hydroxylase activity. Clinically aggressive neuroblastomas express N-myc oncogene amplification in several chromosomal sites (Abramowsky *et al.*, 1989) and a relationship between N-myc amplification and DNA ploidy has been reported.

Treatment

Thoracic neuroblastoma and ganglioneuroblastoma have generally a low grade of malignancy and a good prognosis, and children usually do well with any type of treatment. Localized tumour can be cured by surgery alone. In children with advanced disease there is little evidence that treatment significantly lowers the mortality, although aggressive combined therapy, including total-body irradiation followed by bone marrow rescue, may result in long-term survival (Carachi *et al.*, 1983; Evans *et al.*, 1987; Sawaguchi *et al.*, 1990; Paul *et al.*, 1991).

In stage IV-s neuroblastoma that tends to regress spontaneously, and that develops in very young patients which are more likely to die of treatment complication, the probability of death from progressive disease must be weighed against the risk of therapy. Thus, neither chemotherapy nor radiation therapy is advised unless local disease compromises vital organ function (Haas *et al.*, 1988).

Ganglioneuroma

Ganglioneuromas are benign tumours composed of nerve fibres and mature ganglion cells. They originate from the line of autonomic nervous system ganglions and, in the thorax, are situated in the posterior medistinum, occupying the paravertebral sulcus. They develop in children and young adults in an age group older than that of patients with neuro- or ganglioneuroblastoma. They are infrequent in children younger than 2 years of age. A family history of neurofibromatosis or a familial occurrence has been described.

Clinically the patients are symptomatic in half of the cases and the symptoms are similar to those of other thoracic nervous tumours. On chest X-ray the tumours appear as large, well-limited, round to oval posterior mediastinal masses. Calcifications are frequent. Intravertebral extension, rib erosion, and spinal cord compression are uncommon findings. Ganglioneuromas are usually biochemically silent, and only occasionally the urine of the patient may contain low concentrations of dopamine metabolites. Ganglioneuromas do not express N-myc oncogene amplification.

Morphologic features

Ganglioneuromas have regular limits and are well encapsulated (Fig. 5.32). The cut section is grey and fibrous (Fig. 5.33). Histologically, they are composed of a variable admixture of Schwann cells, ganglion cells and nerve fibres (Harkin and Reed, 1969; Fig. 5.34). Schwann cells are arranged in interlacing fascicles, that are usually fibrous and resemble those seen in neurofibromas (Fig. 5.35). The ganglion cells are irregularly distributed or arranged in clusters. They are large, with an abundant pink cytoplasm containing Nissl granules. The nucleus is often eccentric, round and dense, with prominent nucleoli (Fig. 5.36). Binucleated ganglion cells are common. Satellite cells, surrounding the ganglion cells, are infrequent, but may occasionally be seen in a more or less normal arrangement. Clusters of calcifications are frequently seen (Fig. 5.37).

The morphological features of ganglioneuroma are characteristic and the differential diagnosis is usually easy. Nevertheless, adequate sampling of the tumours is mandatory in order to avoid missing small foci of immature cells. In the case of immature areas the lesion should be classified as ganglioneuroblastoma or as immature ganglioneuroma.

Prognosis and treatment

Ganglioneuromas are benign tumours that are cured by surgery alone. Some isolated cases may be accompanied with lymph node metastases, composed of undifferentiated neuroblastomatous elements. Such cases are interpreted as neuroblastomas that have matured into ganglioneuroma. The reverse, i.e. neuroblastic transformation of a benign ganglioneuroma, is rather exceptional.

References

Abramowsky, C. R., Taylor, S. R., Anton, A. H., Berk, A. I., Roederer, M. and Murphy, R. F. (1989) Flow cytometry DNA ploidy analysis and catecholamine secretion profiles in neuroblastoma. *Cancer*, **63**; 1752–1756.

Adam, A. and Hochholzer, L. (1981) Ganglioneuroblastoma of the posterior mediastinum: A clinicopathologic review of 80 cases. *Cancer*, **47**, 373–381.

Beckwith, J. B. and Martin, R. F. (1968) Observations on the histopathology of neuroblastomas. *J. Pediatr. Surg.*, **3**, 106–110.

Carachi, R., Campbell, P. E. and Kent, M. (1983) Thoracic neural crest. A clinical review. *Cancer*, **51**, 949–954.

Evans, A. E., D'Angio, G. J., Propert, K., Anderson, J. and Hann, H. L. (1987) Prognostic factors in neuroblastoma. *Cancer*, **59**, 1853–1859.

Evans, A. E., D'Angio, G. J. and Randolph, J. (1971) A proposed staging for children with neuroblastoma: Children's Cancer Study Group A. *Cancer*, **27**, 374–378.

Garvin, J., Bendit, I. and Nisen, P. D. (1990) N-myc oncogene expression and amplification in metastatic lesions of stage IV-S neuroblastoma. *Cancer*, **65**, 2572–2575.

Gonzalez-Angelo, A., Reyes, H. A. and Reyna, A. N. (1965) The ultrastructure of ganglioneuroblastoma. *Neurology*, **15**, 242.

Haas, D., Ablin, A. R., Miller, C., Zoger, S. and Mattay, K. K. (1988) Complete pathologic maturation and regression of stage IVS neuroblastoma without treatment. *Cancer*, **62**, 818–825.

Hajdu, S. I. (1979) *Pathology of Soft Tissue Tumors*. Lea & Febiger, Philadelphia, PA.

Harkin, J. C. and Reed, R. J. (1969) Tumors of the peripheral nervous system, *Atlas of Tumor Pathology*, 2nd series, fasc. 3. Armed Forces Institute of Pathology, Washington, DC.

Henderson, D. W. and Papadimitriou, J. M. (1982) *Ultrastructural Appearances of Tumours*. Churchill Livingstone, Edinburgh.

Kaye, J. A., Warhol, M. J., Kretschmar, C., Landsberg, L. and Frei, E. III (1986) Neuroblastoma in adults. Three case reports and a review of the literature. *Cancer*, **58**, 1149–1157.

Laug, W. E., Siegel, S. E., Shaw, K. N. F., Landing, B., Baptista, J. and Gutenstein, M. (1978) Initial urinary catecholamine metabolites and prognosis in neuroblastoma. *Pediatrics*, **62**, 77–83.

Nakagawara, A., Sasazuki, T., Akiyama, H. *et al.* (1990) N-myc oncogene and stage IV-S neuroblastoma. Preliminary observations on ten cases. *Cancer*, **65**, 1960–1967.

Oppedal, B. R., Storm-Mathisen, I., Lie, S. O. and Brandtzaeg, P. (1988) Prognostic factors in neuroblastoma. Clinical, histopathologic, and immunohistochemical features and DNA ploidy in relation to prognosis. *Cancer*, **62**, 772–780.

Paul, S. R., Tarbell, N. J., Korf, B. *et al.* (1991) Stage IV neuroblastoma in infants. *Cancer*, **67**, 1493–1497.

Romansky, S. G., Crocker, D. W. and Shaw, K. N. F. (1978) Ultrastructural studies on neuroblastoma. Evaluation of cytodifferentiation and correlation of morphology and biochemical and survival data. *Cancer*, **42**, 2392–2398.

Sawaguchi, S., Kaneko, M., Uchino, J-I. *et al.* (1990) Treatment of advanced neuroblastoma with emphasis on intensive induction chemotherapy. *Cancer*, **66**, 1879–1887.

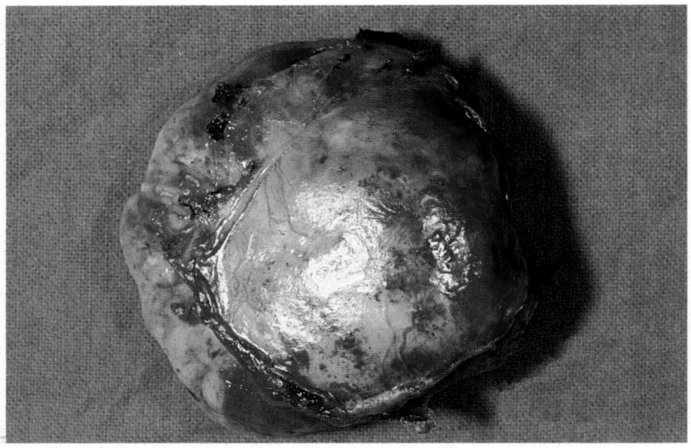

Figure 5.32 Ganglioneuroma. Large well-encapsulated tumour

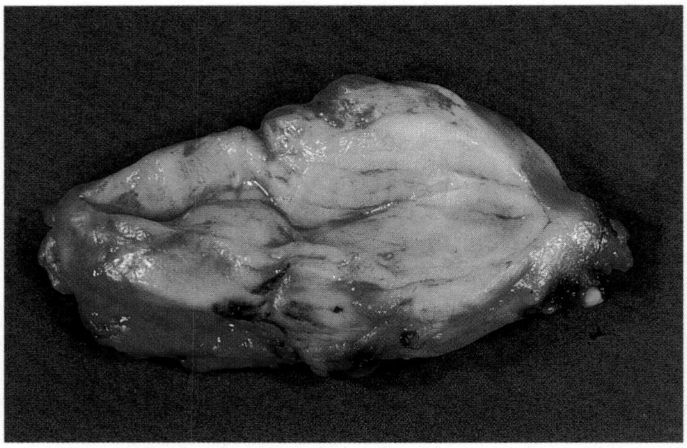

Figure 5.33 Ganglioneuroma. Fibrous, slightly lobated, encapsulated tumour

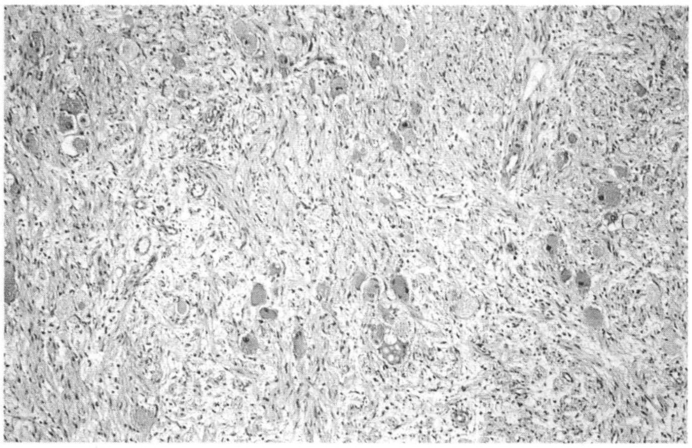

Figure 5.34 Ganglioneuroma. The tumour is composed of Schwann cells, ganglion cells and nerve fibres

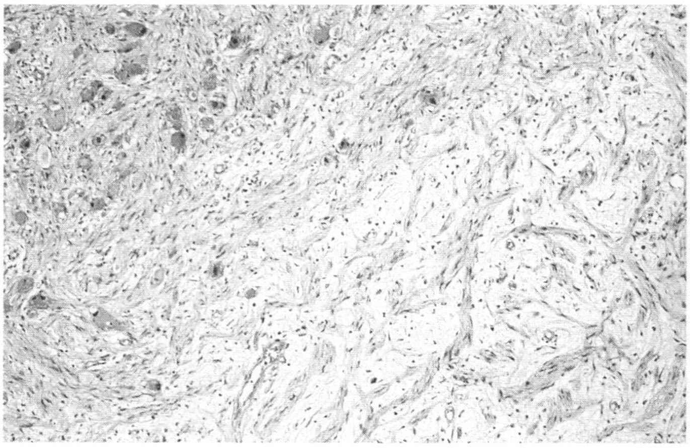

Figure 5.35 Ganglioneuroma. Same tumour. On the right, note the resemblance to a neurofibroma

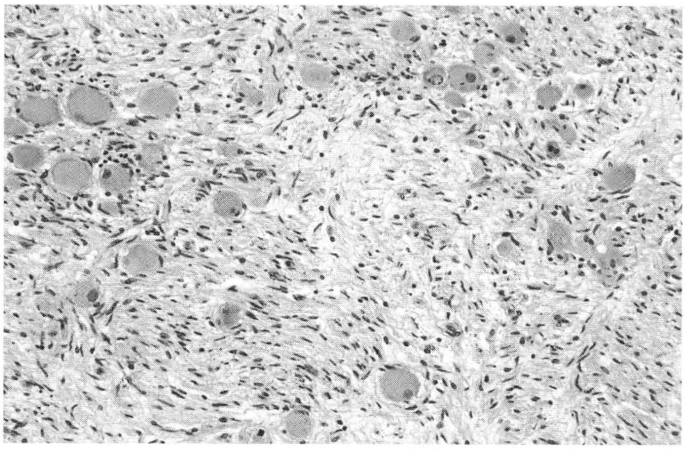

Figure 5.36 Ganglioneuroma. Mature ganglion cells are large, with an abundant cytoplasm and an eccentric nucleus

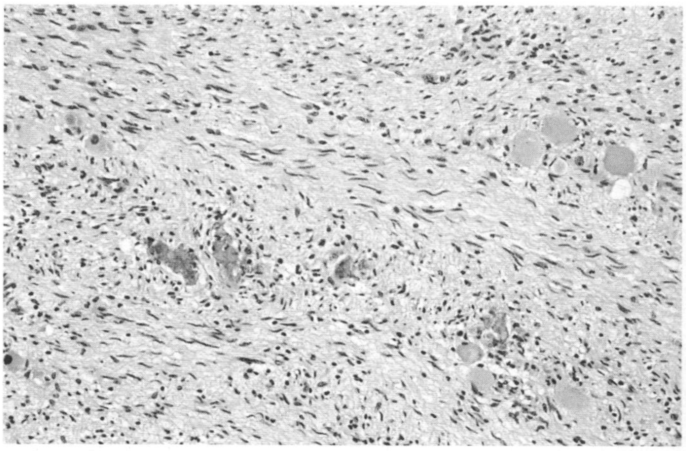

Figure 5.37 Ganglioneuroma. Same tumour. Cluster of calcifications

Tomisawa, M., Sawada, T., Imashuku, S., Takada, H., Inui, A. and Kusunoki, T. (1975) Ultrastructural observations of functional neural tumor. *Acta Paed. Jpn*, **79**, 313.
Tsuda, T., Masanobu, O., Hirano, H. *et al.* (1987) Analysis of N-myc amplification in relation to disease stage and histologic types in human neuroblastomas. *Cancer*, **60**, 820–826.
Yokoyama, M., Okada, K., Tokue, A., Takayasu, H. and Yamada, R. (1971) Ultrastructural and biochemical study of neuroblastoma and ganglioneuroblastoma. *Invest. Urol.*, **9**, 156.

Tumours of paraganglionic origin or paragangliomas: chemodectoma and phaeochromocytoma

Intrathoracic paragangliomas are infrequent tumours. Most of them are non-secreting chemodectomas originating from the aorticopulmonary paraganglia and developing in the superior or anterior mediastinum (Olson and Salyer, 1978; Lack *et al.*, 1979). These tumours usually present as incidentally discovered asymptomatic masses or more rarely in patients with symptoms of an intrathoracic mass, such as respiratory distress. They occur in patients over the age of 40, with an equal sex ratio.

Functioning paragangliomas or phaeochromocytoma are very uncommon and are likely to be localized in the posterior mediastinum (Nigam *et al.*, 1981; Ogawa *et al.*, 1982; Sheps and Brown, 1985). Patients with functioning tumours have paroxysmal or persistent hypertension, palpitation, headaches, and flushing or sweating spells in various combinations, with increased urinary vanilmandelic acid and other catecholamine metabolites. These tumours are more common in males (sex ratio 2:1), occur in younger patients, and often develop in children (one-third of the incidence).

Mediastinal paragangliomas are sometimes multiple, or arise in familial clusters with an autosomal dominant genetic transmission. They may also be associated with neurofibromatosis, or von Hippel-Lindau disease (Pritchett, 1982; Glenner and Grimley, 1974). Carney's triad is a very rare syndrome characterized by the association of functioning paraganglioma, pulmonary chondroma and gastric leiomyosarcoma.

On chest radiograph paragangliomas appear as a lobated mass situated either in the aorticopulmonary area (Figs 5.38 and 5.39) or in the paravertebral region, along the sympathetic chains. The tumours are highly vascularized at aortography. Computerized tomographic (CT) scan shows the rich vascular supply and gives better definition of the relationship of the tumour to adjacent tissues.

Morphological features

Mascroscopically, paragangliomas are circumscribed lobated tumours. The cut surface is pink-grey or red (Fig. 5.40). Haemorrhages, cystic areas, calcifications, or dense fibrous scarring areas occasionally occur. Chromaffin test on fresh tissue may reveal a dark-brown colour in the secreting tumours*.

Histologically, branchiomeric paragangliomas closely resemble the normal paraganglion tissue and appear to derive principally from the chief cell component. They are composed predominantly of large polygonal and ovoid cells with an abundant eosinophilic granular cytoplasm and vesicular nuclei. In some areas there is an admixture of large and small cells with a dark cytoplasm and hyperchromatic nuclei (the so-called light and dark cells). The tumour cells are arranged in nests or alveoli with a highly vascularized interstitial stroma (Figs 5.41 and 5.42). They show some nuclear pleomorphism and occasional mitoses, but no morphological features clearly distinguish a malignant from a benign paraganglioma. Sustentacular cells are rare or absent (Fig. 5.43). Intracytoplasmic granules comparable to those in normal chief cells are positively stained by the Masson Fontana and Grimelius techniques. In the branchiomeric paragangliomas the chromaffin reaction is usually negative whereas the formalin-induced fluorescence method depicts many cells as having a green to yellow–green colour consistent with the presence of catecholamine. According to Glenner and Grimley (1974), there is no relationship between the abundance of granules, catecholamine storage, catecholamine secretion, and a positive chromaffin reaction.

The aorticosympathetic paragangliomas may resemble a branchiomeric paraganglioma or an adrenal phaeochromocytoma, or have an intermediate feature of both. Most, however, are similar to the adrenal phaeochromocytomas. They are composed of small, polygonal or slightly spindly cells, arranged in irregular anastomosing sheets surrounded by a delicate vascular network. Chromaffin reaction is positive in about half of the cases.

Ultrastructurally, three distinct cell types are present within the tumours: endothelial cells, pericytes and neoplastic chief cells. Sustentacular cells are infrequent and difficult to distinguish from pericytes. The neoplastic chief cells are characterized by the presence of intracytoplasmic membrane-bound neurosecretory granules measuring 100–200 nm in diameter (Lack *et al.*, 1979; Fig. 5.44).

The immunological profile of paraganglioma is that of tumours of neuronal origin. The chief cells are positive for neuron-specific enolase and neurofilament protein. Chromogranin, one of the matrix proteins of the dense core granule, may also be localized in these cells. The sustentacular cells, which are considered as modified Schwann cells, are positively stained with S-100 protein.

Differential diagnosis

It is necessary to distinguish paragangliomas from other endocrine tumours, of primary or metastatic origin, that have a similar alveolar pattern. In the mediastinum, medullary carcinoma of the thyroid and thymic carcinoid must be considered. Carcinoid tumours are characterized by typical features such as ribbons, festoons, and rosettes. The cells are more uniform in appearance and the nuclei are polarized to the vascular margin of the cell nest. In order to elucidate the differential diagnosis, immunohistochemistry and electron microscopy are of great value. In the case of a catecholamine-producing tumour, CT scan is a very useful tool to eliminate a tumour located in the adrenal medulla, and is helpful to localize an extra-adrenal secreting tumour.

Prognosis and treatment

The mediastinal paragangliomas have a rather aggressive course (Olson and Salyer, 1978), but the incidence of malignancy is not well established. It is estimated by Lack *et al.* (1979) at approximately 10% and ranges as widely as 3% to 50% in different series (Ogawa *et al.*, 1982). The most useful information in terms of prognosis derives from the degree of invasiveness of the tumours, and the outcome is more related to residual local spread of the neoplasm than to the effect of metastatic tumours (Odze and Bégin, 1989). However, the incidence of metastasis appears to be related to the length of the follow-up period.

The treatment of choice is surgical resection but the

*The chromaffin reaction is the dark-brown colour produced by a dichromate solution in the presence of catecholamines. Glenner and Grimley (1974) discuss the value of this reaction in the classification of paragangliomas as chromaffin and non-chromaffin. Indeed the chromaffinity is altered by fixation, and the typical dark-brown colour is produced by epinephrine, whereas norepinephrine yields only a yellow or yellow-brown non-characteristic colour. Thus, the chromaffin reaction may be negative in cases of catecholamine-secreting tumours.

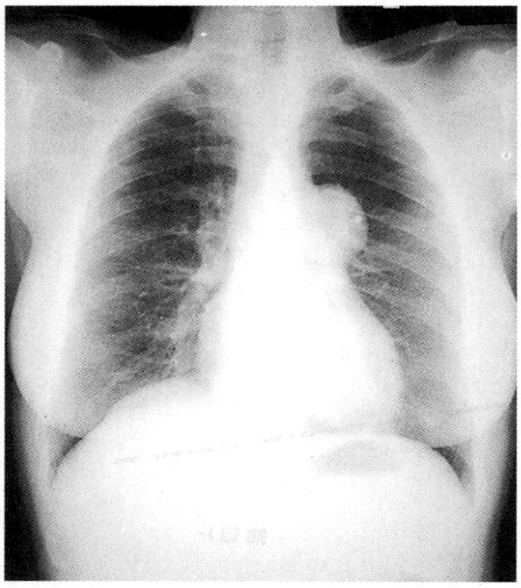

Figures 5.38 and 5.39 Aorticopulmonary paraganglioma. Chest radiographs demonstrate a well-delimited mass in the aorticopulmonary area. **Fig. 5.38**: Posteroanterior view; **Fig. 5.39**: lateral view

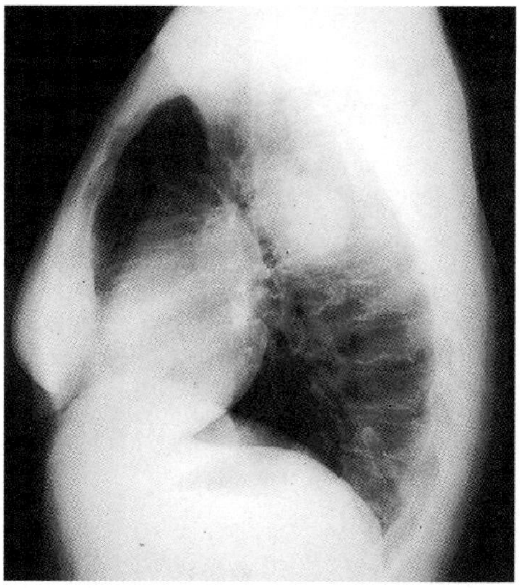

Figure 5.39

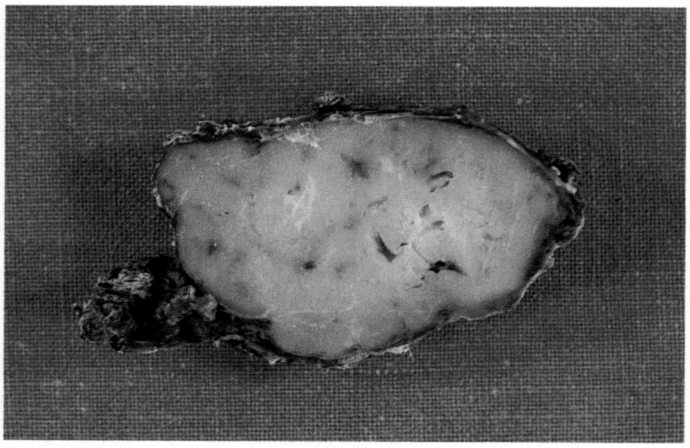

Figure 5.40 Aorticopulmonary paraganglioma. The tumour is well-circumscribed and pink–yellow (Figs 5.38 through 5.40 are from the same patient.)

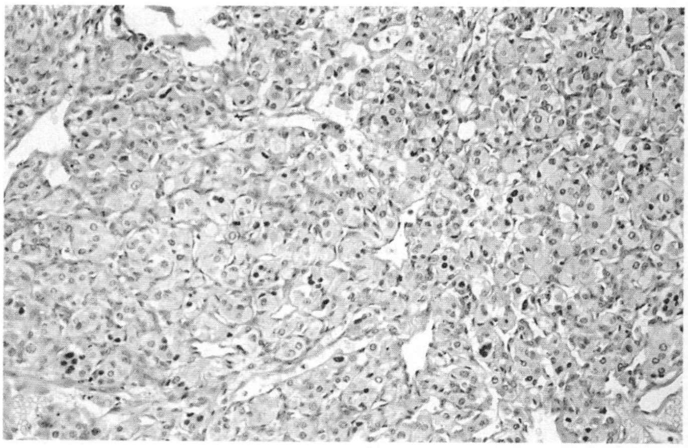

Figure 5.41 Aorticopulmonary paraganglioma. The tumour is composed of nests of large cells (chief cells) surrounded by a prominent vascular network

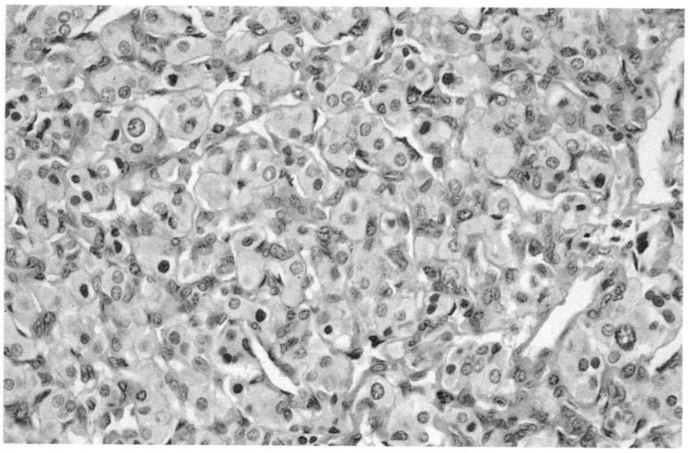

Figure 5.42 Aorticopulmonary paraganglioma. The tumour cells have an abundant clear eosinophilic cytoplasm and vesicular nuclei

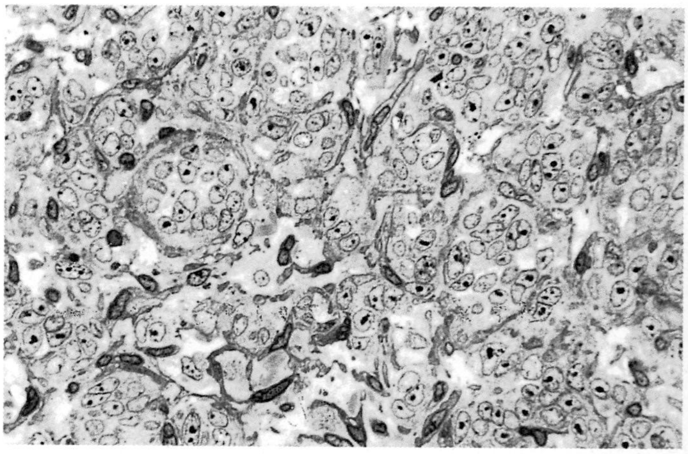

Figure 5.43 Aorticopulmonary paraganglioma. A half-thin section of the same tumour illustrates the presence of well-defined sustentacular cells

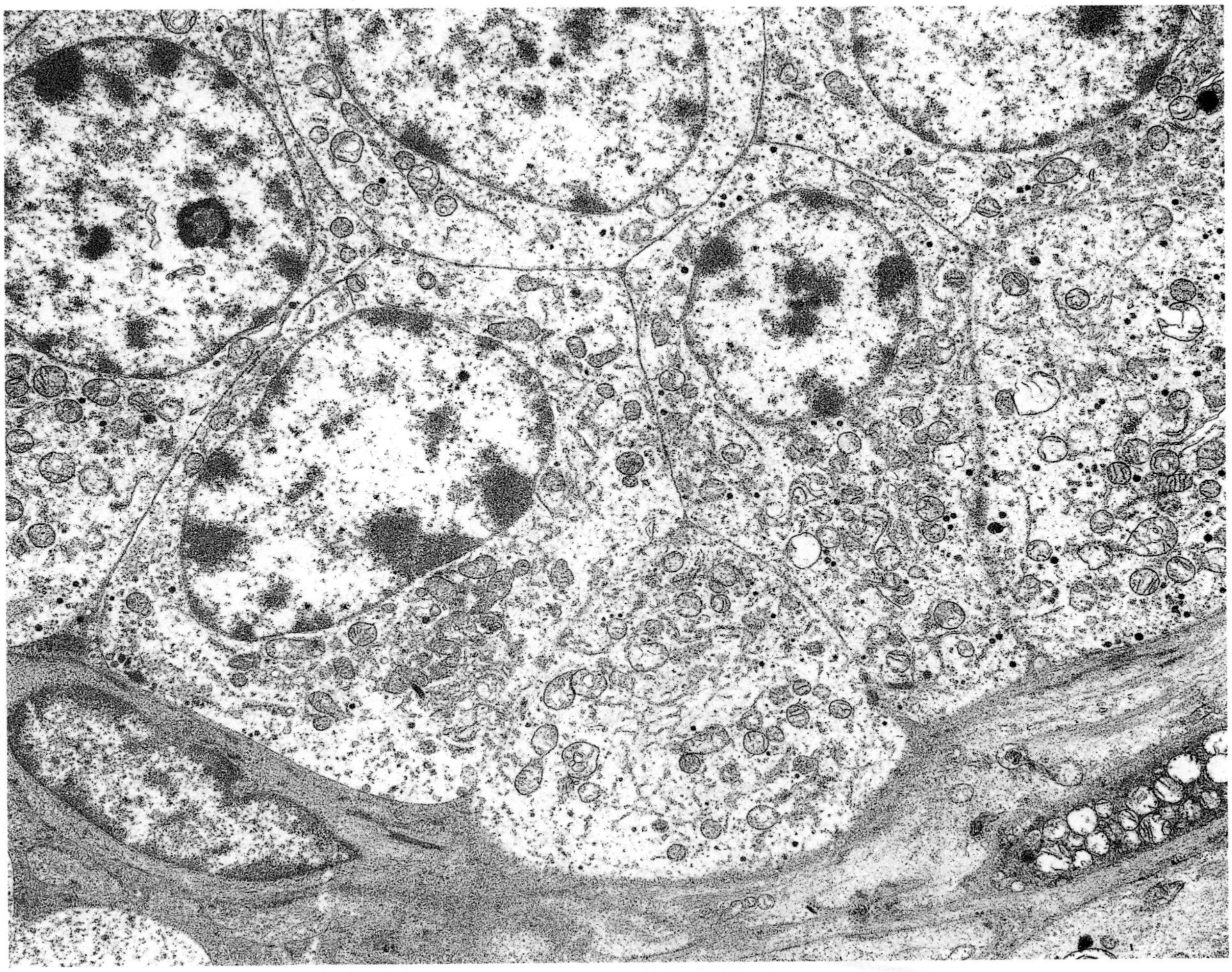

Figure 5.44 Aorticopulmonary paraganglioma. The electron microscopic study shows the characteristic features of the neoplastic chief cells containing intracytoplasmic neurosecretory granules. At the bottom, sustentacular cells are present

intimate relation of the tumours to the great vessels, their rich vascular supply and the neoplastic invasion of vital structures in the mediastinum may preclude a complete excision. When complete resection is impossible, complementary radiotherapy may be of value.

References

Glenner, G. G. and Grimley, P. M. (1974) Tumors of the extra-adrenal paraganglion system (including chemoreceptors). In *Atlas of Tumor Pathology*, 2nd series, fasc. 9. Armed Forces Institute of Pathology, Washington, DC.

Lack, E. E., Stillinger, R. A., Colvin, D. B., Groves, R. M., and Burnette, D. G. (1979) Aortico-pulmonary paraganglioma. Report of a case with ultrastructural study and review of the literature. *Cancer*, **43**, 269–278.

Nigam, B. K., Hyer, S. L., Taylor, E. J. and Guha, T. (1981) Intrathoracic chemodectoma with noradrenaline secretion. *Thorax*, **36**, 66–68.

Odze, R. and Bégin, L. R. (1990) Malignant paraganglioma of the posterior mediastinum. A case report and review of the literature. *Cancer*, **65**, 564–569.

Ogawa, J., Inoue, H., Koide, S., Kawada, S., Shohtsu, A. and Hata, J. (1982) Functioning paraganglioma in the posterior mediastinum. *Ann. Thorac. Surg.*, **33**, 507–510.

Olson, J. L. and Salyer, M. W. R. (1978) Mediastinal paragangliomas (aortic body tumor). A report of four cases and a review of the literature. *Cancer*, **41**, 2405–2412.

Pritchett, J. W. (1982) Familial concurrence of carotid body tumor and pheochromocytoma. *Cancer*, **49**, 2578–2579.

Sheps, S. G. and Brown, M. L. (1985) Localization of mediastinal paragangliomas (pheochromocytoma). *Chest*, **87**, 807–809.

PRIMITIVE NEUROECTODERMAL TUMOURS OF PERIPHERAL NERVE AND RELATED NEOPLASMS

Although the existence of Askin's tumour as a separate entity is controversial and the histogenesis of Ewing's sarcoma is still debated, modern investigations strongly indicate that peripheral neuroepithelioma, Askin's tumour and Ewing's sarcoma are related tumours of neuroectodermal origin, Ewing's sarcoma representing the most immature form of these neoplasms. The three tumours possess common histological and ultrastructural aspects, immunohistochemical neural expression, and the same cytogenetic abnormalities. They are separate clinicopathological entities from conventional neuroblastomas because of different predilections for site and age, absence of urinary excretion of catecholamine, lack of N-myc oncogene expression, and presence of 11:22 chromosomal translocation (Llombart-Bosch *et al.*, 1987; Fujii *et al.*, 1989; Pappo *et al.*, 1989; Pinto *et al.*, 1989; Ushigome *et al.*, 1989; Table 5.9).

Peripheral neuroectodermal tumour

(neuroepithelioma, peripheral neuroblastoma)

Neuroepitheliomas are rare tumours of adolescents and young adults with a median of 11–21 years according to the different series. They arise from peripheral nerves in soft tissues of lower extremity, trunk, and retroperitoneum. A thoracopulmonary location is predominant, involving the posterior chest wall with frequent bone involvement, or the paravertebral region (Jürgens *et al.*, 1988).

Despite localized disease at presentation, the tumour has an unusually aggressive course with high tendency to invade the pleura, lung, and diaphragm and to recur locally. Unlike neuroblastoma or Ewing's sarcoma, widespread or skeletal metastases are uncommon (Gonzalez-Crussi *et al.*, 1984).

The prognosis is poor. The best results are obtained with aggressive combined treatment including radical surgery, chemotherapy and irradiation (Marina *et al.*, 1989). Chemotherapy regimens designed for the treatment of Ewing's sarcoma or soft-tissue sarcoma are superior to those designed for neuroblastoma (anthracyclines and high doses of alkylating agents).

Macroscopically the tumours are often well limited. The cut surface is grey–white and lobulated, showing numerous foci of calcification and yellow discoloration (Fig. 5.45).

Histology

The tumours are morphologically poorly differentiated and composed of sheets of closely aggregated non-cohesive round cells of high nucleocytoplasmic ratio (so-called small blue round-cell tumours; Fig. 5.46). The nuclei are frequently vesicular and the nucleoli indistinct. The mitoses are frequent.

Large areas lack any architectural pattern, whereas others show a semblance of row orientation or a more characteristic interweaving arrangement of the cells within a background of abundant eosinophilic fibrillary and vacuolar material forming a pattern of irregular pseudorosettes (Figs 5.47–5.49). Well-formed rosettes with a central fibrillary core (Homer–Wright rosettes) are generally only focally present in isolated tumour areas. There is a conspicuous absence of blood vessels and foci of necrosis are frequent. Calcifications may be observed. Diastase-sensitive periodic acid-Schiff (PAS) staining for glycogen is positive in most cases.

Immunohistochemistry

Neuron-specific enolase staining is positive in the cytoplasm of isolated tumour cells and in the centre of the rosettes. S-100 protein and neurofilament (NF) are generally positive in most of the tumours. Leu-7 is positive, as well as vimentin. Cytokeratin is sometimes expressed (Table 5.8).

Electron microscopy

Electron microscopic study reveals the poor differentiation of the tumours, but demonstrates features of neuroectodermal lineage. Tumour cells range from 10 to 16 μm and contain abundant free ribosomes, few cytoplasmic organelles and poorly developed cell junctions. Basal laminae are not observed. In the more differentiated areas the cells are larger and possess small cell processes suggestive of dendritic prolongations. The cytoplasm contains microtubules averaging 25 nm in diameter, generally situated in the paranuclear region, and fine filaments, approximately 5 nm in diameter, often placed in the cell processes. Scarce dense-core neurosecretory granules 150–200 nm in diameter are present.

Malignant small-cell tumour of the thoracopulmonary region (Askin's tumour)

The separation of Askin's tumour from peripheral neuroblastoma is the subject of controversy.

Askin's tumour has been initially described as a unique clinicopathologic entity corresponding to a malignant small-cell tumour of the thoracopulmonary region in children and young adults (Askin *et al.*, 1979). Following this first description, tumours with similar features were seen in other localizations.

There is a slight female predilection for this tumour, which appears to originate predominantly in the soft tissues of the chest wall or the peripheral lung. As do peripheral neuroepithelioma, Askin's tumour tends to recur locally and does not seem to disseminate as widely as neuroblastoma or Ewing's sarcoma. In Askin's series the prognosis was poor, the median survival being only 8 months.

Histology

Compact sheets of cells, a nesting arrangement of cells with an intervening fibrovascular stroma, and serpiginous bands of cells with necrosis are the three basic microscopic patterns. Tumour cells are small, measuring 10–14 μm in diameter, and comprise scanty cytoplasm and large oval nuclei with coarse evenly dispersed chromatin (Fig. 5.50). The mitotic activity is moderate. Rosette-like structures are occasionally found, but without neurofibrillary material. Special histological stains for glycogen (PAS with diastase digestion), formerly described as negative by Askin *et al.*, was occasionally positive in other studies.

Immunohistochemistry shows evidence of neural features, such as expression of neuron-specific enolase, S-100 protein, and neurofilaments (Table 5.8). *Electron microscope studies* reveal ultrastructural features suggesting neural differentiation, such as cytoplasmic processes containing microtubules, and scarce dense-core granules.

Ewing's sarcoma

Ewing's sarcoma is an undifferentiated small round-cell neoplasm that may present in typical or atypical forms, and develops in bone or in soft tissue (extraskeletal Ewing's sarcoma).

To date, there is increasing evidence that Ewing's sarcoma may derive from primitive, pluripotential cells that differentiate into cells with mesenchymal, epithelial and neural features, and that there is a continuum from primitive neuroectodermal tumour or Askin's tumour to Ewing's sarcoma that express neural features in various degrees.

Extraskeletal Ewing's sarcoma is a neoplasm of soft tissues in children and young adults that usually involves the soft tissues of the lower extremities, the paravertebral regions, and the chest wall. The lungs and the skeleton are the most common sites of metastases. Prognosis is considered to be good when wide local resection of the tumour is completed at early stages of the disease and combined with radiation therapy and chemotherapy (Rud *et al.*, 1989).

Histology

The tumours are composed of small rounded, closely packed cells showing predominantly a diffuse pattern or, less frequently, a lobular or filigree pattern, with an interspersed fibrovascular stroma (Fig. 5.51). The cells are characterized by scanty cytoplasm containing abundant diastase-sensitive PAS-positive glycogen. The nuclei are round with finely dispersed chromatin and inconspicuous nucleoli. Mitotic figures are occasionally seen. Pseudo-

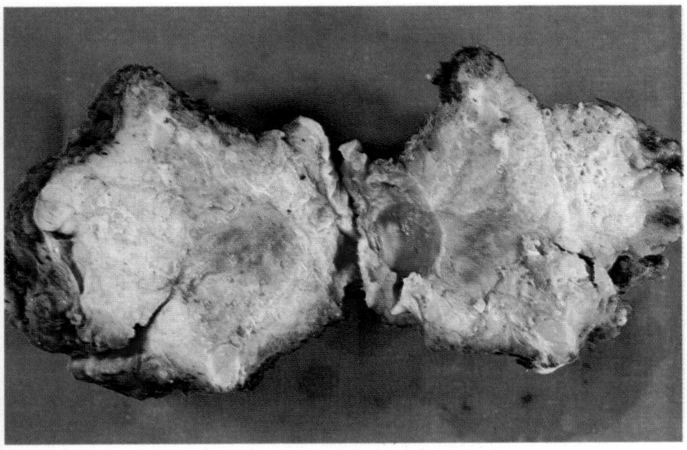

Figure 5.45 Neuroepithelioma. Irregular fleshy tumour with extensive areas of necrosis

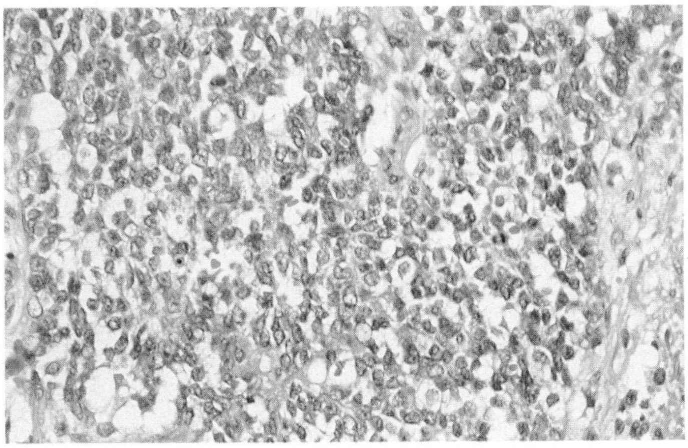

Figure 5.46 Neuroepithelioma. Poorly differentiated tumour composed of sheets of non-cohesive small round cells with hyperchromatic nuclei

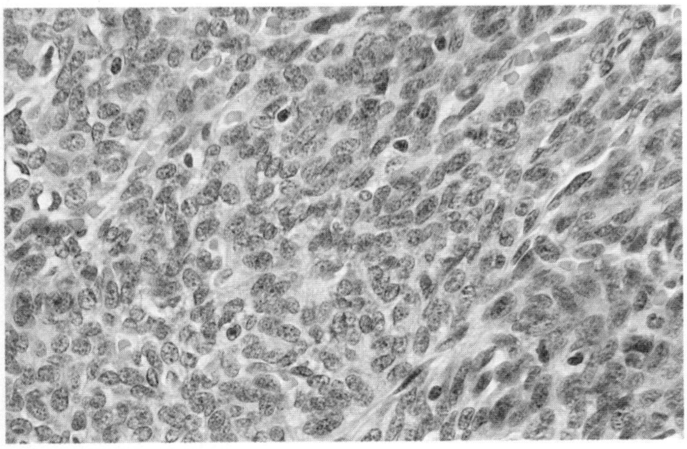

Figures 5.47–5.49 Neuroepithelioma. The figures illustrate different aspects of a slightly differentiated tumour showing areas simulating a small-cell carcinoma (**Fig. 5.47**), row arrangements reminiscent of a carcinoid tumour (**Fig. 5.48**), and a pattern of Homer–Wright rosettes, as seen in neuroblastomas (**Fig. 5.49**)

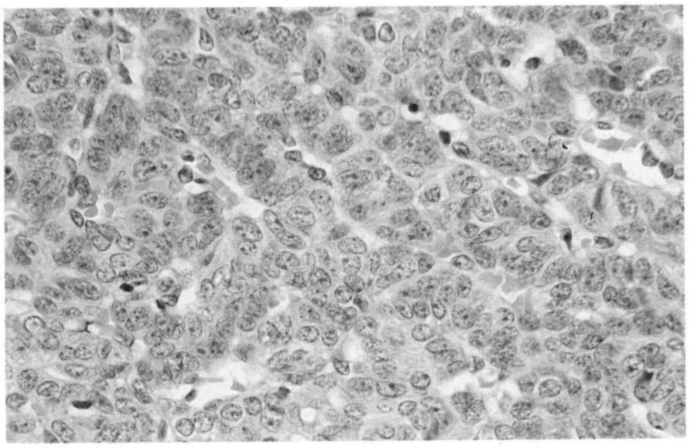

Figure 5.48

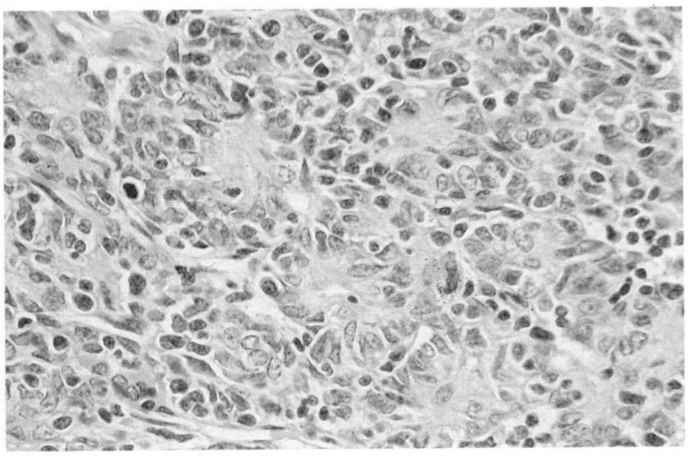

Figure 5.49

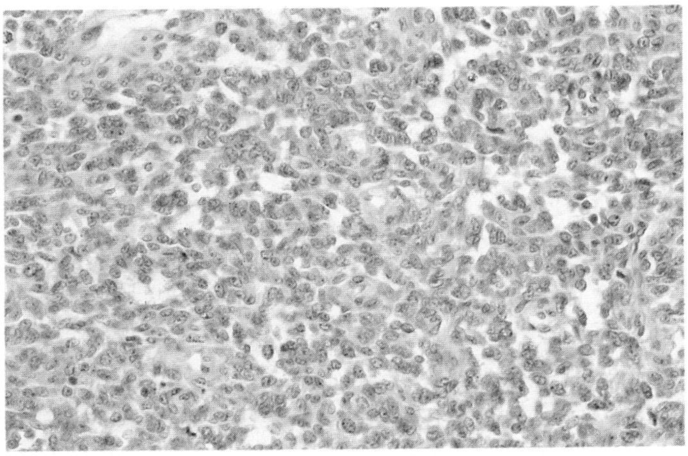

Figure 5.50 Askin's tumour. The tumour is composed of compact sheets of small cells with large hyperchromatic nuclei. The aspect is very similar to that of the poorly differentiated neuroepithelioma illustrated on Fig. 5.46

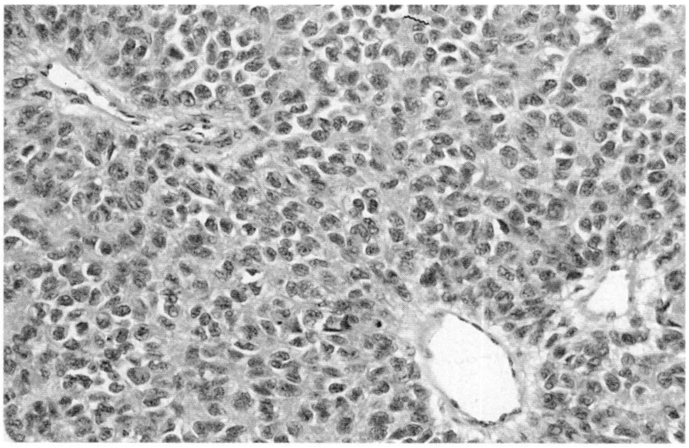

Figure 5.51 Ewing's sarcoma. The tumour has a diffuse pattern and is composed of closely packed small cells with a scanty cytoplasm and large hyperchromatic nuclei

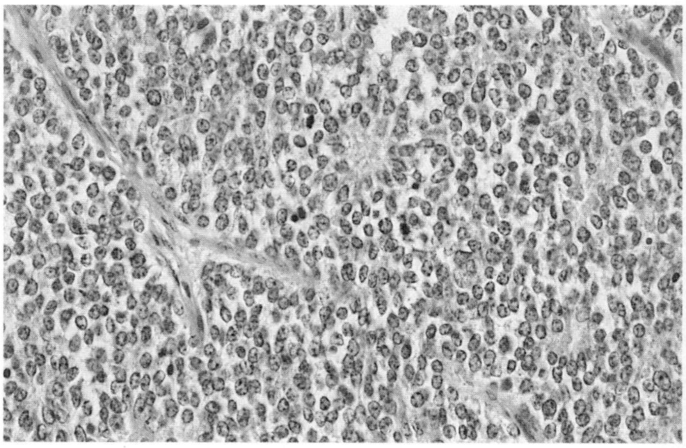

Figure 5.52 Ewing's sarcoma. In another tumour, note the presence of rosettes

rosettes are frequently observed and rosette-like structures with a central fibrillary core (Homer–Wright rosettes) are found in approximately 10% of the cases (Fig. 5.52).

Immunohistochemistry

Immunohistochemical studies demonstrate that neuron-specific enolase, S-100 protein, Leu-7, and neurofilament are inconstantly expressed by the tumour cells. Whereas neuron-specific enolase is positive in only a few cases, vimentin, cytokeratin and epithelial membrane antigens are coexpressed in most cases of Ewing's sarcoma, supporting the concept that Ewing's sarcoma may be derived from primitive, pluripotential cells, differentiating into mesenchymal, epithelial, and neural features in variable proportions (Fujii *et al.*, 1989; Ushigome *et al.*, 1989; Table 5.8). Although immunohistochemical neural expression (NSE, S-100 protein, and neurofilament) is inconsistently found in Ewing's sarcoma, it is noteworthy that undifferentiated Ewing's sarcoma cell lines can be induced to neural differentiation under certain conditions *in vitro*. Ultrastructurally these cells show the characteristics of neurites and dense core granules, and finally begin to express NSE or/and NF reactivity.

Electron microscopy

Electron microscopic studies show predominantly primitive cells with relatively scanty cytoplasm and rather scarce organelles. Glycogen is frequently observed and fine intracytoplasmic filaments of intermediate type are often present, especially around the nuclei. Cell processes, neurosecretory granules, and microtubules are encountered only occasionally.

References

Askin, F. B., Rosai, J., Sibley, R. K., Dehner, L. P. and McAlister, W. H. (1979) Malignant small cell tumor of the thoracopulmonary region in childhood. A distinctive clinicopathologic entity of uncertain histogenesis. *Cancer*, **43**, 2438–2451.

Fujii, Y., Hongo, T., Nakagawa, Y., Nasuda, K., Mizuno, Y., Igarashi, Y., Naito, Y. and Maeda, M. (1989) Cell culture of small round cell tumor originating in the thoracopulmonary region. Evidence for derivation from a primitive pluripotent cell. *Cancer*, **64**, 43–51.

Gonzalez-Crussi, F., Wolfson, S. L., Misugi, K. and Nakajima, T. (1984) Peripheral neuroectodermal tumors of the chest wall in childhood. *Cancer*, **54**, 2519–2527.

Jürgens, H., Bier, V., Harms, D., Beck, J., Brandeis, W., Etspüler, G., Gadner, H., Schmidt, D., Treuner, J., Winkler, K. and Göbel, U. (1988) Malignant peripheral neuroectodermal tumors. A retrospective analysis of 42 patients. *Cancer*, **61**, 349–357.

Llombart-Bosch, A., Lacombe, M. J., Contesso, G. and Peydro-Olaya, A. (1987) Small round blue cell sarcoma of bone mimicking atypical Ewing's sarcoma with neuroectodermal features. An analysis of five cases with immunohistochemical and electron microscopic support. *Cancer*, **60**, 1570–1582.

Marina, N. M., Etcubanas, E., Parham, D. M., Bowman, L. C. and Green, A. (1989) Peripheral primitive neuroectodermal tumor (peripheral neuroepithelioma) in children. A review of the St. Jude experience and controversies in diagnosis and management. *Cancer*, **64**, 1952–1960.

Pappo, A. S., Cheah, M. S. C., Saldivar, V. A., Britton, H. A. and Parmley, R. T. (1989) Disseminated primitive neuroectodermal tumor: Diagnosis using immunocytochemistry, electron microscopy, and molecular probes. *Cancer*, **63**, 2515–2521.

Pinto, A., Grant, L. H., Hayes, F. A., Schell, M. J. and Parham, D. M. (1989) Immunohistochemical expression of neuron-specific enolase and Leu 7 in Ewing's sarcoma of bone. *Cancer*, **64**, 1266–1273.

Rud, N. P., Reiman, H. M., Pritchard, D. J., Frassica, F. J. and Smithson, W. A. (1989) Extraosseous Ewing's sarcoma. A study of 42 cases. *Cancer*, **64**, 1548–1553.

Ushigome, S., Shimoda, T., Takaki, K. *et al.* (1989) Immunocytochemical and ultrastructural studies of the histogenesis of Ewing's sarcoma and putatively related tumors. *Cancer*, **64**, 52–62.

TUMOURS OF THE DIFFUSE NEUROENDOCRINE SYSTEM

The place of neuroendocrine tumours of the mediastinum in the chapter of neural tumours may appear debatable in so far as their endodermal or neural crest histogenesis is still discussed. Moreover, considerable controversy exists concerning the relationship between carcinoid tumour and oat-cell carcinoma. Irrespective of the histogenesis, however, it seems justified to describe these tumours under the heading of neuroendocrine tumours and in the framework of neural tumours, since all of them express morphological, immunohistochemical and biological features of neural crest-derived tumours.

Their nomenclature also remains controversial. The term 'carcinoid tumour' was first introduced by Rosai and Higa (1972) to identify a mediastinal endocrine neoplasm, of probable thymic origin, distinctly different from thymomas. Later, 'oat-cell carcinoma' of the thymus was reported as the malignant counterpart of thymic carcinoid (Rosai *et al.*, 1976; Wick and Scheithauer, 1982), but other authors introduced this neoplasm as a subgroup of thymic carcinomas (Kuo *et al.*, 1990; see Chapter 2).

As in other localizations the mediastinal neuroendocrine neoplasms show a spectrum of morphological aspects and of clinical behaviour. In parallel to the classification proposed by Gould *et al.* (1983) in the cases of neuroendocrine tumours of the lung, it would be more accurate to subdivide the thymic neuroendocrine tumours into (1) the carcinoid tumour as the very well-differentiated variant of these tumours, (2) the well-differentiated neuroendocrine carcinoma that is more atypical histologically and clinically more aggressive, and (3) the poorly differentiated neuroendocrine carcinoma or oat-cell carcinoma showing highly aggressive clinical behaviour. Most of the thymic carcinoids are aggressive tumours with a poor prognosis and would be best classified as differentiated neuroendocrine carcinoma.

Although it is not excluded that neuroendocrine neoplasms may arise in any part of the mediastinum, most of them develop from the thymus. Thymic carcinoid tumours are infrequent, and fewer than 100 cases have been reported in the world literature (Economopoulos *et al.*, 1990). Oat-cell carcinomas of the thymus are considered as exceedingly rare, and very few cases have been reported (Duguid and Kennedy, 1930; Rosai *et al.*, 1976; Wick and Scheithauer, 1982), but their frequency is certainly underestimated.

Clinical features

Neuroendocrine tumours of the thymus have significant clinical features that distinguish them from both thymomas and from carcinoid tumours of other origin. They occur in a wide age range with a predilection for the fourth decade and a strong predominance in males (male to female ratio 4:1).

The most common presentation of a thymic neuroendocrine tumour is that of an anterior mediastinal mass. Clinical symptoms such as pain, cough, dyspnoea, or vena cava syndrome are not distinctive. A major characteristic for these tumours is the presence, in 30–50% of cases, of a number of associated disorders, the most common of which is Cushing's syndrome (Rosai *et al.*, 1972; Lowenthal *et al.*, 1974; Marchevsky and Dikman, 1979; Wick *et al.*, 1980; Gelfand *et al.*, 1981; Pass *et al.*, 1990). The tumours with associated disorders are considered as more aggressive than those without accompanying disorders, except for ectopic ACTH production whose prognostic significance is discussed (Odell, 1990). Table 5.10 indicates the decreasing frequency of these associated diseases. It must be underlined that the tumours are not associated with the carcinoid syndrome.

Cushing's syndrome is characterized by a cushingoid habitus, weakness, weight gain, oedema, hypertension and hyperpigmentation. The patients have hypokalaemic alkalosis, along with elevated cortisol serum levels and urinary free cortisol elevation. Pituitary independence of the ectopic ACTH production is assessed by the dexamethasone suppression test, the metyrapone stimulation test and the ovine corticotropin-releasing hormone stimulation test (Pass *et al.*, 1990).

Multiple endocrine adenomatosis (MEA) is a familial disorder characterized by the presence of neoplasms or hyperplasias of endocrine glands. The organs most often affected are the parathyroids, pancreatic islets, and pituitary gland, followed by the adrenals and thyroid. Lesions in any of these glands may be hormonally active. In MEA I (Wermer) syndrome, hyperparathyroidism and Zollinger–Ellison syndrome are the two most prominent functional manifestations (Wermer, 1963). MEA II (Sipple) syndrome is characterized by the association of medullary carcinoma of the thyroid, phaeochromocytoma, parathyroid enlargement and neuromas (Sipple, 1961). The existence of a thymic carcinoid as a part of a multiple endocrine adenomatosis syndrome, along with the possible coexistence of carcinoid tumours of the bronchus, stomach and ileum (Rosai *et al.*, 1972; Lowenthal *et al.*, 1974, and others) is consistent with the concept of a neural crest origin.

Chest roentgenogram, computed tomography and magnetic resonance imaging show evidence of an anterior mediastinal mass. The tumour may be well limited and encapsulated but more frequently invades the adjacent structure or is accompanied by metastases to the lymph nodes (Figs 5.53—5.56).

Macroscopy

Thymic carcinoid tumours are large, hard, nodular, well-vascularized tumours (Fig. 5.57). The cut section is grey–white or tan, fleshy, lobular, with foci of necrosis and haemorrhagic areas. Focal calcification, with a gross 'sand grain' texture of the cut surface, is often present.

The poorly differentiated neuroendocrine tumours or oat-cell carcinomas are largely invading, highly vascular, soft and pinkish-white masses showing at section extensive areas of necrosis and haemorrhage.

Histology

Carcinoid tumours of the thymus are composed of uniform, round to oval cells of medium size, with a faintly granular, eosinophilic, relatively scanty cytoplasm and a central round or oval vesicular nucleus. The cytoplasm contains argyrophilic granules detected with the Grimelius and Sevier–Munger methods, but argentaffin staining is negative. The nuclear chromatin is finely scattered and nucleoli are inconspicuous. Mitotic figures are always present, their number varying from case to case. The tumour cells are arranged in lobules, sheets or nests growing in a rather loose, well-vascularized connective tissue (Figs 5.58–5.61). The formation of rosettes, ribbons and festoons is also a characteristic feature that confers an endocrine pattern to the neoplasm. Areas of necrosis, calcifications, invasion of lymphatic and blood vessels are other common findings. The thymic carcinoid thus resembles an atypical carcinoid, according to the criteria proposed by Arrigoni *et al.* (1972). A spindle-cell variant is occasinally observed (Levine and Rosai, 1976; Fig. 5.62). A case of pigmented carcinoid containing melanin has also been reported (Ho and Ho, 1977). Unlike thymomas, thymic carcinoids lack features such as association with a lymphocyte component, perivascular spaces and medullary differentiation.

Oat-cell carcinoma of the thymus has the same histological pattern as high-grade malignant neuroendocrine tumours of other origins (Fig. 5.63). The tumour cells are small, anaplastic, round to fusiform, and have a scanty cytoplasm and a large ovoid nucleus with a stippled chromatin and a small nucleolus. The tumour cells grow in large sheets. Mitoses are always numerous, and areas of haemorrhage and necrosis are abundant. A histological transition between oat-cell carcinoma and recognizable carcinoid tumour has been reported by Wick and Scheithauer (1982).

Electron microscopy

Ultrastructurally, the thymic neuroendocrine tumours are similar to those found in other organs (Rosai and Higa, 1972; Wick and Scheithauer, 1982, 1984). In carcinoids, the tumour cells show smooth cytoplasmic borders and a few desmosomes. Nuclei are round to oval, and occasionally indented. They have an even, finely dispersed chromatin and small distinct nucleoli. The cytoplasm contains numerous round mitochondria with well-preserved cristae, a number of ergastoplasmic profiles and a well-developed Golgi apparatus. In addition, the cells contain a variable amount of characteristic dense core neurosecretory granules, 50 to 400 nm in diameter, scattered throughout the cytoplasm (Fig. 5.64) or concen-

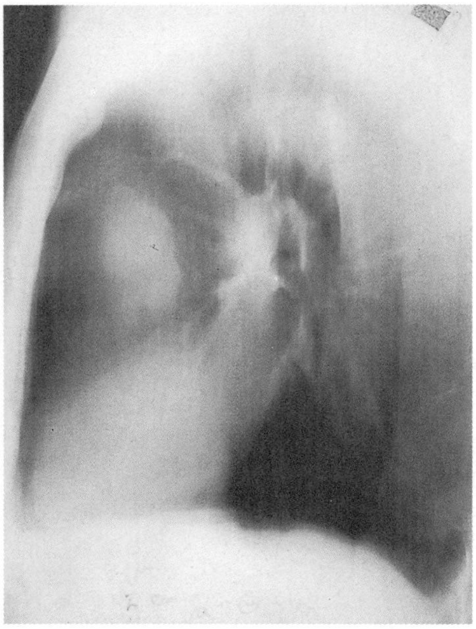

Figure 5.53 Carcinoid tumour of the thymus. Chest lateral tomography showing a well-delimited, medium-sized anterior mediastinal tumour. The histology of the tumour is illustrated on Fig. 5.62

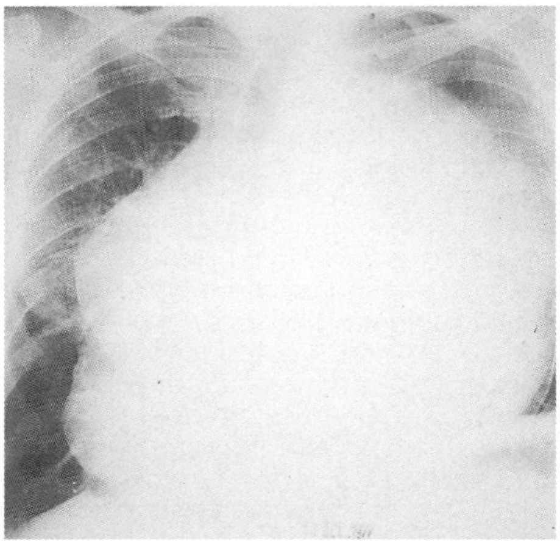

Figures 5.54 and 5.55 Chest radiographs of a patient with a differentiated neuroendocrine carcinoma (atypical carcinoid) of the thymus illustrating a very large anterior mediastinal mass protruding on both sides (**Fig. 5.54**: posteroanterior view; **Fig. 5.55**: lateral view). The histological aspect of the tumour is shown on Figs 5.58 and 5.59

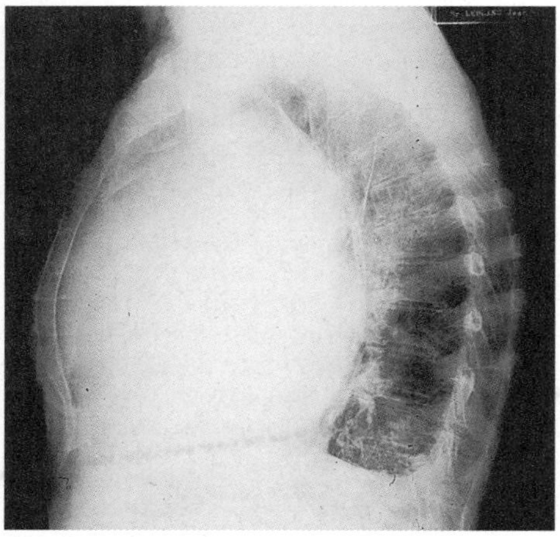

Figure 5.55

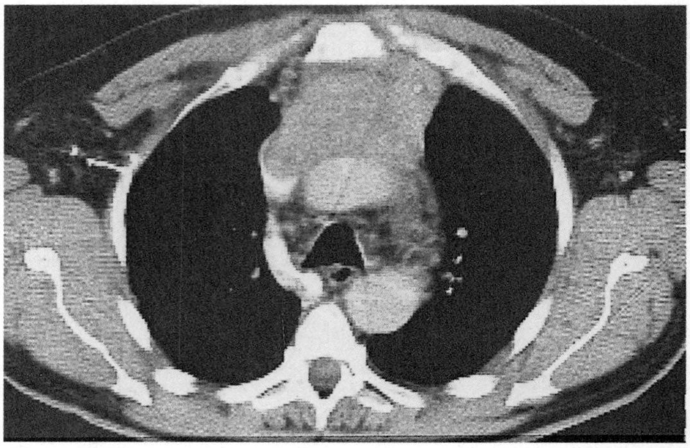

Figure 5.56 Computed tomography scan of a patient with a small-cell carcinoma of the thymus. Although the tumour is medium-sized and well-limited the histology shows a characteristic small-cell carcinoma (Fig. 5.63)

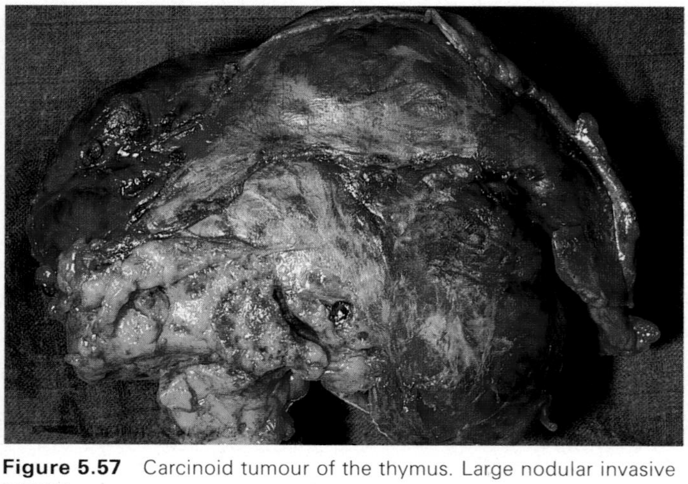

Figure 5.57 Carcinoid tumour of the thymus. Large nodular invasive tumour

trated at a pole. An intermittent basal lamina may be present between tumour cells and stroma. Elongated cytoplasmic processes, and broad tonofilaments, as seen in thymoma, are absent, but aggregates of fine, intertwining cytoplasmic fibrils are sometimes encountered. In oat-cell carcinoma the anaplastic cells are poor in organelles and the small rim of cytoplasm contains smaller and fewer membrane-bound neurosecretory granules (Fig. 5.65).

Immunohistochemistry

Most neuroendocrine tumours of the thymus react positively for specific neuroendocrine markers. Neuron-specific enolase (NSE) is the most likely to stain these tumours, but is the least specific (Fig. 5.66). Chromogranin, a membrane protein of the secretory granules in neuroendocrine cells, is highly specific but does not react with high-grade malignant neuroendocrine tumours because of the paucity of granules (Fig. 5.67). NF proteins are also present in thymic neuroendocrine tumours (Flinner and Hammond, 1989).

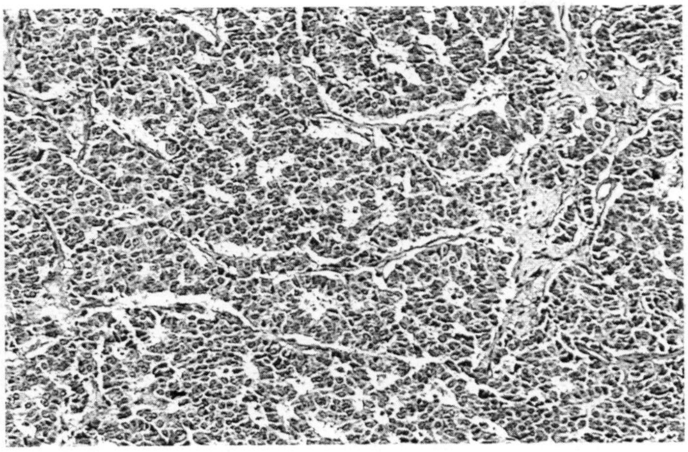

Figure 5.58 Carcinoid tumour of the thymus. The tumour is characteristically composed of ribbons and rosettes, disposed in a well-vascularized connective tissue

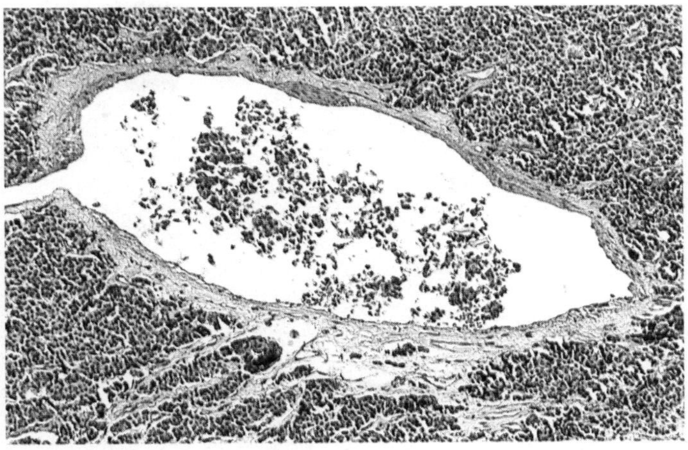

Figure 5.59 Carcinoid tumour of the thymus. The figure shows a more aggressive pattern with a vascular invasion. (Figures 5.54, 5.55 and 5.58 are from the same tumour.)

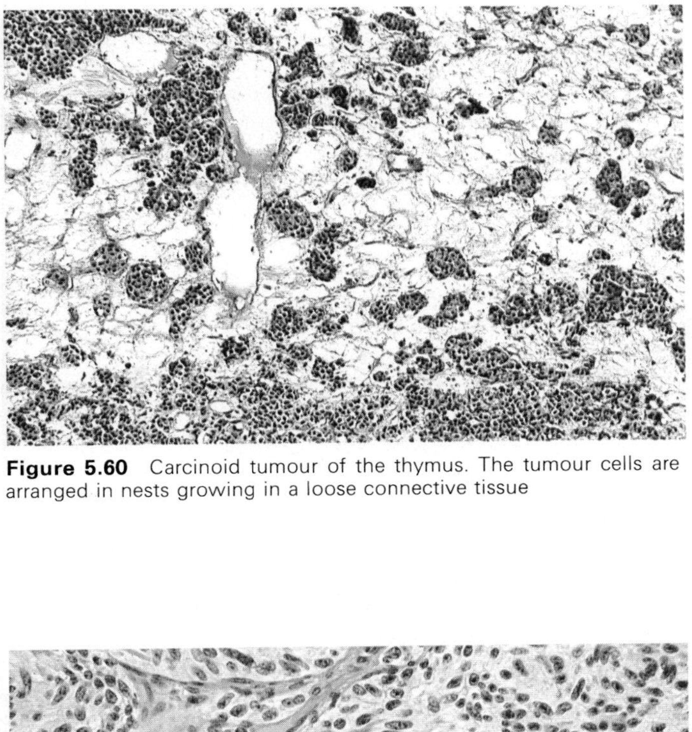

Figure 5.60 Carcinoid tumour of the thymus. The tumour cells are arranged in nests growing in a loose connective tissue

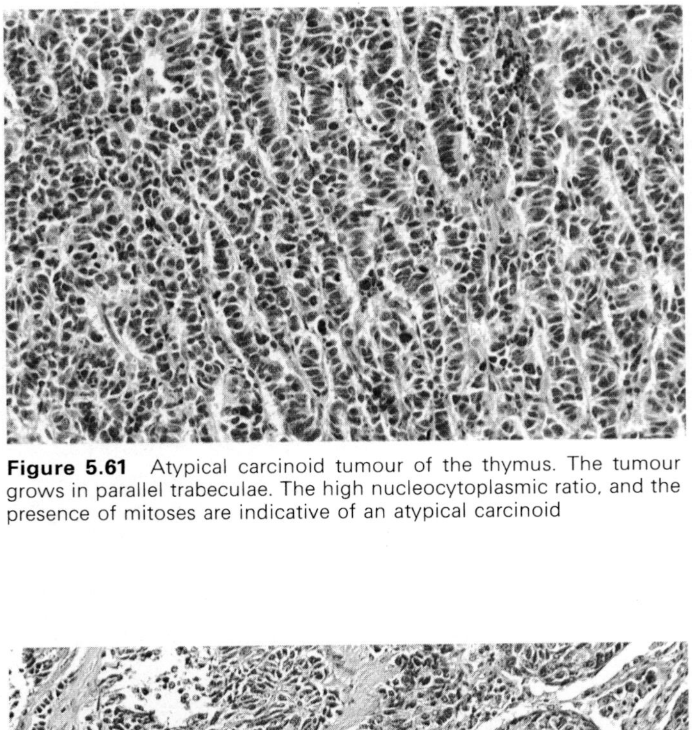

Figure 5.61 Atypical carcinoid tumour of the thymus. The tumour grows in parallel trabeculae. The high nucleocytoplasmic ratio, and the presence of mitoses are indicative of an atypical carcinoid

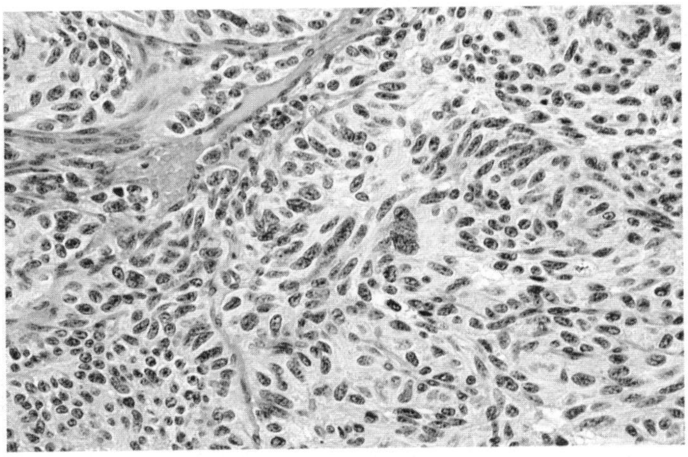

Figure 5.62 Atypical carcinoid tumour of the thymus, spindle-cell variant. Nuclear atypia are obvious. The radiological aspect is presented in Fig. 5.53

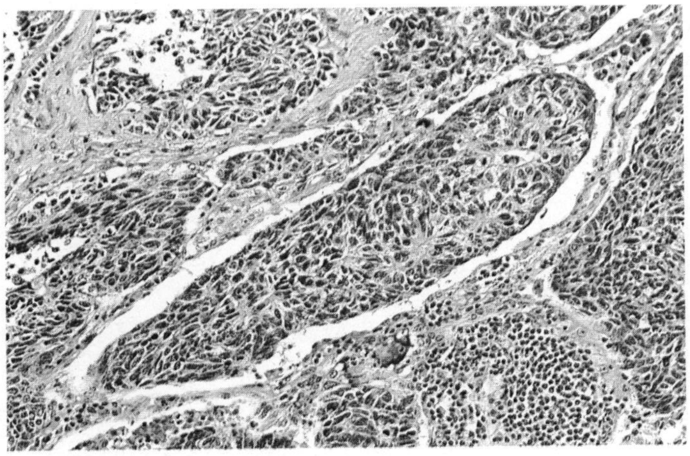

Figure 5.63 Small-cell carcinoma of the thymus: the figure shows small anaplastic cells growing in sheets, with areas of necrosis. The corresponding CT is represented in Fig. 5.56

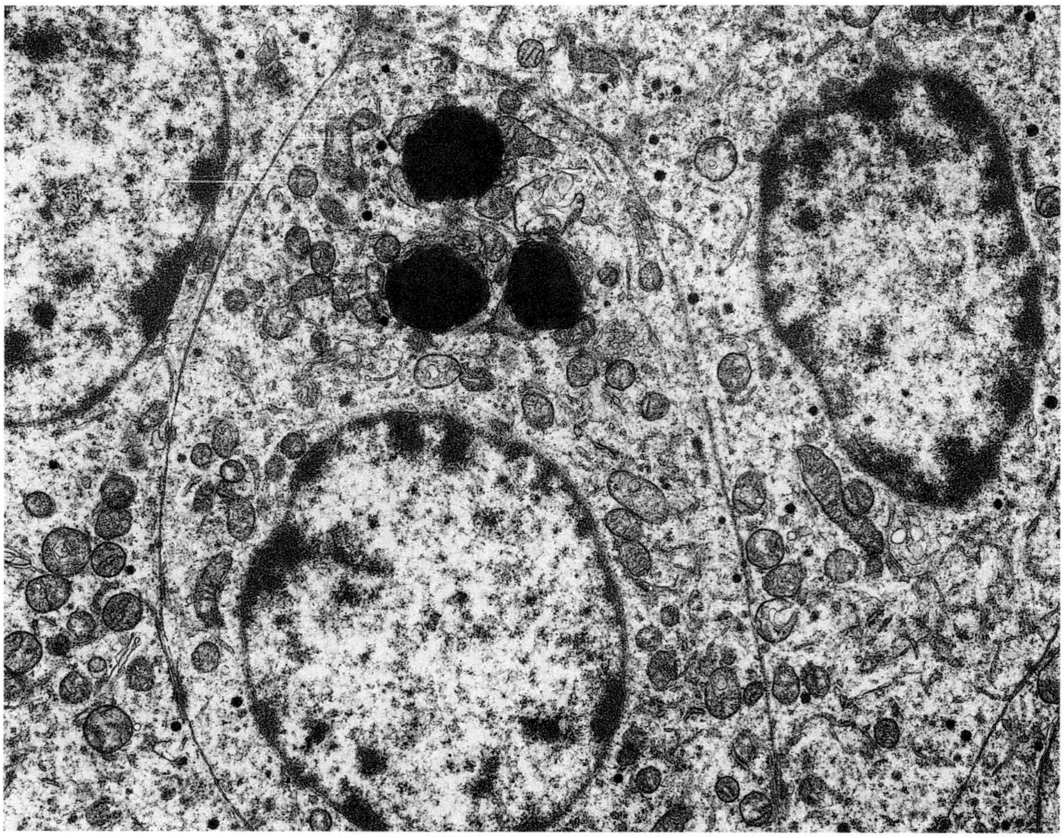

Figure 5.64 Carcinoid tumour of the thymus. The electron micrograph illustrates carcinoid cells with well-developed cytoplasmic organelles, and characteristic neurosecretory granules scattered in the cytoplasm

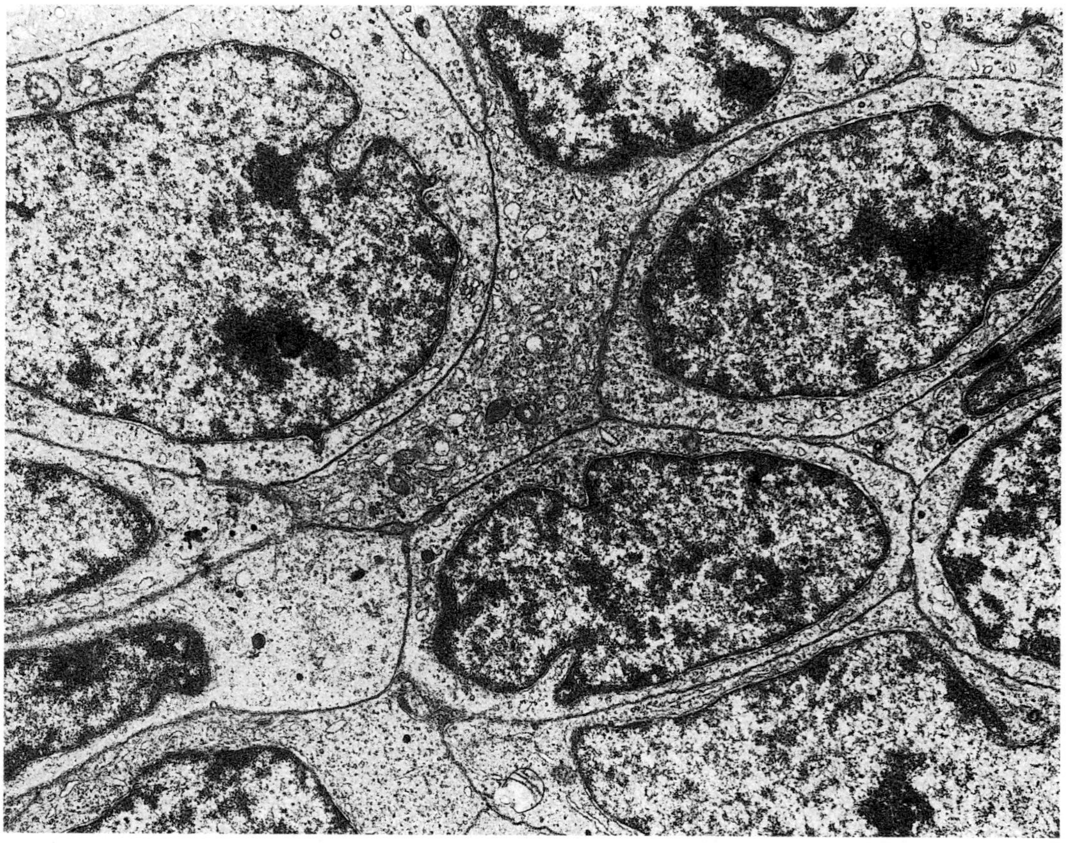

Figure 5.65 Small-cell carcinoma of the thymus. The electron micrograph shows a group of cells with large nuclei and scanty cytoplasm, poor in organelles. The neurosecretory granules are small and very sparse

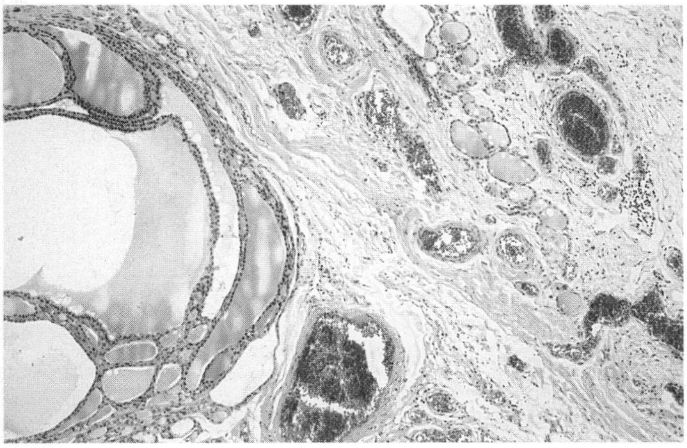

Figure 6.7 Intrathoracic goitre. Follicular hyperplasia (left) and fibrosis (right)

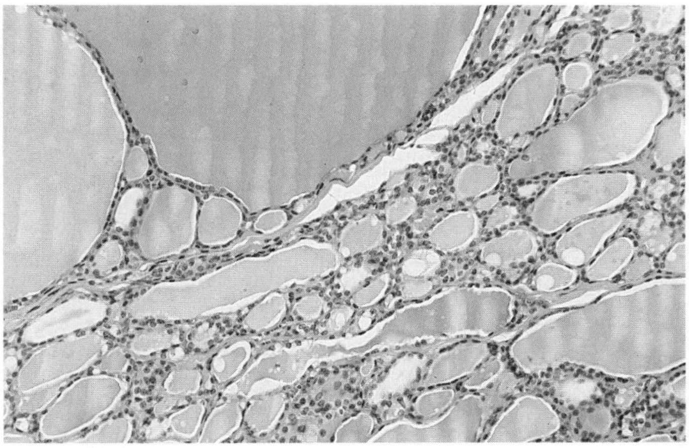

Figure 6.8 Intrathoracic goitre. Follicular hyperplasia of varying degree

Figure 6.9 (below) Thyroid carcinoma presenting as a large bosselated mass of the anterosuperior mediastinum

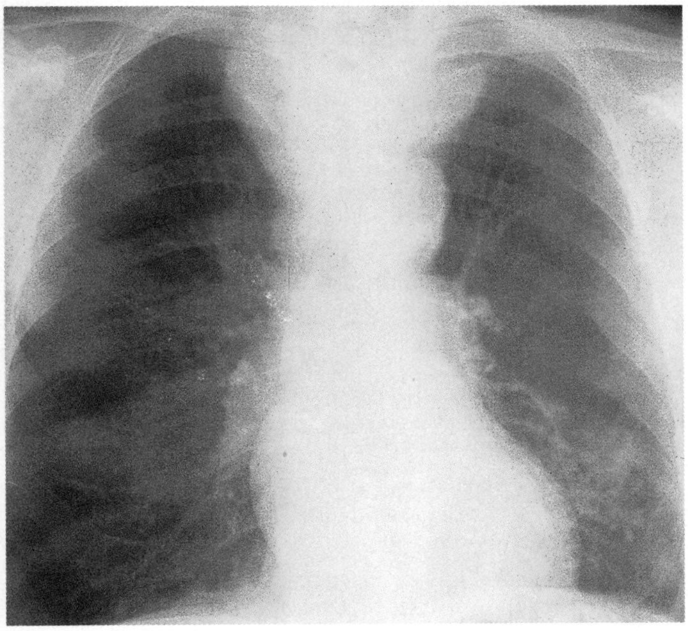

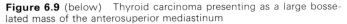

The parathyroid adenoma is an encapsulated, orange-brown, soft, occasionally lobular mass embedded in adipose or often thymic tissue. It may occasionally have a fibrous stalk, and foci of parenchymal or capsular calcification. On section, many tumours show small cysts, 0.1–1 cm in diameter, filled with clear, watery fluid, but large cystic degeneration is infrequent. Histologically the parathyroid adenomas are composed of sheets, nests or acini comprising enlarged chief cells, oxyphil cells, or clear cells (Figs 6.10 and 6.11), that may show various degrees of pleomorphism. Mediastinal parathyroid adenoma should be treated by surgical excision. Preoperative localization, however, is difficult, and usually needs the use of combined techniques (ultrasonography, thallium–technetium scanning, CT, MRI, and selective venous catheterization for parathyroid hormone) (Clark, 1988).

References

Castleman, B. and Roth, S. I. (1978) Tumors of the parathyroid glands. *Atlas of Tumor Pathology*, 2nd series, fasc. 14. Armed Forces Institute of Pathology, Washington, DC

Clark, O. H. (1988) Mediastinal parathyroid tumors. *Arch. Surg.*, **123**, 1096–1100

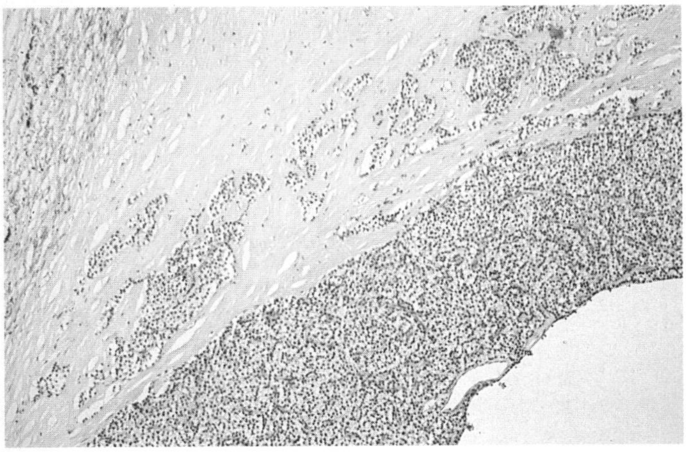

Figures 6.10 and 6.11 Parathyroid clear-cell adenoma of the posterior mediastinum from a patient with primary hyperparathyroidism. The tumour is cystic

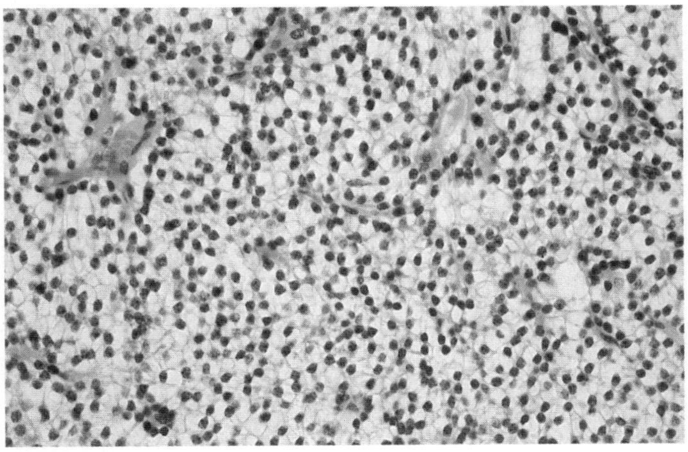

Figure 6.11

Mesenchymal Tumours 7

Mesenchymal tumours constitute 7% of adult primary mediastinal tumours. They are more frequent in children (Sabiston and Oldham, 1983). They usually occur in the anterior mediastinum and they are malignant or benign with equal frequency. A wide variety of these tumours may occur in the mediastinum, the most common types being those of vascular origin and of adipose tissue (Table 7.1). The general features of mediastinal mesenchymal tumours are similar to those of mesenchymal tumours found elsewhere, and only the more frequent neoplasms or peculiar aspects will be detailed in this chapter. For a more comprehensive approach the reader is referred to major texts on soft-tissue tumours (Hajdu, 1979; Enzinger and Weiss, 1988; Nash, 1989). Tumours of neural crest origin are described in Chapter 5, but whenever appropriate these tumours are discussed in the differential diagnosis of neoplasms that bear histological resemblance.

Table 7.1 Mesenchymal tumours of the mediastinum

	Benign	*Malignant*
Adipose	Lipoma Lipoblastoma Hibernoma	Liposarcoma
Vascular	Lymphangioma Haemangioma	Haemangioendothelioma Angiosarcoma Epithelioid variant
	Haemangiopericytoma (benign)	Haemangiopericytoma (malignant)
Fibroblastic	Fibromatosis Solitary fibrous tumour of the mediastinum	Fibrosarcoma
Fibrohistiocytic		Malignant fibrous histiocytoma
Muscular	Leiomyoma Rhabdomyoma	Leiomyosarcoma Rhabdomyosarcoma
Skeletal		Osteosarcoma Chondrosarcoma
Others		

The main histological and immunohistochemical characteristics of the mediastinal soft-tissue sarcomas are summarized in Tables 7.2 and 7.3. As a generality it must be recalled that the clinical behaviour of sarcomas depends on the histological type and grade of the tumour, the size, anatomical site, and the patient's age. In the mediastinum the deep situation of the neoplasms, and subsequently their usually large size at discovery (>5 cm) and the presence of necrosis, correspond to an overall bad prognosis. Another distinct facet of mediastinal sarcomas concerns the variety of histogenesis of the tumours including:

1. *De novo* sarcomas.
2. Radiation-induced tumours, especially following treatment of Hodgkin's disease (Halperin *et al.*, 1984; Boivin and O'Brien, 1988); the radiation-induced sarcomas include fibrosarcomas, liposarcomas, malignant fibrous histiocytomas, leiomyosarcomas and osteosarcomas.
3. Malignant sarcomatous changes within a mediastinal germ-cell tumour, mostly rhabdomyosarcomas but also angiosarcomas and liposarcomas, occurring spontaneously or as a result of therapy (Ulbright *et al.*, 1984, 1985; Manivel *et al.*, 1986).
4. Sarcomatoid variant of thymic carcinomas, and/or sarcomas deriving from myoid cells of the thymus (rhabdomyosarcoma).

Table 7.2 Soft-tissue sarcomas of the mediastinum: histological features

Liposarcoma	
Myxoid	Stellate cells and occasional malignant lipoblasts scattered in a loose mucoid stroma.
Round-cell	Dense infiltrates of round cells with acidophilic cytoplasm intermingled with lipoblasts.
Pleomorphic	Numerous markedly atypical lipoblasts with abundant eosinophilic cytoplasm, and frequent mitoses.
Well-differentiated	Large areas of mature fat containing only occasional scattered malignant lipoblasts and rare mitoses.
Haemangioendothelioma (angiosarcoma)	Formation of atypical vascular spaces by the tumour cells. The microscopic appearance varies widely, depending on the degree of differentiation of the tumour cells and the extent of vascular neoformation.
Epithelioid variant	Spindly epithelioid cells arranged in nests or cords, often mimicking a carcinoma. Subtle degree of vascular differentiation manifested by the formation of small intracellular lumina, but no well-formed vascular spaces.
Haemangiopericytoma	Rich vascular framework of benign-appearing vessels surrounded by a homogeneous population of densely packed, uniform, round to ovoid cells. Lack of significant cellular and nuclear pleomorphism.
Fibrosarcoma	Tumour composed of fibroblastic collagen-producing spindle cells. 'Herring-bone' pattern. General lack of significant cellular pleomorphism.
Malignant fibrous histiocytoma	Tumour composed of both fibroblastic and histiocytic cells. Wide spectrum of varied cellular morphology and histological aspect. Storiform or cartwheel pattern. Presence of inflammatory element and of highly pleomorphic multinucleated giant tumour cells. Stroma either predominantly fibrocollagenous (classical pleomorphic–storiform variant), myxoid (myxoid type), or sparse and moderately dense (giant-cell and inflammatory variant).
Leiomyosarcoma	Interlacing bundles of large spindle cells with elongated hyperchromatic, cigar-shaped nuclei. Intracytoplasmic myofibrils.
Rhabdomyosarcoma	Great variety of histological patterns (embryonal, alveolar, and pleomorphic). Combination of poorly differentiated primitive mesenchymal cells mixed with various types of differentiating rhabdomyoblastic elements.
Malignant schwannoma	Spindle-cell tumours with a spectrum of histological patterns and a wide variation in organization, composed of plump fusiform cells arranged in whorls, interlacing fascicles or in herring-bone pattern. The nuclei are plump or elongated, often twisted with a characteristic wavy or comma shape.

Tumours of adipose tissue

Lipomas account for approximately 2% of all primary mediastinal neoplasms (Mullen and Richardson, 1986). They are usually found in the anterior mediastinum, just above the diaphragm, and can extend into both sides of the pleural cavity. Despite their intrinsic benignity, these

Table 7.3 Soft-tissue sarcomas of the mediastinum: immunohistochemistry

	Vim	*Des*	*Act*	*Myos*	*Myog*	*Factor VIII*	Ulex europ	*S-100*
Liposarcoma	+							
Haemangioendothelioma	+					+	+	
Haemangiopericytoma	+							
Fibrosarcoma	+							
Malignant fibrous histiocytoma	+							
Leiomyosarcoma	+	+	+	+				
Rhabdomyosarcoma	+	+	+	+	+			
Malignant schwannoma	+							+

Vim: vimentin, 57 kD intermediate filament protein found in all forms of mesenchymal and some epithelial tissues.
Des: desmin, 53 kD intermediate filament protein present in all forms of normal and neoplastic muscle tissues.
Act: muscle actin, specific marker for tumours of muscle origin (myofilaments). Skeletal muscle actin is specific for tumour of skeletal muscle origin.
Myos: myosin, marker for normal and neoplastic muscle tissues.
Myog: myoglobin, specific marker for skeletal muscle differentiation.
Factor VIII: factor VIII-related antigen, glycoprotein present in endothelial cell.
Ulex europ: *Ulex europaeus* antigen, endothelial cell marker.
S-100 protein: non-specific marker for tumours derived from Schwann's cells and melanocytes.

tumours tend to grow to enormous proportions and may cause compression to mediastinal structures. They are, however, never invasive. On chest roentgenogram they appear as well-limited, round to oval masses, and they have a characteristic low homogeneous density on CT scan.

Macroscopically, lipomas are encapsulated tumours that appear soft, yellow or slightly fibrous on section (Figs 7.1 and 7.2). On histology the tumours are composed of mature adipose tissue, lobulated by thin fibrous septa, and penetrated by a few lymphocytes. A unique case of *angiolipoma* of the anteroinferior mediastinum has been observed by us (unpublished observation; Fig. 7.3). Lipomas are benign lesions that are cured by surgical resection. Total excision, however, is essential because these tumours have a tendency to recur.

Lipoblastomas are benign but diffuse, infiltrating lesions, which may extend into the neck, the diaphragm, or through the chest wall. Histologically they are composed of lobules of immature fat with lipoblasts at various stages of development that appear as stellate, spindle or round cells with unilocular intracytoplasmic single vacuoles. As lipomas, lipoblastomas are cured by complete surgery. The extent of the lesions, however, may make complete removal difficult. *Hibernomas* are benign tumours derived from brown adipose tissue. Their most common site is the subcutaneous tissues of the back. A single case within the mediastinum has been described recently by Ahn and Harvey (1990).

Liposarcomas, although unusual, are the most frequent malignant mesenchymal tumours of the mediastinum. To date nearly 60 cases have been reported in the world literature (Shibata *et al.*, 1986).

Mediastinal liposarcomas occur in patients ranging from 1 year to 77 years (mean 45 years), without sex predilection. They usually present with dyspnoea, wheezing, chest pain, cough, superior vena caval obstruction, or weight loss, but may be asymptomatic (Schweitzer and Aguam, 1977). On chest roentgenogram, liposarcomas are large and lobulated masses, and show a density similar to fat. On CT scan, however, the density of the sarcomas appears intermediate between fat and water.

The pathological features of liposarcomas range from well-encapsulated, relatively benign tumours to highly malignant neoplasms which grow rapidly and which cause death by direct invasion of the intrathoracic structures. They are subdivided into four histological types: myxoid, round-cell, well-differentiated, and pleomorphic (Enzinger and Weiss, 1988). Myxoid liposarcomas are composed of stellate cells and occasional malignant lipoblasts scattered in a loose mucoid stroma. Round-cell sarcomas contain dense infiltrates of round cells with acidophilic cytoplasm intermingled with lipoblasts. Pleomorphic liposarcomas contain numerous markedly atypical lipoblasts with abundant eosinophilic cytoplasm, and frequent mitoses. Well-differentiated liposarcomas are composed of large areas of mature fat containing only occasional scattered malignant lipoblasts and rare mitoses. The majority of primary mediastinal liposarcomas are of the well-differentiated variety, and a number are found to be well encapsulated. The treatment in all clinical varieties should be as complete a resection as possible, followed by radiotherapy. The role of systemic chemotherapy is yet to be determined. Late recurrences of well-differentiated tumours may be resected again with benefit in some cases (Standerfer *et al.*, 1981).

Tumours of vascular origin

Lymphangiomas

Primary mediastinal lymphangiomas are infrequent. They are congenital anomalies consisting of endothelial-lined spaces that can vary from capillary size to several centimetres in diameter.

Mediastinal lymphangiomas occur in four localizations, presenting separate clinicopathologic features (Brown *et al.*, 1986):

1. *Superior mediastinal lymphangioma* appears as an extension of the more frequent neck lymphangioma. This cervicomediastinal type of lymphangioma occurs mainly in young patients and is usually detected at birth or shortly after. The majority have an infiltrative growth pattern, cannot benefit from complete resection and tend to recur after surgery.
2. *Anterior mediastinal lymphangioma* represents about 30% of intrathoracic lymphangiomas. It arises exclusively in the mediastinum and not from cervical cystic hygroma. It occurs in middle-aged patients, is often asymptomatic, and simulates more common anterior mediastinal lesions such as adenopathy or thymoma. It is often easily enucleated.
3. *Posterior mediastinal lymphangioma* may have the same characteristics as its anterior mediastinum counterpart (Fig. 7.4) or be part of a generalized lymphangiomatosis (cystic angiomatosis) as reported in two cases by Brown *et al.* (1986). *Cystic angiomatosis or generalized lymphangiomatosis* is an extensive process that includes widespread lymphangiomas and haemangiomas of the skeleton, thoracic and abdominal organs, and retroperitoneum, and is usually associated with persistent chylothorax.
4. *Diffuse intrathoracic lymphangioma* is the mediastinal localizaton of cystic angiomatosis

Brown *et al.* (1986) emphasize the relationship of intrathoracic lymphangiomas with Gorham's disease and other related disorders. *Gorham's disease, or disappearing bone disease,* is an extensive lymphatic dysplastic disorder involving both the vertebrae and ribs and the non-skeletal soft tissues of the mediastinum. It is characterized pathologically by lymphangiomatous elements sometimes associated with angiomatosis that lead to osteolysis and destruction of the affected bones that can ultimately lead

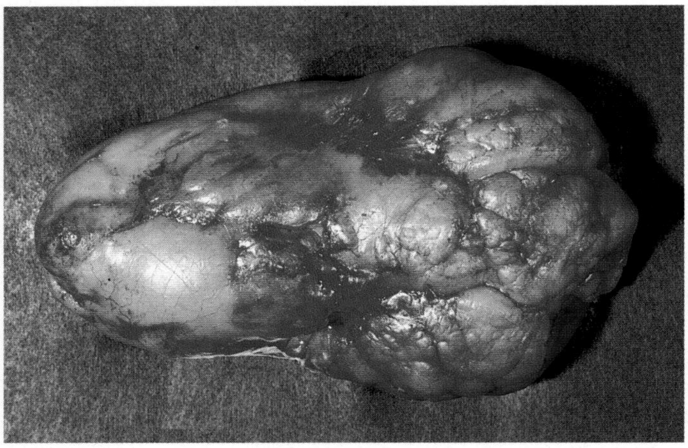

Figure 7.1 Lipoma of the mediastinum. Very large, encapsulated tumour

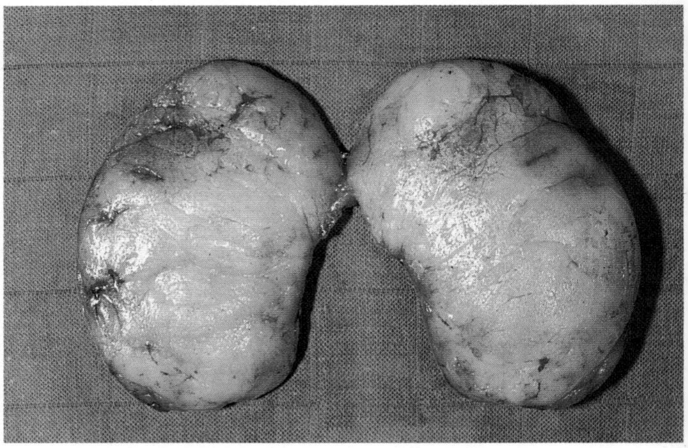

Figure 7.2 Lipoma of the mediastinum. On section, the tumour appears soft yellow

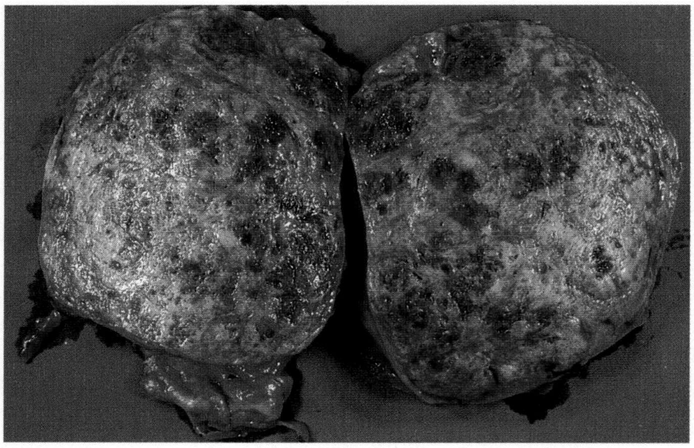

Figure 7.3 Angiolipoma. This large tumour, 15 cm in diameter, was discovered in the anterior mediastinum. At histology the lesion was composed of mature adipose tissue and numerous blood vessels of haemangioma-like pattern, and was benign in appearance

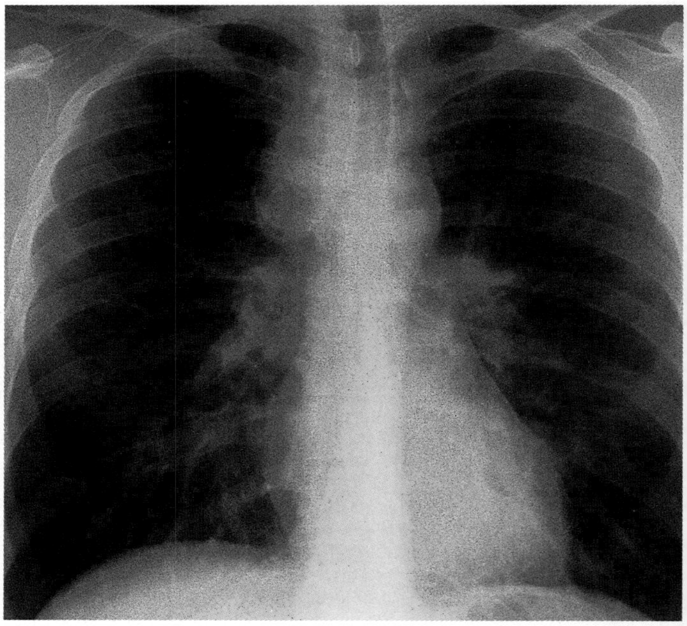

Figure 7.4 (right) Mediastinal lymphangioma. The radiography shows a well-circumscribed posterolatero–tracheal mass of cystic aspect

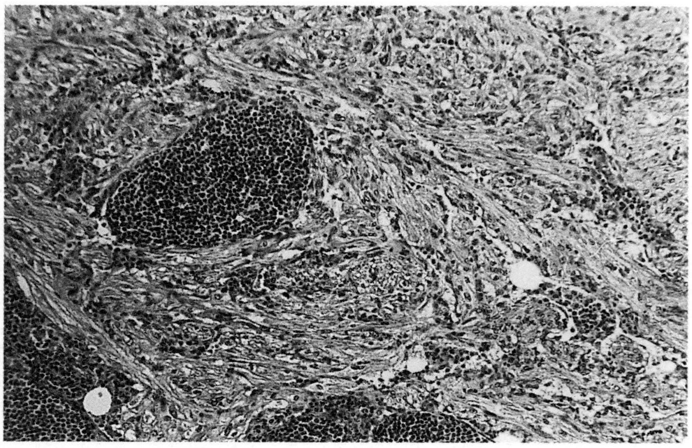

Figure 7.5 Mediastinal lymphangiomyomatosis. The normal lymph node tissue is replaced by proliferating smooth muscle

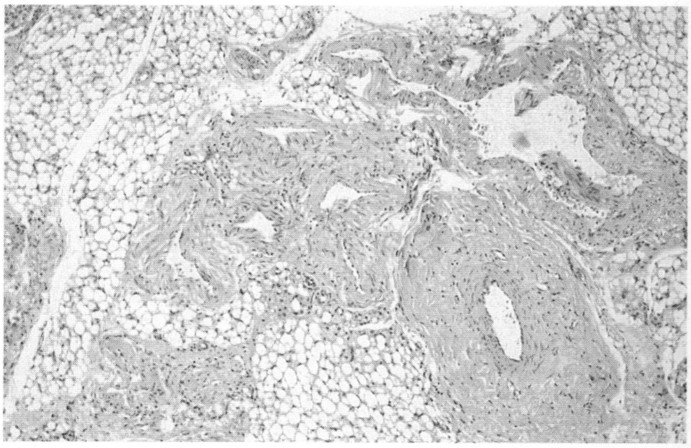

Figure 7.6 Cavernous lymphangioma composed of dilated lymphatic channels with thick smooth muscle walls

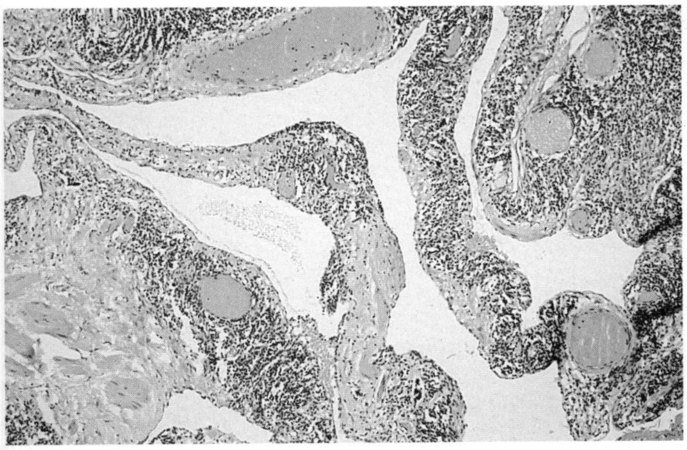

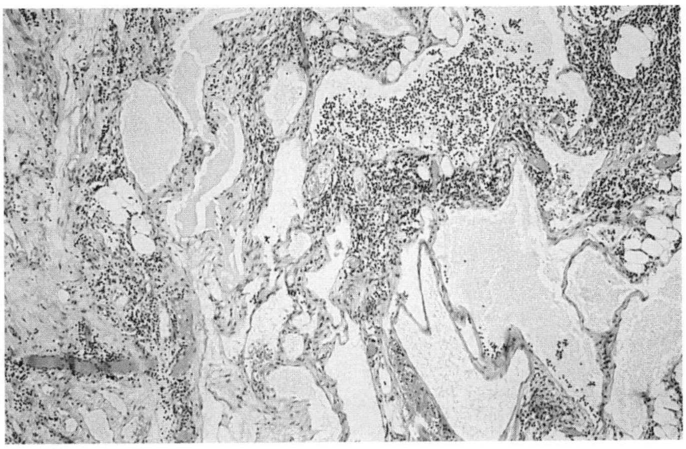

Figures 7.7 and 7.8 Multilocular lymphangioma (hygroma) consisting of interconnecting cavities. The stroma is heavily infiltrated by lymphocytes

Figure 7.8

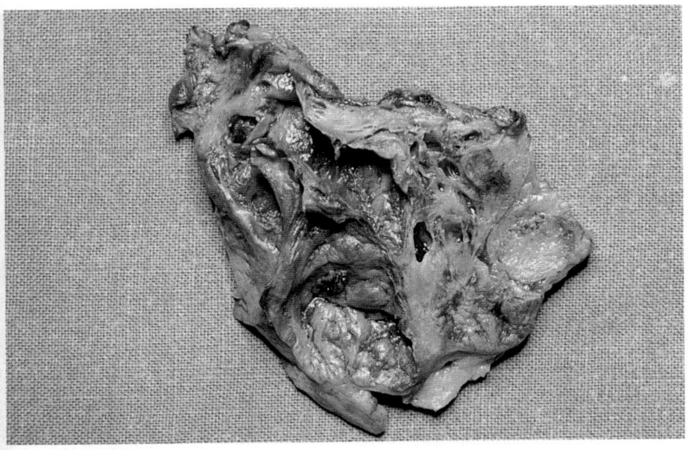

Figure 7.9 Cavernous haemangioma of the anterior mediastinum. The tumour is multicystic, and brown–yellow

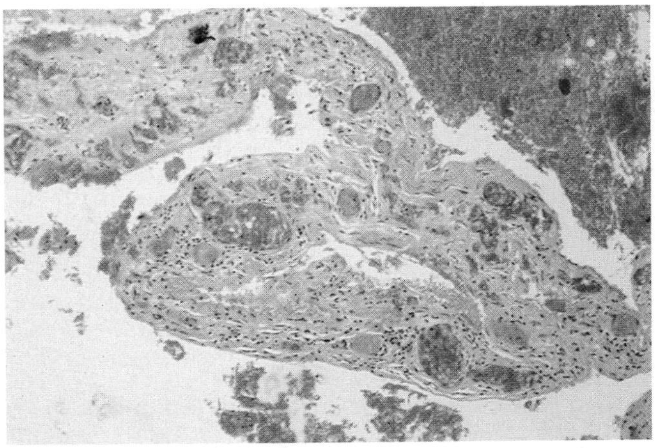

Figure 7.10 Cavernous haemangioma of the anterior mediastinum. Histologically, the lesion is composed of interconnecting vessels containing red blood cells

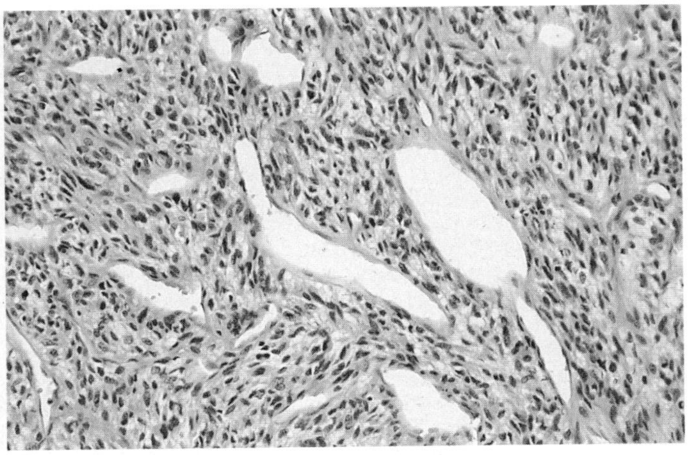

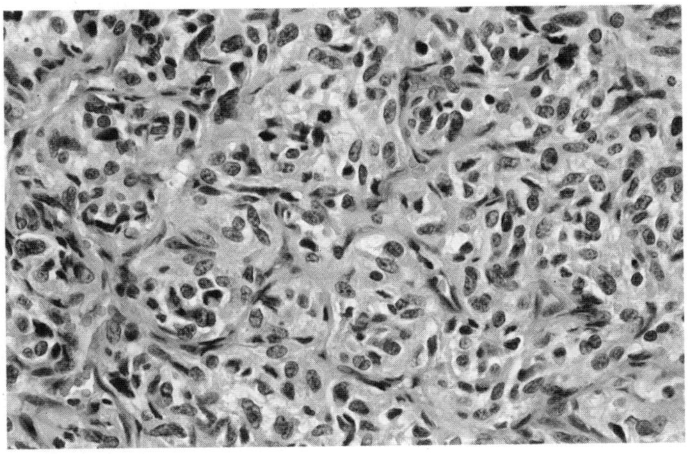

Figures 7.11 and 7.12 Haemangiopericytoma. The tumour consists of a rich vascular framework surrounded by densely packed ovoid cells

Figure 7.12

to death. Chylothorax due to mediastinal lymphangiomatosis is relatively frequent and associated with a poor prognosis. Gorham's disease differs from cystic angiomatosis in that in the former there is involvement of contiguous bones and soft tissue, whereas in cystic angiomatosis the lesions are more diffuse and non-contiguous. Other related disorders are the *Klippel–Trenaunay syndrome* that consists of a triad of soft tissue and bony hypertrophy of the extremities, haemangiomas or lymphangiomas, and varicosities; *Servelle-Noquès disease*, which is characterized by a congenital or early acquired malformation of the lymphatics and absence of the cisterna chyli causing the development of lymphatic collateral pathways; and *lymphangiomyomatosis* which is characterized by the proliferation of lymphatics and smooth muscle in mediastinal lymph nodes (Fig. 7.5), lung parenchyma, and retroperitoneum.

Histologically, lymphangiomas are classified into three groups according to the size of the cavities and to the thickness of the vascular walls: (1) lymphangioma simplex, composed of capillary-sized thin-walled lymphatic channels; (2) cavernous lymphangioma, composed of dilated lymphatic channels with fibrous adventitial coats (Fig. 7.6); and (3) cystic uni- or multilocular lymphangioma with septa, or hygroma (Figs 7.7 and 7.8; Murayama, 1985; Johnson *et al.*, 1986; Brown *et al.*, 1986; Holden *et al.*, 1987). The tumours contain serous or chylous fluid and sometimes blood cells. In such cases the lesion can be mistaken for haemangioma.

The prognosis and treatment depends on the extent of the lesions. Unlike congenital haemangiomas these lesions do not tend to regress spontaneously, and occasionally cause severe complications. Their infiltrative tendency enables them to envelop the nerves and blood vessels in their neighbourhood and to invest other mediastinal structures. Thus, complete surgical removal is difficult, accounting for their high recurrence rate postoperatively.

Haemangiomas

Benign haemangiomas of the mediastinum represent 0.5% or less of mediastinal masses, and fewer than 100 cases have been reported in the literature (Vente and Meiss, 1985; Cohen *et al.*, 1987; Saada *et al.*, 1987; Ceccanti *et al.*, 1989).

Benign haemangiomas are usually well encapsulated and slow-growing tumours, but infiltrative growth is not unusual. They are often discovered on routine chest roentgenogram. Symptoms are related to compression or invasion of adjacent structures. The majority of the tumours are localized in the anterior mediastinum (70%), whereas others arise in the posterior mediastinum. Extension of the tumours to the neck or the supraclavicular area may be observed. Radiologically, haemangiomas are lobed tumours with smooth contours and uniform density. Phleboliths, characteristic of benign haemangiomas, are described in 10% of cases. Angiography usually offers little information and CT scan may demonstrate the mass as solid with attenuation similar to the surrounding vessels, but generally is of no help for diagnosis.

Histologically, haemangiomas are differentiated into cavernous, capillary, venous, or mixed, and are similar to haemangiomas in other locations. Most mediastinal haemangiomas are cavernous (Figs 7.9 and 7.10). They are composed of large vascular spaces with thick smooth muscle walls, as opposed to the capillary haemangiomas, which consist of many fine lumina.

The benign haemangioma should be treated surgically and must be removed as completely as possible. Radiotherapy does not appear to have any benefit. The prognosis is favourable even in subtotal excision. Metastases never occur.

Haemangioendotheliomas are neoplasms of endothelial cell composition arising from either blood vessels or lymphatic vessels. They are a heterogeneous group of tumours ranging from the *highly malignant angiosarcoma* (haemangiosarcoma and lymphangiosarcoma) to the *epithelioid haemangioendothelioma* of low grade malignancy (Enzinger and Weiss, 1988).

Haemangioendotheliomas have been reported only occasionally in the mediastinum (Abratt *et al.*, 1983; Yousem and Hochholzer, 1987; Toursarkissian *et al.*, 1990). They occur in patients over a broad age range and there is no sex predilection. Whereas tumours develop more frequently in the anterior mediastinum, all cases reported as occurring in young children were located in the posterior mediastinum (Bedros *et al.*, 1986). A case of angiosarcoma developed as a result of malignant change within a germ-cell tumour of the mediastinum has been described by Ulbright *et al.* (1985).

Grossly, *angiosarcoma (malignant haemangioendothelioma)* is typically a soft haemorrhagic, ill-defined tumour, partly solid and partly spongy. Histologically, the hallmark of angiosarcoma is the formation of atypical vascular spaces by the tumour cells. The microscopic appearance varies widely, depending on the degree of differentiation of the tumour cells and the extent of vascular neoformation. *Epithelioid haemangioendothelioma* usually arises from a blood vessel and appears solid and pale rather than obviously vascular or haemorrhagic. It is composed of spindly epithelioid cells arranged in nests or cords, often mimicking a carcinoma. A subtle degree of vascular differentiation is manifested only by the formation of small intracellular lumina, but there are no well-formed vascular spaces. In both malignant haemangioendothelioma and epithelioid haemangioendothelioma the silver reticulin stain highlights the neoformed vascular spaces lined by the neoplastic cells. The endothelial nature of the tumour may be confirmed by a positive immunostain for factor VIII-related antigen or lectin binding for *Ulex europaeus* antigen, which are two recognized endothelial cell markers. Electron microscopic studies often demonstrate the presence of intracellular Weibel–Palade bodies, characteristic of endothelial-derived cells.

Mediastinal angiosarcomas are very malignant tumours that necessitate radical local excision, followed by chemotherapy. The more indolent epithelioid haemangioendotheliomas should be treated by wide local excision without adjuvant therapy. Recurrence and metastases may benefit from radiotherapy and chemotherapy.

Haemangiopericytomas are rare soft-tissue tumours originating from pericytes, and their mediastinal localization is quite uncommon (Collet *et al.*, 1985; Biagi *et al.*, 1990). The tumours occur primarily in adults, and both sexes are equally affected. Grossly, they are usually well-circumscribed or encapsulated, with a variable cut section appearance ranging from a solid fleshy texture to a soft, haemorrhagic or cystic aspect. Histologically the tumours consist of a rich vascular framework of benign-appearing vessels surrounded by a homogeneous population of densely packed, uniform, round to ovoid cells (Figs 7.11 and 7.12). A dense reticulin meshwork surrounds the individual tumour cells and outlines the vessels bordered by a single layer of normal endothelial cells. Whereas the endothelial cells are immunostained by factor VIII-related antigen or *Ulex europaeus* I lectin, the tumour cells stain strongly only for vimentin. The electron microscopic studies illustrate the basal lamina completely separating the tumour cells from endothelial cells, and the presence of intracytoplasmic microfilaments (Enzinger and Weiss, 1988).

The differential diagnosis of haemangiopericytoma may be difficult. Reticulin stain and immunohistochemistry are the most useful procedures in the separation of this neoplasm from other tumours with prominent vascular patterns (Nash, 1989). In the mediastinum the distinction from a thymoma with haemangiopericytoma-like pattern is a rare but critical problem. In such a case positive staining for cytokeratin allows an unequivocal diagnosis of thymoma.

The majority of haemangiopericytoma are benign, but the prediction of clinical behaviour on histological grounds remains difficult. The increased mitotic rate, a greater degree of cellularity, the presence of pleomorphic tumour cells, and foci of haemorrhage and necrosis are the best indicators of malignancy (Enzinger and Weiss, 1988). Surgical excision is the primary treatment for these tumours, followed by radiotherapy and chemotherapy in the malignant cases.

Tumours of fibroblastic origin

Fibromatosis is a term that refers to a group of non-neoplastic connective tissue lesions that tend to infiltrate surrounding tissues and often recur after surgical excision (Hajdu, 1979). The aetiology of the disease is unknown.

Mediastinal fibromatosis is an extremely rare occurrence, which affects patients of all ages and which may cause signs of obstruction of the superior vena cava (Kaplan and Davidson, 1986). It consists of a dense and non-encapsulated, collagenous tissue that surrounds the aorta, trachea, bronchi, and heart. Histologically, the fibrous tissue is composed of abundant collagen containing sparse, well-differentiated fibroblasts interspersed with variable numbers of lymphocytes, plasma cells and other inflammatory elements. Fibromatoses are benign but invasive lesions and the treatment should be aimed at relieving the obstruction of vital structures. Their differential diagnosis includes sclerosing mediastinitis and well-differentiated fibrosarcoma.

Solitary fibrous tumours of the mediastinum, identical to solitary fibrous tumours (so-called fibrous mesotheliomas) of the pleura, have been described by Witkin and Rosai (1989).

The lesion may be symptomatic or discovered incidentally at radiography. As its pleural homologue, it is sometimes associated with hypoglycaemia. Most of the tumours arise in the anterosuperior mediastinum, occasionally on a pedicle, and may entrap thymic elements. Macroscopically the tumours are well circumscribed firm masses with a tan–grey whorled cut surface and frequent cystic change (Fig. 7.13). Histologically the neoplasms are composed of spindle cells haphazardly arranged in a patternless appearance in a thick collagenous background. Vessels are prominent and vascular patterns reminiscent of haemangiopericytoma are not uncommon. Some hypercellular regions show high mitotic activity. Tumour cells are immunoreactive for vimentin, but not for keratin, supporting their mesenchymal origin. Ultrastructural studies demonstrate only spindly mesenchymal cells that have features consistent with fibroblasts. A weak and focal positivity for actin may indicate the emergence of a myofibroblastic component. The differential diagnosis includes spindle-cell thymomas that show epithelial differentiation immunohistochemically and ultrastructurally, haemangiopericytoma, and peripheral nerve tumours that are immunoreactive with S-100 protein. Excision of solitary fibrous tumour of the mediastinum is usually curative. Malignant behaviour usually manifests as local recurrence, although distant metastases may occur. Adverse prognostic factors include large size, high cellularity, mitotic activity, and anaplasia, whereas growth on a pedicle has a favourable prognosis.

Fibrosarcoma is a malignant soft-tissue tumour composed of collagen-producing cells capable of exhibiting varying degrees of fibroblastic differentiation. They are extremely rare in the mediastinum, where they occur in patients of both sexes, mostly in the third through fifth decades of life. They may be associated with hypoglycaemia.

Fibrosarcomas tend to be well-circumscribed tumours, with a fleshy to firm appearance, and frequent areas of necrosis or haemorrhages (Fig. 7.14). They are locally invasive, but rarely metastasize. Histologically they are composed of spindle cells with hyperchromatic nuclei, arranged in long interlacing fascicles, producing the characteristic 'herring-bone' pattern. They differ from malignant fibrous histiocytomas by a general lack of significant histological and cellular pleomorphism, with absence of inflammatory elements and of pleomorphic multinucleated giant tumour cells. The well-differentiated fibrosarcomas have to be distinguished from a sclerosing mediastinitis where the fibroblastic cells are less numerous, have a cytological bland appearance and are admixed with numerous inflammatory cells. The clinical behaviour and prognosis depend mostly on the histological grading of the tumour (i.e. cellularity, collagen production, nuclear atypia, and mitoses). The treatment is surgical resection, followed by radiotherapy and chemotherapy. Recurrences are frequent and the prognosis is poor.

Tumours of fibrohistiocytic origin

Malignant fibrous histiocytoma is one of the most common forms of soft-tissue sarcoma in older people, but its origin in the mediastinum is very unusual and less than 10 cases have been reported in the literature (Morshuis *et al.*, 1990). Additional cases of malignant fibrous histiocytoma arise from the major blood vessels (pulmonary artery, pulmonary vein or thoracic aorta) (Van Damme *et al.*, 1987; Kaiser and Urmacher, 1990; Guttentag *et al.*, 1989) or from the heart (Laya *et al.*, 1987), causing thickening or obstruction of the vessels or symptoms of pulmonary embolism (Fig. 7.15).

Histologically, malignant fibrous histiocytomas show a wide morphological and cytological spectrum. They are composed of a mixture of elements resembling histiocytes and fibroblasts, often arranged in a storiform pattern and accompanied by giant cells and inflammatory cells, and five variants are described: (1) pleomorphic–storiform, (2) myxoid (Figs 7.16–7.18), (3) giant-cell (Fig. 7.19), (4) inflammatory, and (5) angiomatoid. Because of the diverse appearance of malignant fibrous histiocytomas the differential diagnosis includes many other types of soft-tissue tumours. In the mediastinum the diagnosis of spindle-cell thymoma, undifferentiated or sarcomatoid thymic carcinoma and polymorphic lymphoma should also be considered. Immunochemistry and electron microscopy are useful in questionable cases. Surgery remains the only hope for treatment of these rare tumours. The prognosis is poor, with a high incidence of local recurrence and of distant metastases.

Tumours of muscle origin

Leiomyomas are among the least frequent primary benign mesenchymal tumours of the mediastinum. In 1990, Shaffer *et al.* reviewed 10 cases and reported one additional case. The tumours develop more frequently in female patients than in male patients, with an age range of 22–67 years. Leiomyomas usually arise from structures having smooth-muscle walls, such as the oesophagus or great vessels, and the posterior mediastinum is the most common location. They are often quite large at the time of diagnosis, due to their slow growing and the relative

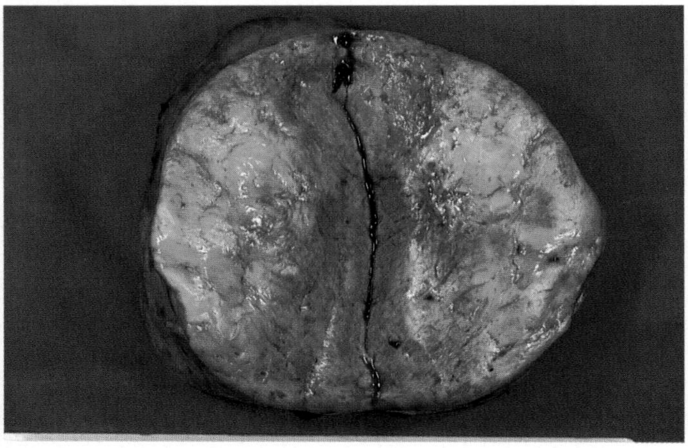

Figure 7.13 Solitary fibrous tumour of the anterior mediastinum. The tumour has all the characteristics described by Witkin and Rosai (1989)

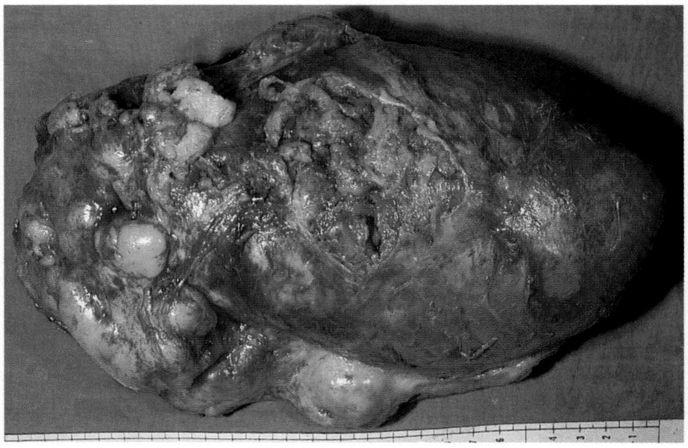

Figure 7.14 Fibrosarcoma of the posterior mediastinum. The neoplasm has a fleshy, necrotic appearance

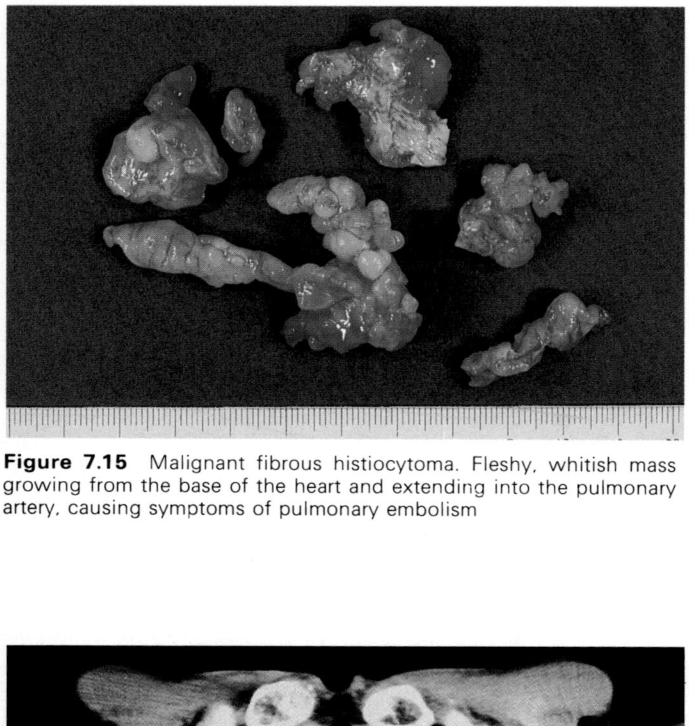

Figure 7.15 Malignant fibrous histiocytoma. Fleshy, whitish mass growing from the base of the heart and extending into the pulmonary artery, causing symptoms of pulmonary embolism

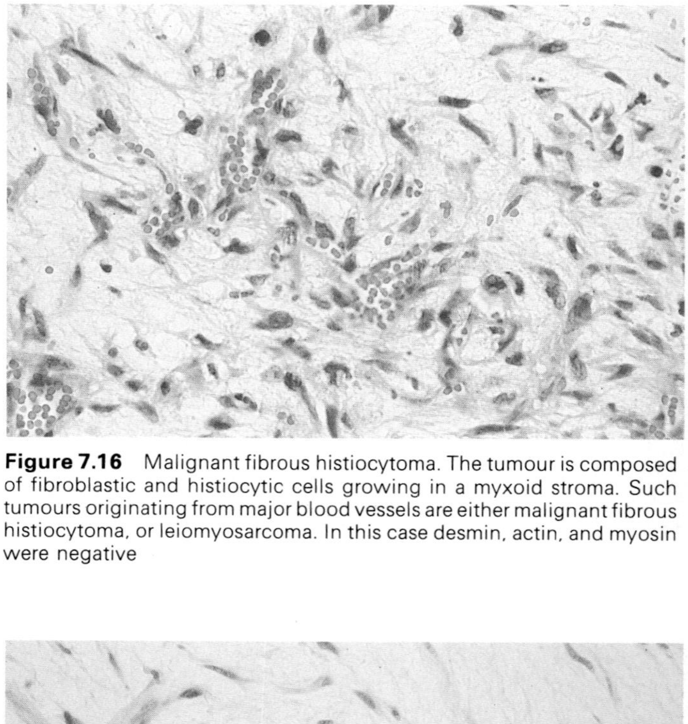

Figure 7.16 Malignant fibrous histiocytoma. The tumour is composed of fibroblastic and histiocytic cells growing in a myxoid stroma. Such tumours originating from major blood vessels are either malignant fibrous histiocytoma, or leiomyosarcoma. In this case desmin, actin, and myosin were negative

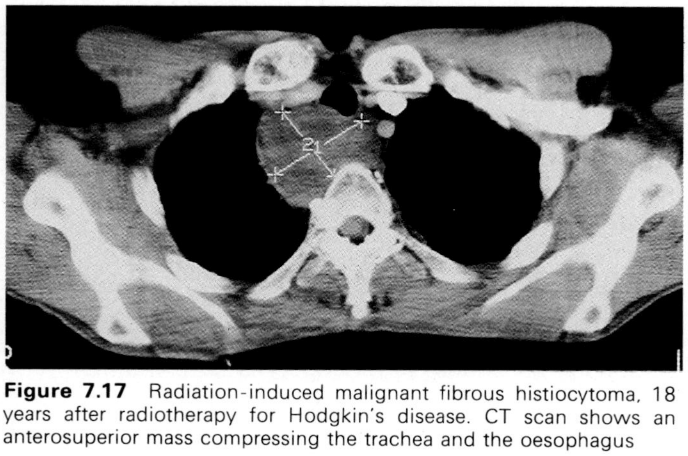

Figure 7.17 Radiation-induced malignant fibrous histiocytoma, 18 years after radiotherapy for Hodgkin's disease. CT scan shows an anterosuperior mass compressing the trachea and the oesophagus

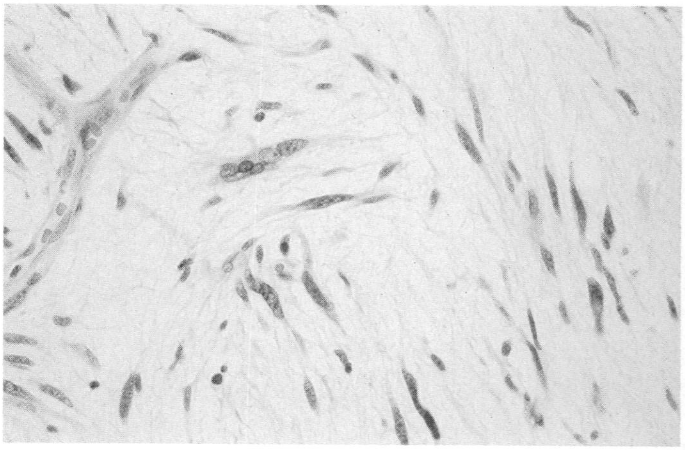

Figure 7.18 Malignant fibrous histiocytoma. Although radiation-induced, the sarcoma displays histologically a low-grade malignancy. Note the characteristic branching of the capillary vessel on the left

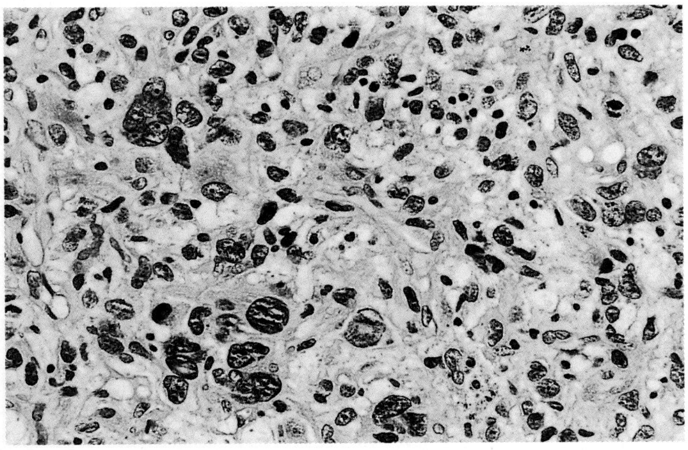

Figure 7.19 Primary malignant fibrous histiocytoma of the superior mediastinum invading the lung. The neoplasm is pleomorphic with numerous giant cells

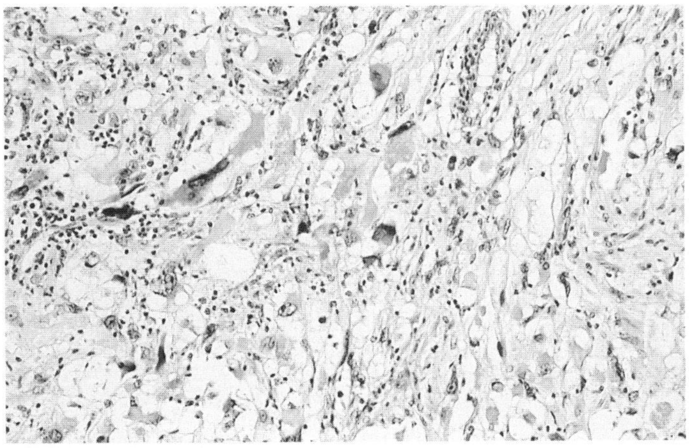

Figures 7.20 and 7.21 Pleomorphic rhabdomyosarcoma arising from a malignant germ-cell tumour of the anterior mediastinum

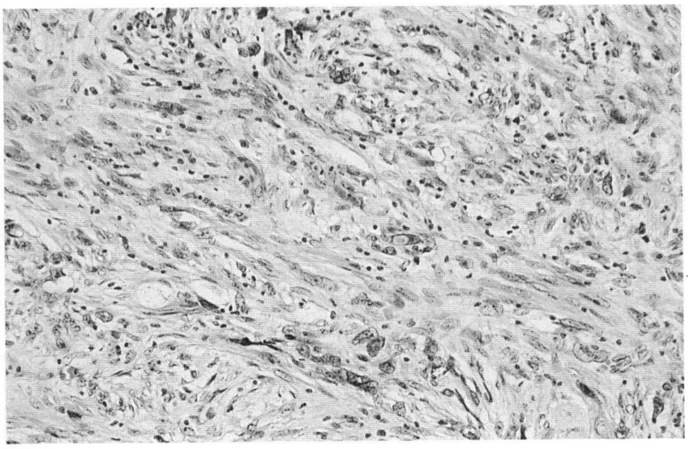

Figure 7.21

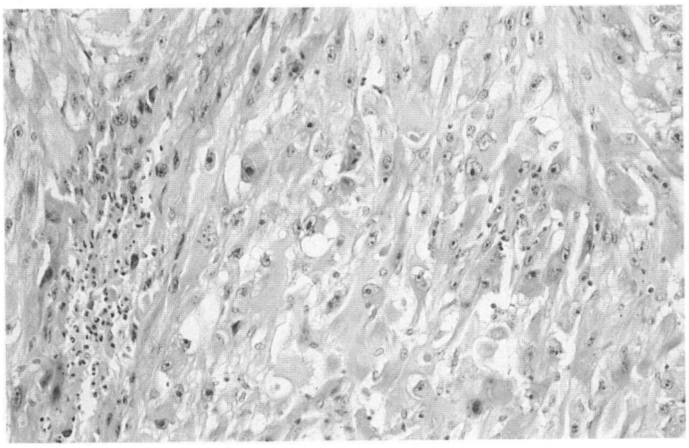

Figure 7.22 Primary rhabdomyosarcoma of the anterior mediastinum

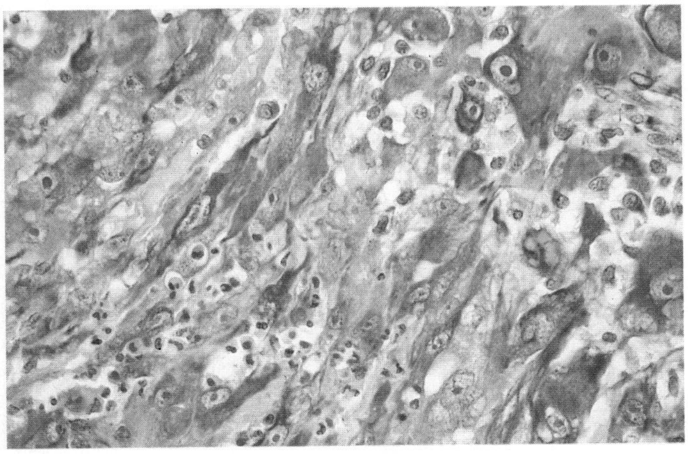

Figure 7.23 Primary rhabdomyosarcoma of the anterior mediastinum. Immunostaining for myoglobin is strongly positive on the cytoplasm of the tumour cells

lack of symptoms. Leiomyomas are cured by surgical excision.

Leiomyosarcomas are relatively rare soft-tissue tumours of smooth muscle origin. In the mediastinum, primary leiomyosarcomas are very unusual neoplasms that may occur in adults of both sexes. The tumours commonly originate from major blood vessels, most of them from the inferior vena cava, less frequently from pulmonary vein or pulmonary artery. They develop into the vascular lumen and appear as a fleshy, whitish-tan mass extending to, or growing from, the base of the heart (Sunderrajan *et al.*, 1984; Kaiser and Urmacher, 1990). Other possible sites of origin include the oesophagus, smaller mediastinal vessels, and mediastinal teratoma. Radiation-induced mediastinal leiomyosarcomas have also been described (Weiss *et al.*, 1987). Histologically, the tumours are composed of long spindled cells arranged in interlacing fascicles. The tumour cells have a distinctly fibrillary cytoplasm and elongated hyperchromatic, cigar-shaped nuclei. Mitoses are always present. Intracytoplasmic myofibrils are better demonstrated by Masson trichrome stain and phosphotungstic acid–haematoxylin stain. Reticulin stain reveals delicate reticulin fibres unwrapping individual tumour cells and cell bundles. Tumour cells are positively immunostained for vimentin, desmin and actin. The electron microscopic study shows a partial or complete basal lamina around individual cells and the presence of variable numbers of thin actin filaments (5–8 nm in diameter), punctuated by dense bodies and attachment plaques in the cytoplasm of the neoplastic cells. These special techniques may be of help in differentiating leiomyosarcoma from other spindle-cell sarcomas of the soft tissue and allow a definite distinction from epithelial spindle-cell tumour of thymic origin.

Rhabdomyoma is a benign neoplasm of striated muscle origin that may occur in cardiac and extracardiac localization. A single case of rhabdomyoma has been described in the anterior mediastinum by Miller *et al.* (1978), and the authors postulate the possible origin of the tumour from the myoid cells of the thymus.

Rhabdomyosarcomas are the most frequent soft-tissue sarcomas in children but a mediastinal primary site is unusual (less than 2% of childhood rhabdomyosarcomas) (Crist *et al.*, 1982). These primary mediastinal sarcomas occur in older children (mean age 9.9 years) and are more frequently of undifferentiated histological types than tumours from most other primary sites. Additionally, this particular primary site is associated with advanced disease at presentation and its attendant high mortality. In adults, mediastinal rhabdomyosarcomas are more likely to occur either as the sarcomatoid component of a thymic carcinoma, putatively deriving from the normal myoid thymic cells, or as the development of sarcoma from a primary mediastinal teratoma. Malignant changes within teratomatous components of germ-cell tumours is a phenomenon of increasing importance in the era of effective chemotherapy for these tumours. According to Ulbright *et al.* (1984) rhabdomyosarcoma is the most common type of non-germ-cell malignancy developing within germ-cell tumours (Figs 7.20 and 7.21).

Rhabdomyosarcomas show a great variety of cytological and histological patterns that lead to the differentiation of three histological types: embryonal, alveolar, and pleomorphic (Fig. 7.22). Regardless of the histological subtype, the hallmark of the tumours is the combination of poorly differentiated primitive mesenchymal cells mixed with various types of differentiating rhabdomyoblastic elements. Trichrome stain colours the cytoplasm of differentiating rhabdomyoblasts bright red, and highlights myofibrils and cross-striations. Antibodies to desmin and myosin give a positive reaction in most partially differentiated rhabdomyosarcomas, but they are not specific for skeletal muscle differentiation. Myoglobin is a specific marker for striated muscle (Fig. 7.23), but is less sensitive than desmin. Antiskeletal muscle actin appears to be the most specific and sensitive marker to date (Nash, 1989). Ultrastructurally, rhabdomyosarcomas are characterized by the presence of thin (actin) and thick (myosin) cytoplasmic filaments, with, in addition, the presence of spots (wisps) of Z-band substance.

Tumours of skeletal tissues

Intrathoracic osteosarcomas, chondromas and chondrosarcomas usually arise from the thoracic skeleton, and mediastinal extraskeletal occurrences are exceedingly rare. Three cases of primary osteogenic sarcoma of the mediastinum (including their own) are reported by Valderrama *et al.* (1983) and another case is described by Catanese *et al.* (1988) following radiotherapy for Hodgkin's disease. Chondrosarcomas arise from the tracheobronchial tree (Daniels *et al.*, 1967).

Other mesenchymal tumours

Occasional cases of mesenchymoma may occur in the mediastinum (Marchevsky and Kaneko, 1984). Recently, Witkin *et al.* (1989) described four cases of a biphasic mediastinal tumour histologically identical to synovial sarcoma of soft tissue. All cases were composed of a mixture of keratin-positive epithelial cells and vimentin-positive spindle cells, raising the differential diagnosis of mesotheliomas. Other differential diagnoses include thymoma, germ-cell tumour, malignant peripheral nerve sheath tumour with glandular differentiation, and metastatic carcinoma.

References

Abratt, R. P., Williams, M., Raff, M., Dodd, N. F. and Uys, C. J. (1983) Angiosarcoma of the superior vena cava. *Cancer*, **52**, 740–743.

Ahn, C. and Harvey, J. C. (1990) Mediastinal hibernoma, a rare tumor. *Ann. Thorac. Surg.*, **50**, 828–830.

Bedros, A. A., Munson, J. and Toomey, F. E. (1986) Hemangioendothelioma presenting as posterior mediastinal mass in a child. *Cancer*, **46**, 801–803.

Biagi, G., Gotti, G., Di Bisceglie, M. *et al.* (1990) Uncommon intrathoracic extrapulmonary tumor: Primary hemangiopericytoma. *Ann. Thorac. Surg.*, **49**, 998–999.

Boivin, J-F. and O'Brien, K. (1988) Solid cancer risk after treatment of Hodgkin's disease. *Cancer*, **61**, 2541–2546.

Brown, L. R., Reiman, H. M., Rosenow III, E. C., Gloviczki, P. M. and Divertie, M.B. (1986) Intrathoracic lymphangioma. *Mayo Clin. Proc.*, **61**, 882–892.

Catanese, J., Dutcher, J. P., Dorfman, H. D., Andres, D. F. and Wiernik, P. H. (1988) Mediastinal osteosarcoma with extension to lungs in a patient treated for Hodgkin's disease. *Cancer*, **62**, 2252–2257.

Ceccanti, J. P., Chauvin, G., Guendon, R. and Burelle, H. (1989) Hémangiome tumoral malformatif géant du médiastin. A propos d'une observation. *Ann. Chir. Thorac. Cardio-vasc.*, **43**, 157–160.

Cohen, A. J., Sbaschnig, R. J., Hochholzer, L., Lough, F. C. and Albus, R. A. (1987) Mediastinal hemangiomas. *Ann. Thorac. Surg.*, **43**, 656–659.

Collet, Ph., Loire, R., Guérin, J. C. and Brune, J. (1985) Hémangiopéricytomes thoraciques apparemment primitifs. *Rev. Pneumol. Clin.*, **41**, 151–154.

Crist, W. M., Raney, R. B., Newton, W. *et al.* (1982) Intrathoracic soft tissue sarcomas in children. *Cancer*, **50**, 598–604.

Daniels, A. C., Conner, G. H. and Straus, F. H. (1967) Primary chondrosarcoma of the tracheobronchial tree. Report of a unique case and brief review. *Arch. Pathol.*, **84**, 615–624.

Enzinger, F. M. and Weiss, S. W. (1988) *Soft Tissue Tumours*, 2nd edn. C.V. Mosby, St Louis, MI.

Guttentag, A., Lazar, H. L., Franklin, P. *et al.* (1989) Malignant fibrous histiocytoma obstructing the thoracic aorta. *Ann. Thorac. Surg.*, **47**, 775–777.

Hajdu, S. I. (1979) *Pathology of Soft Tissue Tumours*, Lea & Febiger, Philadelphia, PA.

Halperin, E. C., Greenberg, M. S. and Suit, H. S. (1984) Sarcoma of bone and soft tissue following treatment of Hodgkin's disease. *Cancer*, **53**, 232–236.

Holden, W. E., Morris, J. F., Antonovic, R., Gill, T. H. and Kessler, S. (1987) Adult intrapulmonary and mediastinal lymphangioma causing haemoptysis, *Thorax*, **42**, 635–636.

Johnson, D. W., Klazynski, P. T., Gordon, W. H. and Russell, D. A. (1986) Mediastinal lymphangioma and chylothorax: The role of radiotherapy. *Ann. Thorac. Surg.*, **41**, 325–328.

Kaiser, L. R. and Urmacher, C. (1990) Primary sarcoma of the superior pulmonary vein. *Cancer*, **66**, 789–795.

Kaplan, J. and Davidson, T. (1986) Intrathoracic desmoids: report of two cases. *Thorax*, **41**, 894–895.

Laya, M. B., Mailliard, J. A., Bewtra, C. and Levin, H. S. (1987) Malignant fibrous histiocytoma of the heart. *Cancer*, **59**, 1026–1031.

Manivel, C., Wick, M. R., Abenoza, P. and Rosai, J. (1986) The occurrence of sarcomatous components in primary mediastinal germ cell tumors. *Am. J. Surg. Pathol.*, **10**, 711–717.

Marchevsky, A. M. and Kaneko, M. (1984) *Surgical Pathology of the Mediastinum*. Raven Press, New York.

Miller, R., Kurtz, S. M. and Powers, J. M. (1978). Mediastinal rhabdomyoma. *Cancer*, **42**, 1983–1988.

Morshuis, W. J., Cox, A. L., Lacquet, L. K., Mravunac, M. and Barentsz, J. O. (1990) Primary malignant fibrous histiocytoma of the mediastinum. *Thorax*, **45**, 154–155.

Mullen, B. and Richardson, J. D. (1986) Primary anterior mediastinal tumors in children and adults. *Ann. Thorac. Surg.*, **42**, 338–345.

Murayama, S. (1985) Retrocrural cystic lymphangioma. *Chest*, **88**, 930—931.

Nash, A. D. (1989) *Soft Tissue Sarcomas: histological diagnosis*. Raven Press, New York.

Saada, J., Almosni, M., Bakdach, H. and Toty, L. (1987) Hémangiomes bénins du médiastin. *Rev. Mal. Resp.*, **4**, 141–143.

Sabiston, D. C. Jr and Oldham, H. N. Jr (1983) The mediastinum. In Sabiston, D. C. Jr and Spencer, F. C. (eds) *Gibbons Surgery of the Chest*, 4th edn, Saunders, Philadelphia, PA.

Schweitzer, D. L. and Aguam, A. S. (1977) Primary liposarcoma of the mediastinum. Report of a case and review of the literature. *J. Thorac. Cardiovasc. Surg.*, **74**, 83–97.

Shaffer, K., Pugatch, R. D. and Sugarbaker, D. J. (1990) Primary mediastinal leiomyoma. *Ann. Thorac. Surg.*, **50**, 301–302.

Shibata, K., Koga, Y., Onitsuka, T. *et al.* (1986) Primary liposarcoma of the mediastinum – a case report and review of the literature. *Jpn. J. Surg.*, **16**, 277–283.

Standerfer, R. J., Armistead, S. H. and Paneth, M. (1981) Liposarcoma of the mediastinum: report of two cases and review of the literature. *Thorax*, **36**, 693–694.

Sunderrajan, E. V., Luger, A. M., Rosenholtz, M. J. and Maltby, J. D. (1984) Leiomyosarcoma in the mediastinum presenting as superior vena cava syndrome. *Cancer*, **53**, 2553–2556.

Toursarkissian, B., O'Connor, W. N. and Dillon, M. L. (1990) Mediastinal epithelioid hemangioendothelioma. *Ann. Thorac. Surg.*, **49**, 680–685.

Ulbright, T. M., Loehrer, P. J., Roth, L. M. *et al.* (1984) The development of non-germ cell malignancies within germ cell tumors. A clinicopathologic study of eleven cases. *Cancer*, **54**, 1824–1833.

Ulbright, T. M., Clark, S. A. and Einhorn, L. H. (1985) Angiosarcoma associated with germ cell tumors. *Hum. Pathol.*, **16**, 268–272.

Valderrama, E., Kahn, L. B. and Wind, E. (1983) Extraskeletal osteosarcoma arising in an ectopic hamartomatous thymus. Report of a case and review of the literature. *Cancer*, **51**, 1132–1137.

Van Damme, H., Vaneerdeweg, W. and Schoofs, E. (1987) Malignant fibrous histiocytoma of the pulmonary artery. *Ann. Surg.*, **205**, 203–207.

Vente, J. P. and Meiss, J. H. (1985) Hemangioma of the mediastinum, *Netherlands J. Surg.*, **37**, 24–26.

Weiss, K. S., Zidar, B. L., Wang, S. *et al.* (1987) Radiation-induced leiomyosarcoma of the great vessels presenting as superior vena cava syndrome. *Cancer*, **60**, 1238–1242.

Witkin, G. B. and Rosai, J. (1989) Solitary fibrous tumor of the mediastinum. A report of 14 cases. *Am. J. Surg. Pathol.*, **13**, 547–557.

Witkin, G. B., Miettinen, M. and Rosai, J. (1989) A biphasic tumor of the mediastinum with features of synovial sarcoma. A report of four cases. *Am. J. Surg. Pathol.*, **13**, 490–499.

Yousem, S. A and Hochholzer, L. (1987) Unusual thoracic manifestations of epithelioid hemangioendothelioma. *Arch. Pathol. Lab. Med.*, **111**, 459–463

Castleman's disease

8

Castleman's disease (giant lymphoid hamartoma, angiofollicular mediastinal lymph node hyperplasia, angiomatous lymphoid hamartoma) was originally described as a localized benign mediastinal lymph node enlargement characterized by angiofollicular hyperplasia and interfollicular capillary proliferation (Castleman *et al.*, 1956). Since this first description, Keller *et al.* (1972) reported the occurrence of extrathoracic unifocal lymph node presentation of the disease and divided the lesion histologically into the hyaline vascular type and the plasma cell type. The hyaline vascular variant accounts for about 80% of cases and has a predilection for the mediastinum. It is usually asymptomatic. In contrast to the hyaline vascular type, the plasma-cell variant is frequently found outside the mediastinum and is often associated with systemic manifestations. A multicentric variant of the disease has also been described, regularly associated with systemic symptoms (systemic Castleman's disease) (Frizzeria *et al.*, 1983).

Localized Castleman's disease of the hyaline vascular type is a large solitary, encapsulated mass of lymphoid tissue involving lymph nodes in various locations, predominantly in the mediastinum (70% of cases). It occurs in all age groups but more often in the adult 20–40 years of age. There is no sex predominance. The disease is essentially asymptomatic and the thoracic lesion is usually discovered incidentally on chest radiographs, as a single rounded or, less frequently, multinodular well-outlined mediastinal or hilar mass 5–15 cm in diameter. The lesions are hypervascular on angiography, and show postcontrast enhancement on CT (Meisel *et al.*, 1988).

Macroscopically, the lesion is encapsulated, with a hard elastic consistency (Fig. 8.1). The cut surface is solid, homogeneous, yellow–grey or brown, finely granular or nodular (Fig. 8.2). Except for size, the gross appearance is quite reminiscent of a hyperplastic lymph node (Rosai and Levine, 1976). Some haemorrhagic areas may occur, but there is no cystic degeneration or necrosis. Calcifications may be present.

On histology the lesion is composed of lymphoid tissue containing numerous enlarged lymphoid follicles regularly distributed throughout the mass. The normal structure of the lymph node has disappeared, because there is no corticomedullary pattern, medullary cords, hilum, or subcapsular sinuses. The follicle centres are small, surrounded by concentric cuffs of lymphocytes (Figs 8.3 and 8.4). They are centred on one or more blood vessels with plump endothelial cells and thick walls (Fig. 8.5). They also contain a varying amount of eosinophilic hyaline material that tends to dispose in parallel strands arranged in an onion-like pattern (Fig. 8.6). The interfollicular areas show an extensive vascular proliferation, and contain lymphocytes, a variable number of plasma cells, and scattered eosinophils. The concentric arrangement of the follicle results in a picture suggestive of a Hassall's corpuscle, and is responsible for the misdiagnosis of the lesion as thymoma (Rosai and Levine, 1976).

Mediastinal Castleman's disease of the hyaline vascular type is a localized benign disorder, and surgical excision is curative. However, an occasional association with a vascular neoplasia has recently been described by Gerald *et al.*, (1990).

The plasma cell variant of Castleman's disease is less common. It differs clinically from the hyaline vascular type by its tendency to arise more commonly in extramediastinal locations, involving the neck, lung, retroperitoneum, intrapelvic cavity, axilla, or mesentery. It is often correlated with fever, anaemia, hyperglobulinaemia, increased erythrocyte sedimentation rate, or a number of unusual clinical entities (amyloidosis, nephrotic syndrome, and thrombocytopenia). Histologically the distinguishing feature is the massive accumulation of plasma cells in the interfollicular areas. The germinal centres are larger, and the vascular hyaline changes are inconspicuous.

As for the hyaline vascular type, the lesions are benign and grow slowly. Surgical excision of the lesion often results in cure and disappearance of the symptoms (Maier and Sommers, 1980).

Although related to the plasma cell type of localized Castleman's disease, *systemic Castleman's disease* is a distinct clinicopathological entity (Frizzeria, 1988, 1991).

1. Patients are older and the clinical presentation is predominantly lymphadenopathic, with consistent involvement of multiple and peripheral nodes. Abdominal and mediastinal disease is uncommon at presentation.
2. There is evidence of multisystem involvement (bone marrow: anaemia, thrombocytopenia; liver and kidney: heptomegaly, hypoalbuminaemia, proteinuria, oedema; skin; and nervous system), with or without fully developed POEMS syndrome (Chan *et al.*, 1990). In addition, systemic symptoms are very common.
3. The histological features of the lesion in lymph nodes are those of Castleman's disease of the plasma cell type. They are non-specific and can be observed in a variety of autoimmune disease, especially rheumatoid arthritis, in an increasing number of HIV-related lymphadenopathies (Lowenthal *et al.*, 1987), in lymph nodes involved by a primary Kaposi's sarcoma, etc. Hodgkin's disease presenting with the histological features of Castleman's disease has also been reported (Maheswaran *et al.*, 1991).
4. The disease behaves like a systemic immunological disorder with a high risk of either immune deficiency or development of lymphoid or other neoplasms

References

Castelman, B., Iverson, L. and Menendez, V. P. (1956) Localized mediastinal lymph node hyperplasia resembling thymoma. *Cancer*, **9**, 822–830.

Chan, J. K. C., Fletcher, C. D. M., Hicklin, G. A. and Rosai, J. (1990) Glomeruloid hemangioma. A distinctive cutaneous lesion of multicentric Castleman's disease associated with POEMS syndrome. *Am. J. Surg. Pathol.*, **14**, 1036–1046.

Frizzeria, G. (1988) Castleman's disease and related disorders. *Semin. Diagn. Pathol.*, **5**, 346–364.

Frizzeria, G. (1991) Systemic Castleman's disease. *Am. J. Surg. Pathol.*, **15**, 192.

Frizzeria, G., Banks, P. M., Massarelli, G. *et al.* (1983) A systemic lymphoproliferative disorder with morphologic features of Castleman's disese. Pathological findings in 15 patients. *Am. J. Surg. Pathol.*, **7**, 211–231.

Gerald, W., Kostianovsky, M. and Rosai, J. (1990) Development of vascular neoplasia in Castleman's disease. Report of seven cases. *Am. J. Surg. Pathol.*, **14**, 603–614.

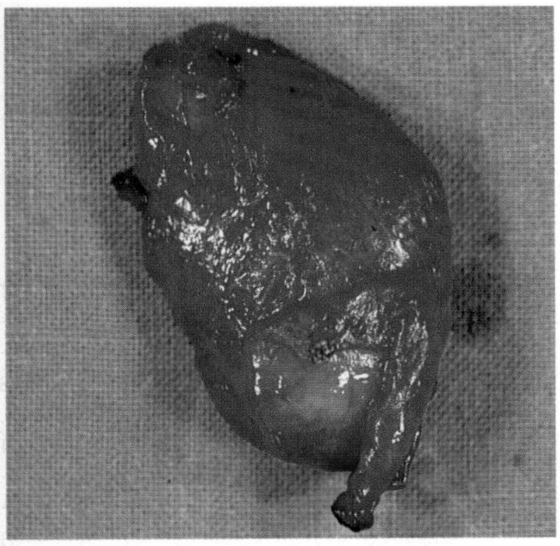

Figure 8.1 Castleman's disease. Well-encapsulated, ovoid tumour, 4 × 2.5 cm in size

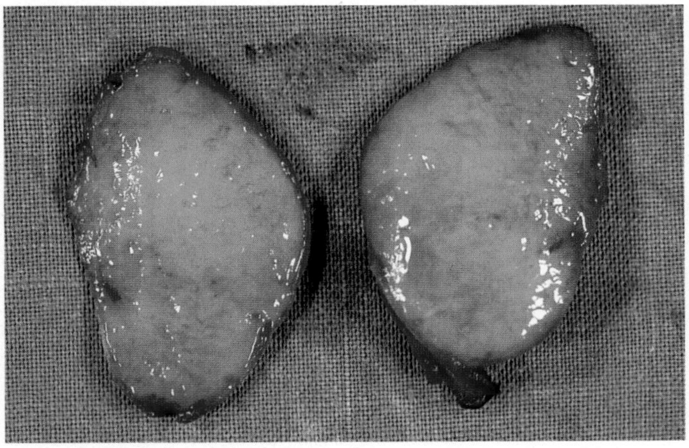

Figure 8.2 Castleman's disease. On section the tumour is pink–yellow, and homogeneous

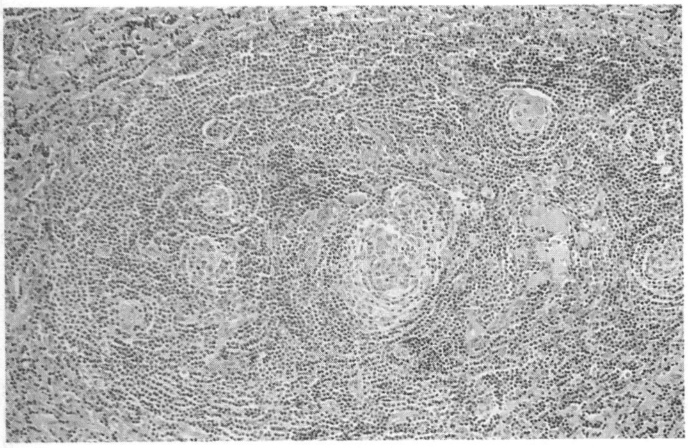

Figure 8.3 Castleman's disease. Several lymphoid follicles are surrounded by concentric cuffs of lymphocytes

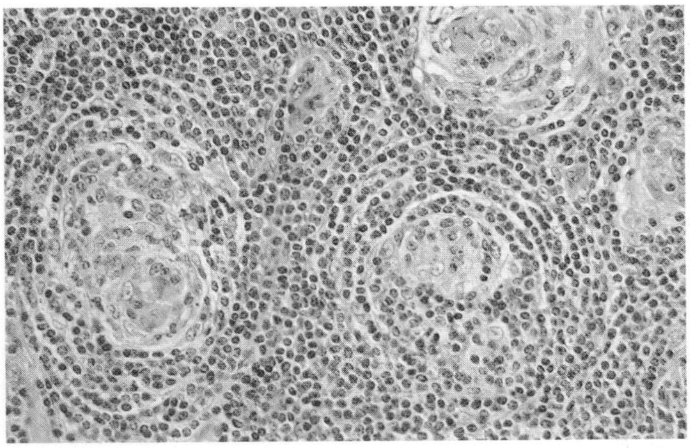

Figure 8.4 Castleman's disease. A higher magnification illustrates the small follicle centres and the concentric arrangement of lymphocytes

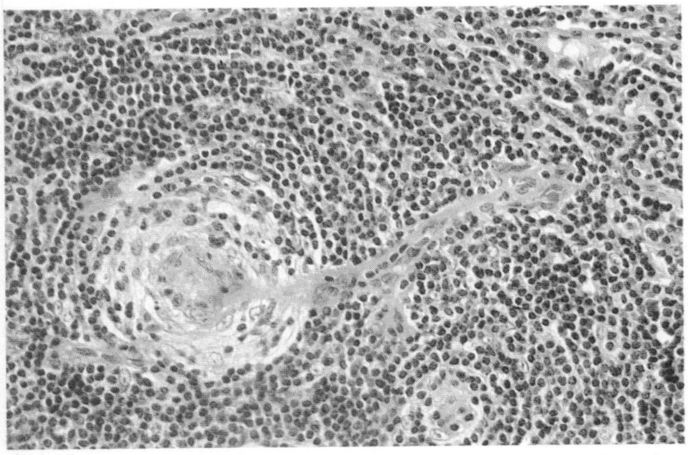

Figure 8.5 Castleman's disease. A blood vessel penetrates into the follicle centre

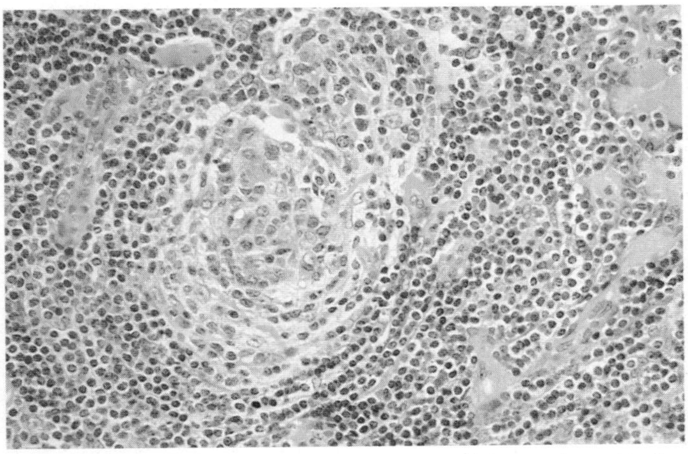

Figure 8.6 Castleman's disease. Hyaline material, together with the lymphocytes, surrounds the follicle centre

Keller, A., Hochholzer, L. and Castleman, B. (1972) Hyaline vascular and plasma-cell types of giant lymph node hyperplasia of the mediastinum and other locations. *Cancer*, **29**, 670–681.

Lowenthal, D. A., Filippa, D. A., Richardson, M. E., Bertoni, M. and Strauss, D. J. (1987) Generalized lymphadenopathy with morphologic features of Castleman's disease in an HIV-positive man. *Cancer*, **60**, 2454–2458.

Maheswaran, P. R., Ramsay, A. D., Norton, A. J. and Roche, W. R. (1991) Hodgkin's disease presenting with the histological features of Castleman's disease. *Histopathology*, **18**, 249–253.

Maier, H. C. and Sommers, S. C. (1980) Mediastinal lymph node hyperplasia, hypergammaglobulinemia, and anemia. *J. Thorac. Cardiovasc. Surg.*, **79**, 860–863.

Meisel, S., Rozenman, J., Yellin, A. *et al.* (1988) Castleman's disease. An uncommon computed tomographic feature. *Chest*, **93**, 1306–1307.

Rosai, J. and Levine, G. D. (1976) Tumors of the thymus. In *Atlas of Tumor Pathology*, 2nd series, fasc 13. Armed Forces Institute of Pathology, Washington, DC.

Cysts (other than thymic) 9

The mediastinal cysts constitute 18–25% of tumours or tumour-like conditions of the mediastinum. The most frequent are bronchogenic, enterogenous, pericardial, lymphatic, and non-specific cysts (Morrison,1958; Vidne and Levy, 1973; Luosto *et al.*, 1978; Øvrum and Birkeland, 1979; Sabiston and Oldham, 1983; Davis *et al.*, 1987) (Table 9.1).

Table 9.1 Mediastinal cysts, other than thymic

Cysts of foregut origin (endodermal cysts)
Bronchogenic
Enterogenous
Oesophageal
Gastroenteric (duplication cyst)
Non-specific cysts
Coelomic cysts
Pericardial
Mesothelial
Other mediastinal cysts
Thoracic duct cyst
Pancreatic pseudocyst
Intrathoracic meningocele
Hydatid cyst
Thyroid and parathyroid cysts

BRONCHOGENIC AND ENTEROGENOUS CYSTS OF FOREGUT ORIGIN

Bronchogenic and enterogenous cysts arise from an abnormal budding of the primitive foregut, the former from the ventral tracheobronchial anlage, and the second from the dorsal division, which develops into the gastrointestinal tract. Since the two lesions share a common foregut origin they are often termed broncho-oesophageal cysts. Foregut cysts are the most common cysts of the mediastinum and account for 3–18% of mediastinal masses. Bronchogenic cysts are more frequent than the enteric ones.

Bronchogenic cysts

These occur mainly in the mediastinum. When attachment to the primitive foregut persists, bronchogenic cysts are associated with the tracheobronchial tree. Their predominant site is the hilar region, followed by subcarinal, paratracheal (Figs 9.1 and 9.2) and para-oesophageal (Figs 9.3 and 9.4). Complete separation can give rise to unusual locations, presumably by migration. Thus, bronchogenic cysts have been reported within the diaphragm, presternal tissues, pericardium, or skin and subcutaneous tissues. There have been reports of 'dumbell' bronchogenic cysts that extend from the mediastinum through the diaphragm into the abdomen. There are also three reports of bronchogenic cysts located exclusively beneath the diaphragm (Snyder *et al.*, 1985). Since bronchogenic cysts originate from the embryonic lung bud before mesodermal differentiation of the splanchnopleure into bronchial cartilage, these cysts may communicate with the bronchial lumen or, rarely, occur in endobronchial locations.

Bronchogenic cysts are usually asymptomatic and found incidentally during routine chest radiography, unless secondarily infected or sufficiently large to cause compression of vital structures. Subcarinal cysts are the more likely to cause serious symptoms by obstruction of a major bronchus.

The radiograhic appearance of the lesion depends on the location and size of the cyst. Typically, the cyst is visible as a regular, solitary round mass contiguous with the mediastinal silhouette. CT scans aids in localizing, determining the cystic structure and differentiating the cyst from other mediastinal mass. Evaluation of the para-oesophageal group may include an oesophagogram and oesophagoscopy (Snyder *et al.*, 1985; Coselli *et al.*, 1987) (Figs 9.1–9.4).

Grossly, bronchogenic cysts are smooth and spherical, ranging from 2 to 10 cm in diameter (Figs 9.5 and 9.6). They contain clear or mucous fluid. Histologically they are lined by ciliated columnar epithelium with occasional squamous metaplasia. The walls contain fibrous connective tissue sometimes intermingled with normal bronchial elements, i.e. mucous glands, smooth muscle, hyaline cartilage, and elastic tissue (Figs 9.7 and 9.8).

Enterogenous cysts

These are divided into oesophageal and gastroenteric.

Oesophageal cysts probably result from the persistence of vacuoles in the wall of the dorsal foregut during its solid stage of formation. They are situated intramurally in the oesophagus and do not normally penetrate into the mucosa. They are not related to vertebral or neural crest anomalies. Although oesophageal cysts are rare, they represent probably the second most common benign oesophageal tumours. Gastroenteric (or duplication) cysts are anomalies that arise from a diverticulum of the developing foregut at the time of notochordal development, but the exact mechanism is not clear. The currently accepted theory implicates a developmental anomaly of the splanchnic mesoderm, which is to form the oesophageal musculature, and of the dorsal mesoderm, representing the notochord. By contrast to oesophageal cysts, gastroenteric cysts are usually not connected with the oesophagus, but are frequently firmly attached to the sixth to eighth dorsal vertebrae and are often associated with vertebral anomalies. They are located paravertebrally and are, in infants, the commonest cause, after neuroblastoma, of a posterior mediastinal mass.

Enterogenous cysts are usually discovered by chest roentgenogram showing a round to oval, well-delineated mass, located mainly in the middle part of the posterior mediastinum. In the case of oesophageal cysts, barium oesophagogram and oesophagoscopy delineate the intramural location of the lesion, with compression of the oesophageal lumen but with intact mucosa, simulating a leiomyoma. CT scan, showing a mass of low density, suggests a cystic lesion and allows a better approach to diagnosis.

Although enterogenous cysts may present as asymptomatic radiographic shadows, they frequently cause symptoms, due to pressure, ulceration, or infection. Fever and chest pain are observed when the cyst becomes infected. When the cyst is lined by gastric mucosa, pain due to

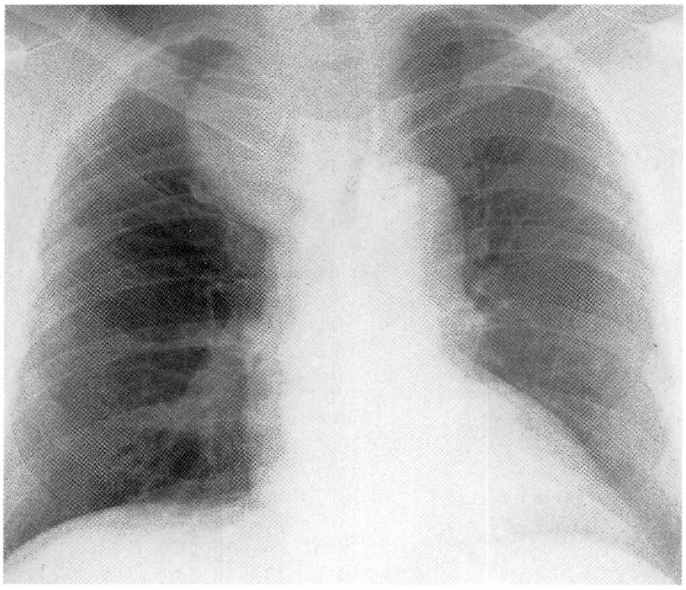

Figure 9.1 Bronchogenic cyst. Regular round mass of the superior mediastinum displacing the trachea

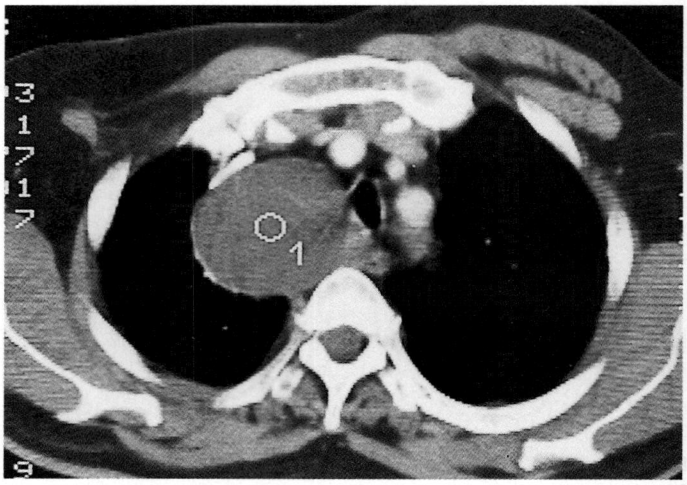

Figure 9.2 Bronchogenic cyst. CT scan delineates a homogeneous, well-delimited mass of low density

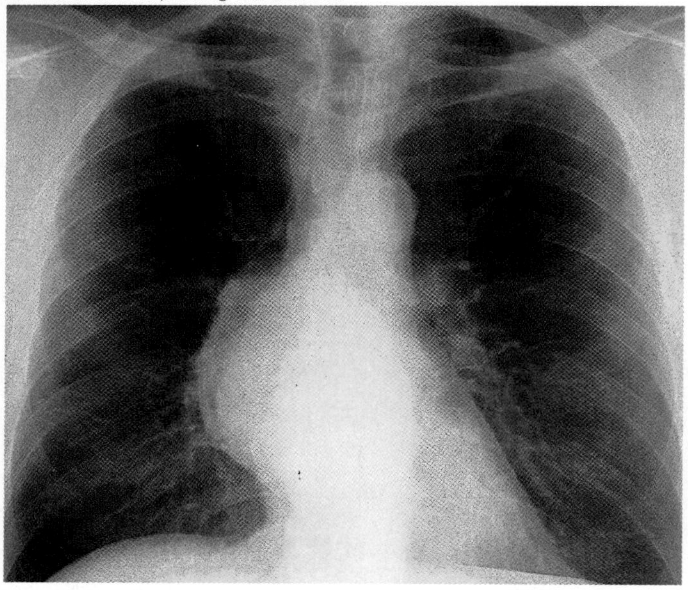

Figures 9.3 and 9.4 Bronchogenic cyst. The cyst presents as a large mass displacing the oesophagus

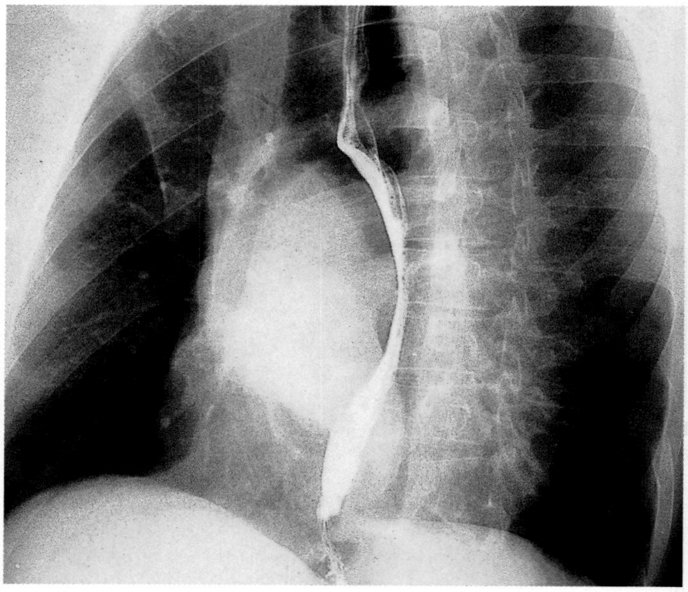

Figure 9.4

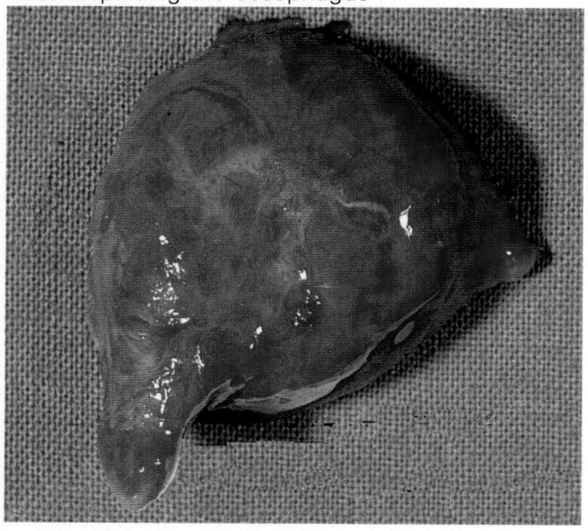

Figure 9.5 Bronchogenic cyst. Grossly, the cyst is smooth and ovoid

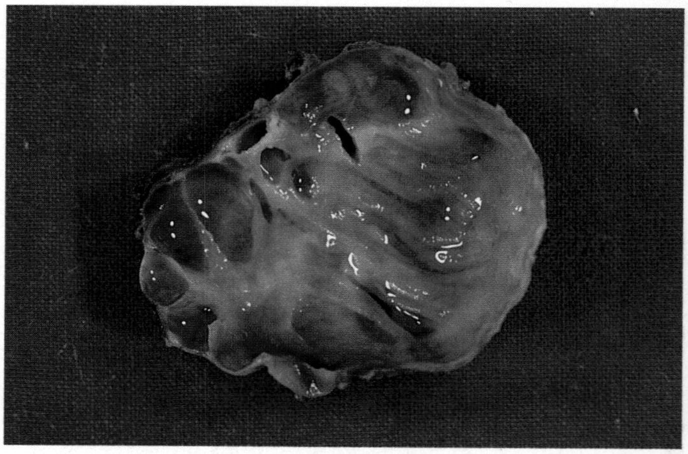

Figures 9.6 Bronchogenic cyst. The opened cyst shows a typical multilocular aspect

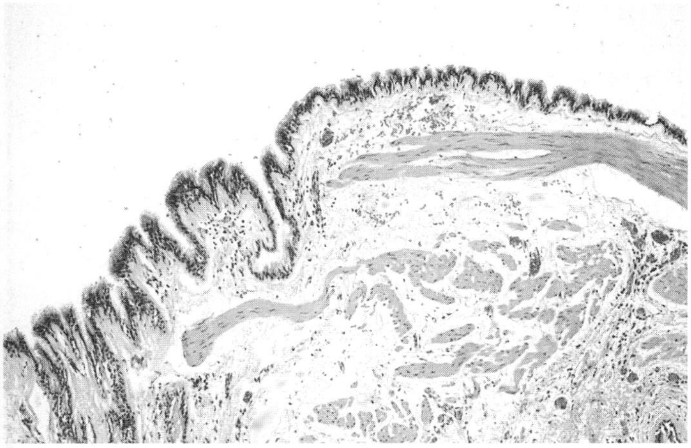

Figures 9.7 and 9.8 Bronchogenic cyst. The cyst is lined by a ciliated columnar epithelium of respiratory type. The cyst wall contains smooth muscle (**Fig. 9.7**) and bronchial glands (**Fig. 9.8**)

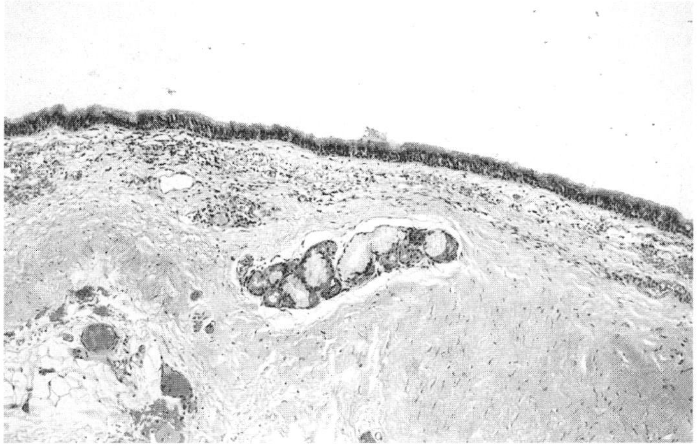

Figure 9.8

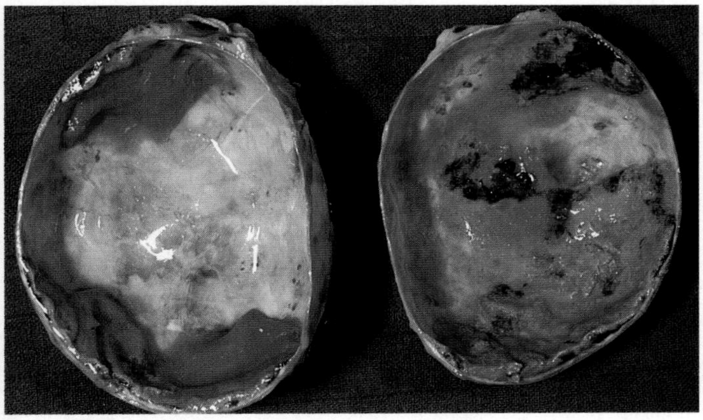

Figure 9.9 Non-specific cyst. The cyst has a fibrous wall and contains a brownish material resulting from haemorrhage

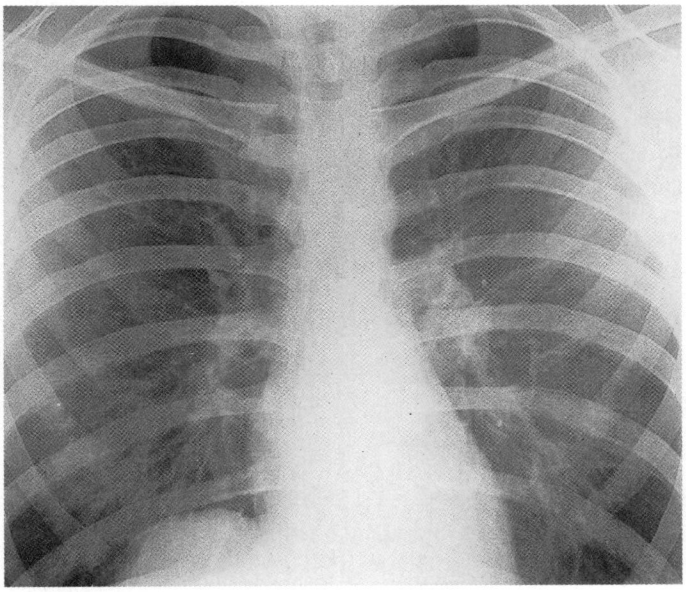

Figure 9.10

Figure 9.10–9.12 Typical radiological aspect of a pericardial cyst presenting as an ovoid, well-delimited opacity of low density situated in the right cardiophrenic angle

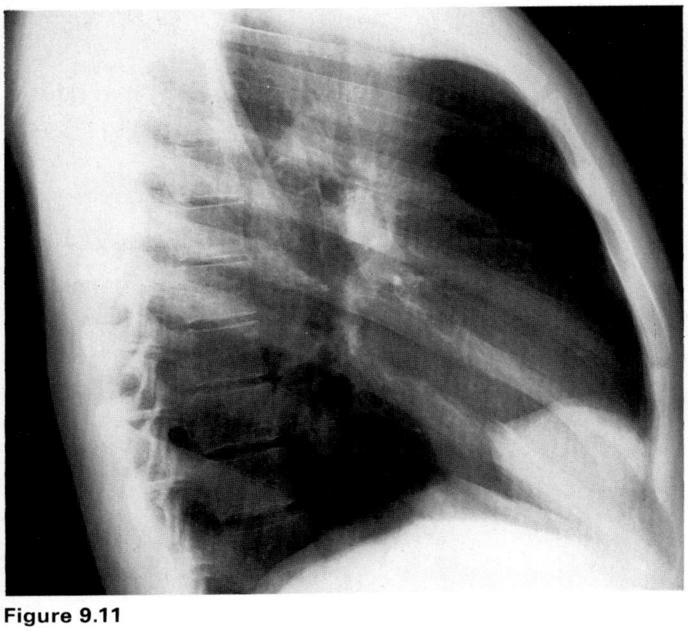

Figure 9.11

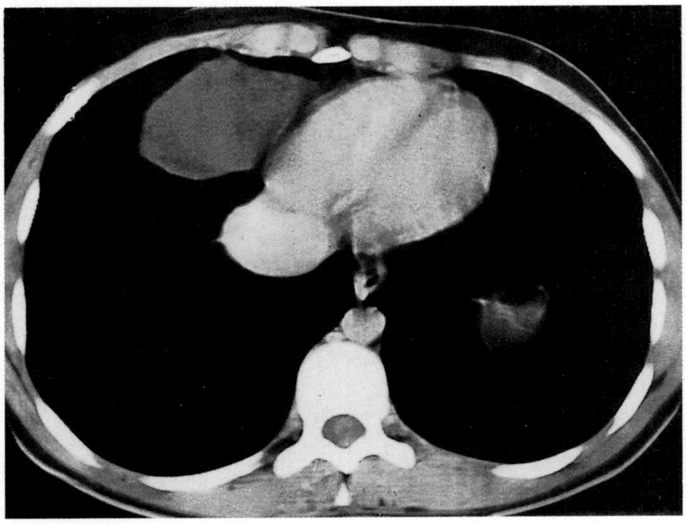

Figure 9.12

ulceration is common. Malignant changes are exceptional and occur mainly in intra-abdominal foregut cysts. One case of adenocarcinoma arising in an intrathoracic duplication cyst has been described by Chuang *et al.* (1981). However, the usual clinical course of these cysts is benign.

Macroscopically, the cysts appear as encapsulated saccular structures measuring from 2 to 10 cm in diameter. The external surface is usually shaggy and pinkish-grey in colour. On section the cysts contain a yellow-greenish, thick and viscous material and the inner surface is smooth.

Histologically oesophageal cysts are lined with squamous or respiratory epithelium, or a mixture of both, whereas gastroenteric cysts are bordered by a mucosa of gastric or enteric type. They are surrounded by two layers of smooth muscle. The epithelium is frequently altered and the wall infiltrated by inflammatory cells. Distinction from bronchial cyst may be difficult, since the latter can be found entirely within the wall of the oesophagus. The best evidence for a cyst of bronchial origin is the presence of cartilage in the wall, whereas the presence of a definite double-layer of smooth muscle favours the enterogenous type of the cyst.

The treatment of bronchogenic and enterogenous cysts is surgical excision. Although the large majority are asymptomatic, removal is recommended to establish diagnosis and prevent complications. In oesophageal cysts the lesion may usually be enucleated without entering the oesophageal lumen. The prognosis after complete resection is excellent.

Non-specific cysts

These are considered to be the result of inflammation and haemorrhage in the various types described above (Fig. 9.9). The walls are fibrous or collagenous, or lined with granulation tissue, without recognizable specific epithelium or mesothelium. They may be included as derivatives of the foregut when they share typical relation to the tracheobronchial tree and oesophagus and signs of infection, a common complication in foregut cysts.

COELOMIC (PERICARDIAL AND MESOTHELIAL) CYSTS

Pericardial and mesothelial cysts arise as a result of failure of fusion of the primitive pericardial lacunae or from abnormal folds in the embryonic pleura. Although regarded as developmental in origin they are rare in childhood and occur most frequently in adults in the fourth to fifth decades of life (Morrison, 1958; Øvrum and Birkeland, 1979).

The pericardial cysts are situated in one of the cardiophrenic angles, more typically in the right angle (Figs 9.10–9.13). They rarely communicate with the pericardial cavity but are attached to the anterior pericardium directly or by a pedicle. The pleural (mesothelial) cysts are located higher up in the anterior mediastinum without anatomical relationship to the pericardium. Most of the patients are asymptomatic and, according to the location, a differential diagnosis between hernia of the foramen of Morgagni and lipoma must be considered.

The coelomic cysts are unilocular, single, ovoid, measuring up to 25–30 cm in diameter. Their walls are thin and semitranslucent (Figs 9.14 and 9.15). They contain a clear and watery fluid. Microscopically, the walls consist of a thin connective tissue lined by one layer of flat or cuboidal cells (Fig. 9.16).

Pericardial and mesothelial cysts are always benign and rarely cause compression. After surgical excision the prognosis is excellent.

OTHER MEDIASTINAL CYSTS

Lymphatic cysts

These vary from unilocular through multilocular to cavernous lymphangioma. Except for thoracic duct cysts they are better described in the chapter on mesenchymal tumours.

Thoracic duct cysts are usually an incidental finding in patients in their fourth or fifth decade of life. They appear as round or oval sharply circumscribed cystic masses situated in the posterior mediastinum and exhibit a clear communication with the thoracic duct. They have a thin wall lined by a layer of flat endothelial cells, and are filled with chyle. They are cured by surgery.

Pancreatic pseudocysts

Pancreatic pseudocysts with a mediastinal extension are very rare (Johnston *et al.*, 1986; Zeilender *et al.*, 1990). They present as a posteroinferior mediastinal mass and occur in two groups of patients. Trauma is the cause of pseudocysts in patients under 20 years of age, whereas alcoholic pancreatitis is responsible for most pseudocysts in adults in the fourth decade of life.

The pseudocyst results from the obstruction of the pancreatic duct. It enters the mediastinum through the oesophageal or aortic hiatus, or less frequently by direct penetration through the diaphragm or through the foramen of Morgagni. The symptoms of mediastinal pseudocyst include a combinatiion of thoracic and abdominal complaints. Pleural effusion is frequent. Elevated serum amylase levels are of diagnostic value. Abdominal ultrasound and computed tomography facilitate the diagnosis. Although pancreatic pseudocyst of the mediastinum presents primarily as a mediastinal lesion, an accurate diagnosis is essential since surgical approach by laparotomy is the treatment of choice for this condition.

The intrathoracic meningocele

The intrathoracic meningocele, which arises by extension of dura and subarachnoid through a spinal nerve foramen, creates a large cystic dilatation beneath the pleura. It appears on chest roentgenograms as a posterior mediastinal mass. Its wall is of delicate vascular connective tissue resembling arachnoid, usually containing nerve tissue, nerve roots, and/or neuroglial tissue (Marchevsky and Kaneko, 1984).

Other cysts

Hydatid cysts of the thymus (Figs 9.17–9.19) (Novick *et al.*, 1987; Zargouni *et al.*, 1988), mediastinal *thyroid cysts* (Minni *et al.*, 1990), and *parathyroid cysts* (Ramos-Gabatin *et al.*, 1985) have occasionally been reported.

References

Chuang, M. T., Barba, F. A., Kaneko, M. *et al.* (1981) Adenocarcinoma arising in an intrathoracic duplication cyst of foregut origin: a case report with review of the literature. *Cancer*, **47**, 1887–1890

Coselli, M. M., Ipoliu, P. (de), Bloss, R. S., Diaz, R. F. and Fitzgerald, J. B. (1987) Bronchogenic cysts above and below the diaphragm: report of eight cases. *Ann. Thorac. Surg.*, **44**, 491–494

Davis, R. D., Oldham, H. N. and Sabiston, D. C. (1987) Primary cysts and neoplasms of the mediastinum: Recent changes in clinical presentation, methods of diagnosis, management, and results. *Ann. Thorac. Surg.*, **44**, 229–237

Johnston, R. H., Owensby, L. C., Vargas, G. M. and Garcia-Rinaldi, R. (1986) Pancreatic pseudocyst of the mediastinum. *Ann. Thorac. Surg.*, **41**, 210–212

Luosto, R., Koikkalainen, K., Jyrälä, A. and Franssila, K. (1978) Mediastinal tumours. A follow-up study of 208 patients. *Scand. J. Thorac. Cardiovasc. Surg.*, **12** 253–259

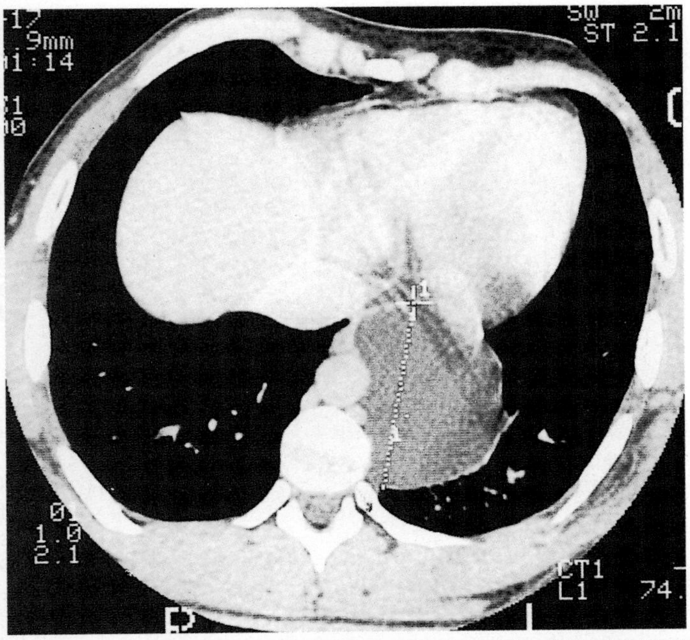

Figure 9.13 (left) Unusual left retrocardiac localization of a pericardial cyst

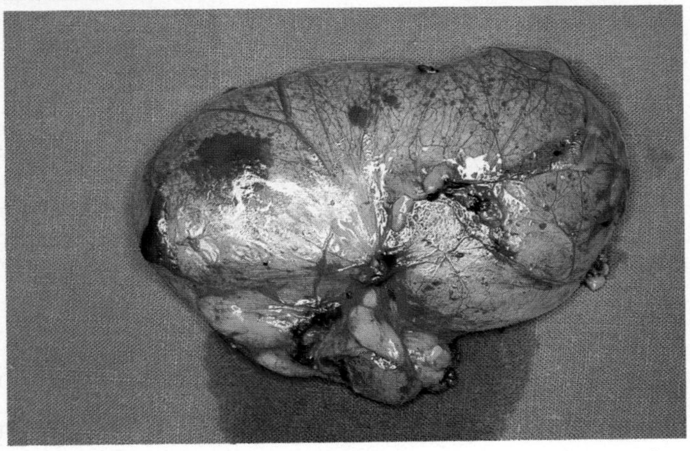

Figure 9.14 Pericardial cyst. Large unilocular cyst with a thin, translucent wall

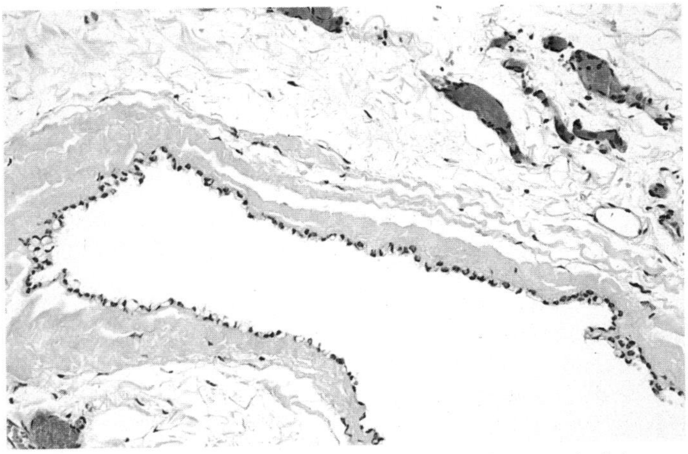

Figure 9.16 Pericardial cyst. The cyst is lined by flat mesothelial-type cells

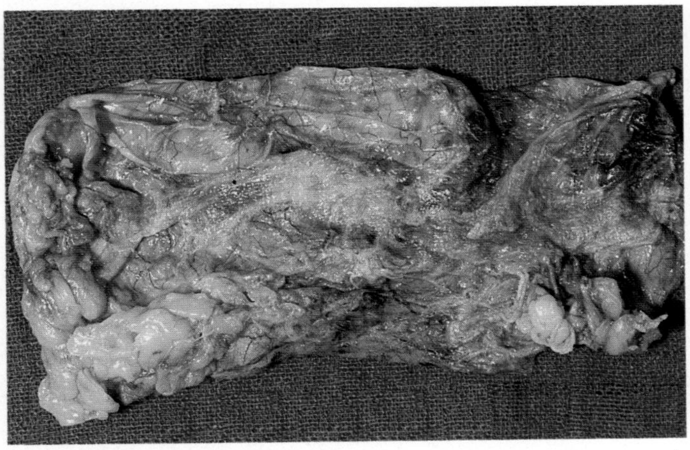

Figure 9.15 Pericardial cyst. When opened the cyst flattens, and shows internal trabeculation

Marchevsky, A. M. and Kaneko, M. (1984) *Surgical Pathology of the Mediastinum*. Raven Press, New York

Minni, F., DiSesa, V. J., Masetti, P. and Marrano, D. (1990) Management of a large mediastinal cyst of thyroid origin. *Chest*, **98**, 487–488

Morrison, I. M. (1958) Tumours and cysts of the mediastinum. *Thorax*, **13**, 294–307

Novick, R. J., Tchervenkov, C. I., Wilson, J. A., Munro, D. D. and Mulder, D. S. (1987) Surgery for thoracic hydatid disease: a North American experience. *Ann. Thorac. Surg.*, **43**, 681–686

Øvrum, E. and Birkeland, S. (1979) Mediastinal tumours and cysts. A review of 91 cases. *Scand. J. Thorac. Cardiovasc. Surg.*, **13**, 161–168

Ramos-Gabatin, A., Mallette, L. E., Bringhurst, F. R. and Draper, M. W. (1985) Functional mediastinal parathyroid cyst. *Am. J. Med.*, **79**, 633–639

Sabiston, D. C. Jr and Oldham, H. N. Jr. (1983) The mediastinum. In Sabiston, D. C. Jr and Spencer, F. C. (eds) *Gibbons Surgery of the Chest*, 4th edn. Saunders, Philadelphia, PA

Snyder, M. E., Luck, S. R., Hernandez, R., Sherman, J. O. and Raffensperger, J. G. (1985) Diagnostic dilemmas of mediastinal cysts. *J. Ped. Surg.*, **20**, 810–815

Vidne, B. and Levy, M. J. (1973) Mediastinal tumours. Surgical treatment in forty-five consecutive cases. *Scand. J. Thorac. Cardiovasc. Surg.*, **7**, 59–65

Zargouni, M. N., Zargouni, A., Mestiri, T., Thameur, M. H., El Gharbi, B. and Abib, A. (1988) Kystes hydatiques du thymus. A propos de trois nouvelles observations. *Ann. Chir. Thorac. Cardiovasc.*, **42**, 610–616

Zeilender, S., Turner, M. A. and Glauser, F. L. (1990) Mediastinal pseudocyst associated with chronic pleural effusions. *Chest*, **97**, 1014–1016

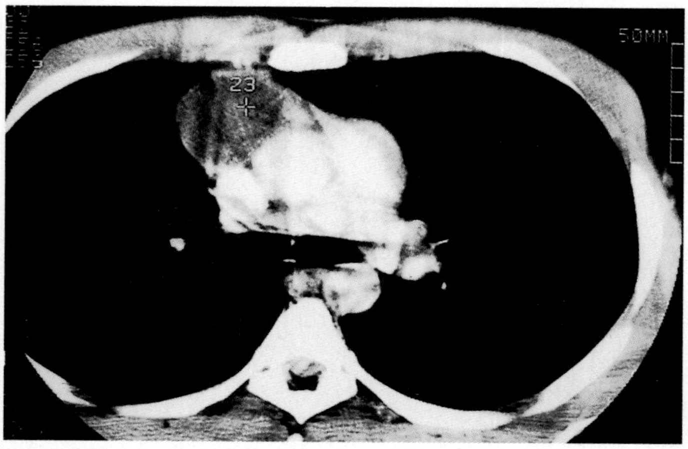

Figure 9.17 Hydatid cyst. CT scan illustrates the cyst that involves the thymus

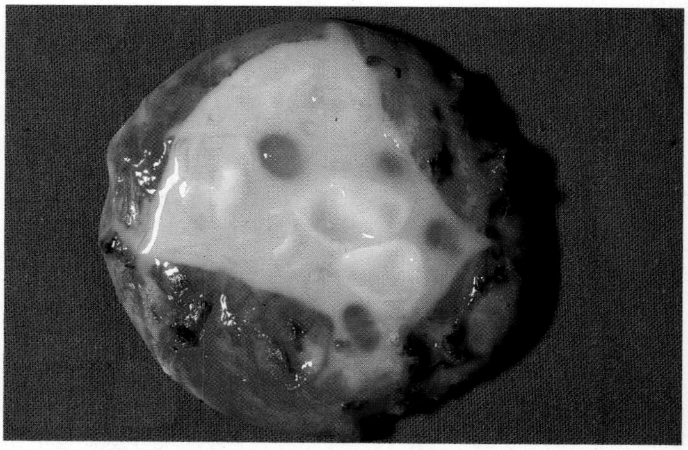

Figure 9.18 Hydatid cyst. The opened cyst displays the typical aspect of the inner germinal layer

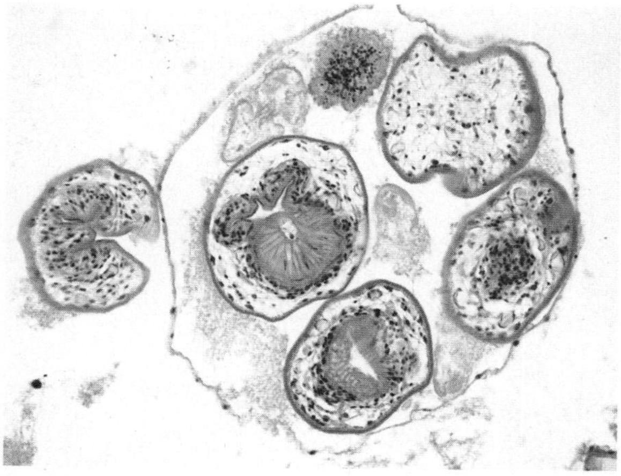

Figure 9.19 Hydatid cyst. The cyst is filled with daughter cysts and scolices of the parasite with characteristic hooklets

Metastases and miscellaneous rare tumours 10

METASTASES

Mediastinal lymph node metastases from bronchogenic carcinomas frequently occur and have a significant prognostic value (Kirsh and Sloan, 1982). They occur more often from adenocarcinomas (Figs 10.1 and 10.2) than from squamous-cell carcinomas (Fig. 10.3), and they are found almost constantly in small-cell carcinomas. Oesophageal carcinomas are another cause of mediastinal involvement, but thymic carcinomas infrequently spread to the lymph nodes. In all cases the primary tumour is apparent.

Mediastinal metastases from extrathoracic neoplasms are less frequent (Figs 10.4 and 10.5) and are usually observed in association with evidence of lymphangitic or haematogenous spread in the lungs. They develop mostly from head and neck, breast, and genitourinary cancers (King *et al.*, 1982). Mediastinal metastases secondary to gastrointestinal carcinomas are observed rarely (Libson *et al.*, 1987), and the metastatic involvement of the mediastinum by all types of soft-tissue sarcomas is distinctly uncommon (McLean *et al.*, 1989). Metastases from malignant melanomas, or as the initial manifestation of malignant mesotheliomas (Sussman and Rosai, 1990) have also been described.

References

King, T. E., Fisher, J., Schwarz, M. I. and Patzelt, L. H. (1982) Bilateral hilar adenopathy: an unusual presentation of renal cell carcinoma. *Thorax*, **37**, 317–318

Kirsh, M. M. and Sloan, H. (1982) Mediastinal metastases in bronchogenic carcinoma: influence of postoperative irradiation, cell type, and location. *Ann. Thorac. Surg.*, **33**, 459–463

Libson, E., Bloom, R. A., Halperin, I., Peretz, T. and Husband, J. E. (1987) Mediastinal lymph node metastases from gastrointestinal carcinoma. *Cancer*, **59**, 1490–1493

McLean, T. R., Hossein Almassi, G., Hackbarth, D. A., Janjan, N. A. and Potish, R. A. (1989) Mediastinal involvement by myxoid liposarcoma. *Ann. Thorac. Surg.*, **47**, 920–921

Sussman, J. and Rosai, J. (1990) Lymph node metastasis as the initial manifestation of malignant mesothelioma. Report of six cases. *Am. J. Surg. Pathol.*, **14**, 819–828

MISCELLANEOUS

Thoracic splenosis

Splenosis is defined as the autotransplanation of splenic tissue, usually after rupture of the spleen. It occurs most commonly in the abdominal cavity but, when the diaphragm and spleen are lacerated simultaneously, seeding of the pleural cavities can occur after a period of up to 32 years. The implants appear as solitary or multiple well-circumscribed purple lesions that may simulate haemangioma, endometriosis, metastatic carcinoma, or angiosarcoma on gross examination. Since splenosis is a benign condition its recognition by technetium radionuclide scanning is recommended, to avoid unnecessary operation (Yousem, 1987).

Intrathoracic extramedullary haematopoiesis

Intrathoracic extramedullary haematopoiesis is a rare tumour occurring predominantly in the posterior mediastinum. It usually occurs as a compensatory phenomenon in patients with chronic haemolytic anaemia or hereditary spherocytosis. Single or multiple masses of bone marrow, up to 6 or 7 cm in diameter, are found lying predominantly paraspinally in the postero-inferior mediastinum (Fig. 10.6). Since the lesion is asymptomatic it is most often detected initially by routine chest roentgenogram. The condition is benign and the excision of the tumour is not necessary when the characteristic location, the associated haemolytic anaemia, and radionuclide scanning or biopsy allow a definitive diagnosis (Catinella *et al.*, 1985).

Mediastinal ependymoma

Two cases of mediastinal ependymoma were reported in the literature (Doglioni *et al.*, 1988; Nobles *et al.*, 1991). The tumours were located in the paravertebral area, without connection with the spinal canal. In the case of Nobles *et al.* the diagnosis was confirmed by immunoperoxidase staining for glial fibrillary protein and by electron microscopic study.

References

Catinella, F. P., Boyd, A. D. and Spencer, F. C. (1985) Intrathoracic extramedullary hematopoiesis simulating anterior mediastinal tumor. *J. Thorac. Cardiovasc. Surg.*, **89**, 580–584

Doglioni, C., Bontempini, L., Izzolino, P., *et al.* (1988) Ependymoma of the mediastinum. *Arch. Pathol. Lab. Med.*, **112**, 194–196

Nobles, E., Lee, R. and Kircher, T. (1991) Mediastinal ependymoma. *Hum. Pathol.*, **22**, 94–96

Yousem, S. A. (1987) Thoracic splenosis. *Ann. Thorac. Surg.*, **44**, 411–412.

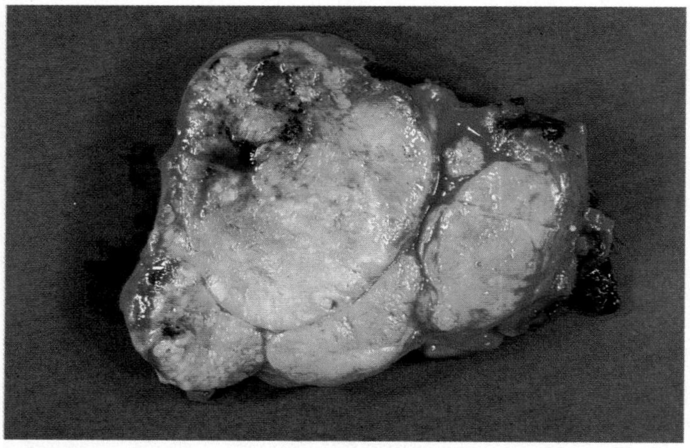

Figure 10.1 Mediastinal lymph node metastasis from adenocarcinoma of the lung. Gross photograph

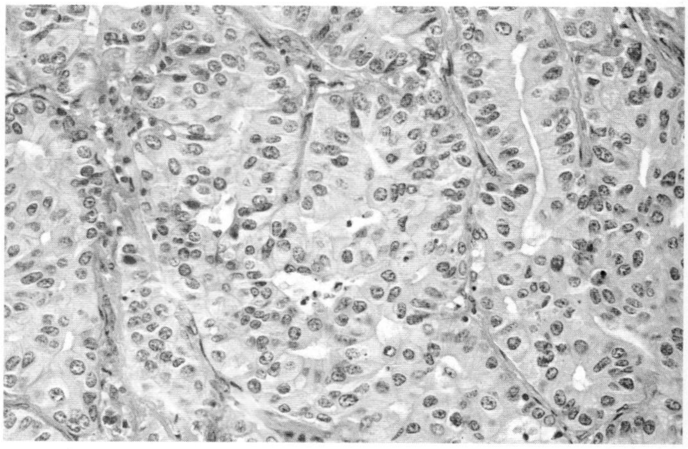

Figure 10.2 Mediastinal lymph node metastasis from adenocarcinoma of the lung. Histologically the tumour is a well-differentiated adenocarcinoma

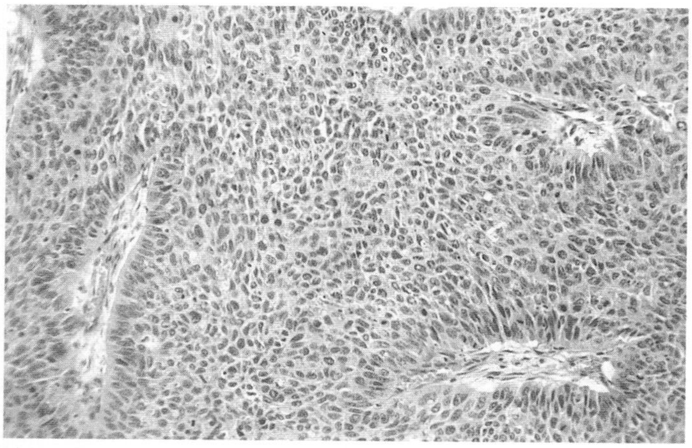

Figure 10.3 Mediastinal lymph node metastasis from a squamous-cell carcinoma of the lung

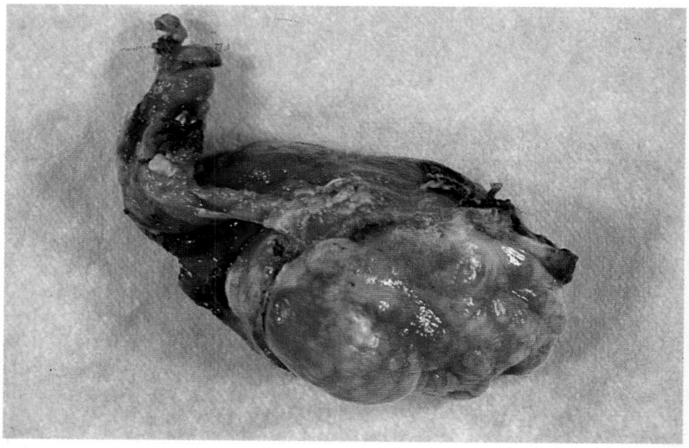

Figures 10.4 and 10.5 Mediastinal lymph node metastasis from hepatosarcoma. The metastatic involvement of the mediastinum by a hepatosarcoma is distinctly unusual

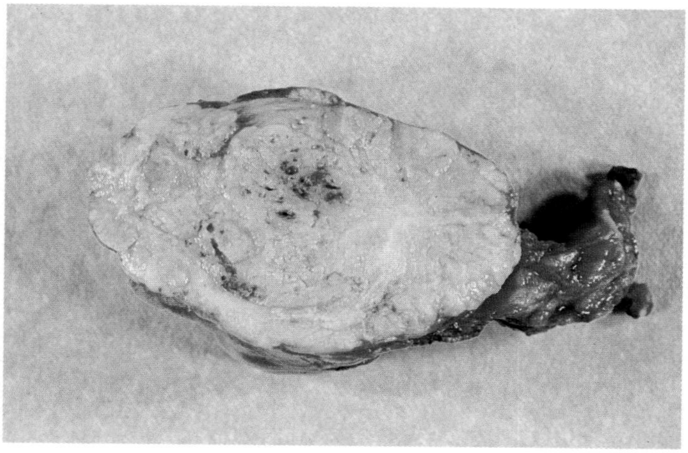

Figure 10.5

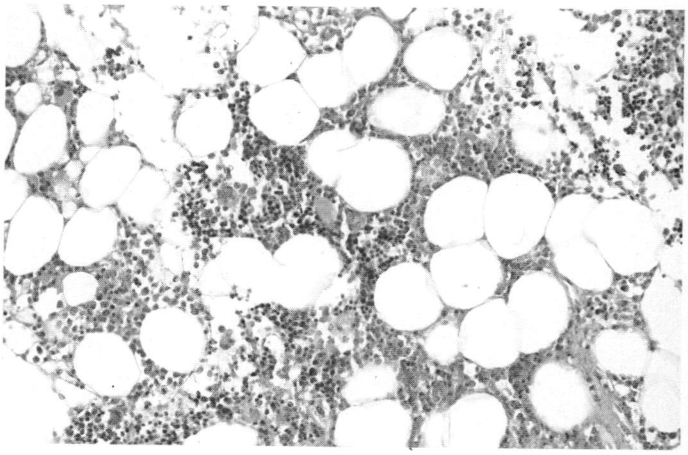

Figure 10.6 Intrathoracic extramedullary haematopoiesis. The lesion was discovered incidentally in the posterior mediastinum

Index

Italic page references are to figures.